NEW VISTAS IN THERAPEUTICS
FROM DRUG DESIGN TO GENE THERAPY

Edited by Sonia I. Skarlatos, Paul Velletri, and Mariana Morris

---

DRUG-RESISTANT TUBERCULOSIS
FROM MOLECULES TO MACRO-ECONOMICS

Edited by Peter Davies

ANNALS OF THE NEW YORK ACADEMY OF SCIENCES
Volume 953

NEW VISTAS IN THERAPEUTICS
FROM DRUG DESIGN TO GENE THERAPY

Edited by Sonia I. Skarlatos, Paul Velletri, and Mariana Morris

———————

DRUG-RESISTANT TUBERCULOSIS
FROM MOLECULES TO MACRO-ECONOMICS

Edited by Peter Davies

The New York Academy of Sciences
New York, New York
2001

Copyright © 2001 by the New York Academy of Sciences. All rights reserved. Under the provisions of the United States Copyright Act of 1976, individual readers of the Annals are permitted to make fair use of the material in them for teaching or research. Permission is granted to quote from the Annals provided that the customary acknowledgment is made of the source. Material in the Annals may be republished only by permission of the Academy. Address inquiries to the Permissions Department (editorial@nyas.org) at the New York Academy of Sciences.

Copying fees: For each copy of an article made beyond the free copying permitted under Section 107 or 108 of the 1976 Copyright Act, a fee should be paid through the Copyright Clearance Center, Inc., 222 Rosewood Drive, Danvers, MA 01923 (www.copyright.com).

⊗ The paper used in this publication meets the minimum requirements of the American National Standard for Information Sciences—Permanence of Paper for Printed Library Materials, ANSI Z39.48-1984.

Library of Congress Cataloging-in-Publication Data has been applied for.

GYAT / PCP
Printed in the United States of America
ISBN 1-57331-335-1 (cloth)
ISBN 1-57331-336-X (paper)
ISSN 0077-8923

ANNALS OF THE NEW YORK ACADEMY OF SCIENCES
Volume 953
December 2001

NEW VISTAS IN THERAPEUTICS
FROM DRUG DESIGN TO GENE THERAPY

Editors
SONIA I. SKARLATOS, PAUL VELLETRI, AND MARIANA MORRIS

Conference Organizers
MARIANA MORRIS, C. FRANK BENNET, PAUL A. VELLETRI, AMY TRAINOR,
SONIA SKARLATOS, AND VICTOR J. DZAU

DRUG-RESISTANT TUBERCULOSIS
FROM MOLECULES TO MACRO-ECONOMICS

Editor
PETER DAVIES

Advisory Board
PETER DAVIES, MARTY ADAIR, FRANCIS DREBNIEWSKI, JANE LEESE,
JOHN MOORE-GILLON, PETER ORMEROD, JOHN PORTER, ANTON POZNIAK,
AND JACK TINKER

[This volume is the result of two conferences: **New Vistas in Therapeutics: From Drug Design to Gene Therapy,** sponsored by the American Society for Biochemistry and Molecular Biology (ASBMB) and the American Society for Pharmacology and Experimental Therapeutics (ASPET) and held as a FASEB satellite meeting on June 3–4, 2000 in Boston, Massachusetts; and **Tuberculosis Drug Resistance: From Molecules to Macro-Economics,** sponsored by Royal Society of Medicine, Liverpool Medical Institution, and TB Focus and held on March 29–30, 2001 in London.]

CONTENTS

Financial assistance for New Vistas in Therapeutics: From Drug Design to Gene Therapy was received from:

- DUPONT PHARMACEUTICALS COMPANY
- ISIS PHARMACEUTICALS
- ASTRAZENECA
- VERTEX PHARMACEUTICALS INCORPORATED

Financial assistance for Drug-Resistant Tuberculosis: From Molecules to Macro-Economics was received from:

- DEPARTMENT FOR INTERNATIONAL DEVELOPMENT, UNITED KINGDOM
- DEPARTMENT OF HEALTH, UNITED KINGDOM
- ROCHE
- MERCK SHARP & DOHME
- SWEDISH ORPHAN
- BOEHRINGER ENGELHEIM
- ORGANON
- 3M
- INTERMUNE PHARMACEUTICALS, INC.

The New York Academy of Sciences believes it has a responsibility to provide an open forum for discussion of scientific questions. The positions taken by the participants in the reported conferences are their own and not necessarily those of the Academy. The Academy has no intent to influence legislation by providing such forums.

NEW VISTAS IN THERAPEUTICS
FROM DRUG DESIGN TO GENE THERAPY

Introduction

SONIA I. SKARLATOS[a] AND VICTOR DZAU[b]

[a]Vascular Biology Research Program, Division of Heart and Vascular Diseases, National Heart, Lung and Blood Institute, Bethesda, Maryland 20892-7956, USA

[b]Harvard Medical School, Brigham and Womens's Hospital, Boston, Massachusetts 02115, USA

In June 2000, the American Society for Pharmacology and Experimental Therapeutics and the American Society for Biochemistry and Molecular Biology cosponsored a conference entitled "New Vistas in Therapeutics: From Drug Design to Gene Therapy" that was held over a day and a half in Boston. This is an important and timely topic, particularly given the rapid advance in novel therapeutic approaches that are being developed both in industry and in academic laboratories. The meeting was organized into three major areas: (1) Natural Products, Rational Drug Design, and Combinatorial Chemistry; (2) Antisense; and (3) Gene Therapy. Following is a brief summary of the papers presented at the meeting.

Gordon Cragg gave an overview of the history of medicinals and emphasized the importance of utilizing natural products to develop effective chemotherapeutics and other bioactive agents. This session led the way to discussing the many opportunities for application of antisense and gene transfer techniques to prevention and treatment of cardiovascular, pulmonary, and hematologic diseases. The introduction of genetic material into human cells with successful expression of the inserted gene is a historic technological advance. Conceptually, gene therapy can be used to correct or replace defective genes. Current approaches for gene therapy employ gene augmentation—that is, methods to restore or enhance normal cellular activities or to confer new cellular activities by introducing functional new genes without the removal or correction of resident, nonfunctional mutant genes. The introduction of genetic material to prevent the expression of disease-causing genes is also another promising gene therapy approach.

As noted by Dr. Roland Scollay, however, molecular genetic interventions for cardiovascular, pulmonary, and hematologic diseases face many difficult technical hurdles. The field started in the early seventies and eighties with two unapproved trials, followed in the nineties with the first approved gene therapy trial in the United States. None of these trials was successful, and the decade of the nineties ended with the tragic death of an eighteen-year-old man undergoing gene therapy for a liver disease. As a result of this event, a serious shadow of doubt was cast on the gene therapy field. It was obvious that critical basic science issues needed to be addressed and the highest standards and care must be achieved as gene transfer technology is being evaluated in human subjects. Fortunately, in the past two years, there have been encouraging results in several trials involving adenosine deaminase deficiency and hemophilia. It is hoped that gene therapy is on its way to reaching its potential in the near future.

The use of antisense to target disease-related genes is another promising area. Indeed, this has been quite successful in blocking the expression of specific genes involved in the regulation of vascular tone, thereby in decreasing blood pressure and preventing experimental hypertension. In this conference, Mohan Raizada and his colleagues describe the use of antisense DNA delivered by retroviral vectors, specifically blocking expression of genes involved in the renin–angiotensin system.

Although there have been several promising advances in the use of gene therapy approaches for cystic fibrosis, major barriers to further progress still exist. The presentation by Larry Johnson highlighted the limitations of current retroviral gene transfer vectors and strategies to improve retroviral gene transfer efficiency to airway epithelial cells *in vitro*. In addition, expanded and new research efforts are necessary to ensure regulated, stable, and cell-specific expression of transferred genes in targeted cells. James Wilson reviewed the importance of regulated gene expression in diseases that require cellular and host homeostasis and/or transient pharmacological levels of protein expression. Such control of transgene transcription is essential for the success of clinical gene therapy.

For gene therapy to be successful in treating lifelong diseases such as hemophilia and cystic fibrosis, it is essential to develop new and effective vectors that can efficiently deliver therapeutic genes and achieve stable transgene integration into the host genome with long-term expression. As described by Katherine High, advances in vector development have paved the way to the first gene transfer clinical trial for hemophilia B. Dose escalation studies utilizing adeno-associated, vector-mediated, muscle-directed gene transfer have shown evidence of gene transfer and lack of toxicity. Since the meeting, Dr. High and her colleagues have been successful in delivering factor IX both intramuscularly and directly into the liver.

Finally, in addition to treating inherited and systemic illnesses such as hemophilia and hypertension, an emerging approach is to use gene transfer as a means of delivering a high concentration of therapeutic gene product in a localized disease area to treat the pathophysiological process. An example of this approach is in the treatment of vascular ischemic disease. Jeffrey Isner and his colleagues have reported encouraging early data on the use of VEGF for therapeutic angiogenesis in treating peripheral and coronary ischemic disorders. His presentation indicated that understanding cell differentiation and blood vessel development during embryogenesis and postnatal neovascularization is essential to improve the outcome of therapeutic neovascularization.

In summary, gene therapy is a powerful technology that has the potential for novel medical applications. As evidenced in these papers, considerable progress has been made in several areas. Within the next five to ten years, gene therapy is likely to reach clinical importance, particularly in the treatment of local pathologic conditions (ischemic vascular disease) that require only a temporary expression of the transferred gene to achieve a beneficial biological effect and possibly also in therapy for monogenic diseases (such as hypertension, cystic fibrosis, and hemophilia) for which the replacement of a mutated single gene may be curative.

Medicinals for the Millennia

The Historical Record

GORDON M. CRAGG AND DAVID J. NEWMAN

Natural Products Branch, DTP, DCTD, National Cancer Institute,
Frederick, Maryland 21702-1201, USA

ABSTRACT: Nature has been a source of medicinal agents for thousands of years, and an impressive number of modern drugs have been isolated from natural sources, many based on their use in traditional medicine. The use of herbal drugs is once more escalating in the form of complementary and alternative medicine. The past century, however, has seen an increasing role played by microorganisms in the production of the antibiotics and other drugs for the treatment of some serious diseases. With less than 1% of the microbial world currently known, advances in procedures for microbial cultivation and the extraction of nucleic acids from environmental samples from soil and marine habitats, and from symbiotic and endophytic microbes associated with terrestrial and marine macro-organisms, will provide access to a vast untapped reservoir of genetic and metabolic diversity. By use of combinatorial chemical and biosynthetic technology, novel natural product leads will be optimized on the basis of their biological activities to yield effective chemotherapeutic and other bioactive agents.

KEYWORDS: anticancer agents; biodiversity; combinatorial biosynthesis/chemistry; drug discovery; herbal drugs; natural products; synthesis; traditional medicine

MEDICINALS

Recorded History

Throughout the ages, humans have relied on nature for their basic needs—for the production of foodstuffs, shelters, clothing, means of transportation, fertilizers, flavors and fragrances, and, not least, medicines. Plants have formed the basis of sophisticated traditional medicine systems that have been in existence for thousands of years.[1] The first records, written on clay tablets in cuneiform, are from Mesopotamia and date from about 2600 B.C.; among the substances that they used were oils of *Cedrus* species (cedar) and *Cupressus sempevirens* (cypress), *Glycyrrhiza glabra* (licorice), *Commiphora* species (myrrh), and *Papaver somniferum* (poppy juice), all of which are still in use today for the treatment of ailments ranging from coughs and

Address for correspondence: Gordon M. Cragg, Natural Products Branch, Developmental Therapeutics Program, Division of Cancer Treatment and Diagnosis, National Cancer Institute, P. O. Box B, Frederick, MD 21702-1201. Voice: 301-846-5387; fax: 301-846-6178.
cragg@dtpax2.ncifcrf.gov

colds to parasitic infections and inflammation. Egyptian medicine dates from about 2900 B.C., but the best known Egyptian pharmaceutical record is the "Ebers Papyrus" dating from 1500 B.C.; this documents some 700 drugs (mostly plants) and includes formulas, such as gargles, snuffs, poultices, infusions, pills, and ointments, with beer, milk, wine, and honey being commonly used as vehicles. The Chinese Materia Medica has been extensively documented over the centuries, with the first record dating from about 1100 B.C. (Wu Shi Er Bing Fang, containing 52 prescriptions), followed by works such as the Shennong Herbal (~100 B.C., 365 drugs) and the Tang Herbal (659 A.D., 850 drugs). Likewise, documentation of the Indian Ayurvedic system dates from about 1000 B.C. (recorded in Susruta and Charaka),[2] and this system formed the basis for the primary text of Tibetan medicine, Gyu-zhi (Four Tantras), translated from Sanskrit during the eighth century A.D.[3] Further information may be found at www.tibetmedicine.org.

In the ancient Western world, the Greeks contributed substantially to the rational development of the use of herbal drugs. The philosopher and natural scientist, Theophrastus (~300 B.C.), in his "History of Plants," dealt with the medicinal qualities of herbs and noted the ability to change their characteristics through cultivation. The many contributions of Theophrastus are summarized on www.hcs.ohio-state.edu/hort/history/009.html. Dioscorides, a Greek physician (100 A.D.), during his travels with Roman armies throughout the then "known world," accurately recorded the collection, storage, and use of medicinal herbs and is considered by many to be the most important representative of the science of herbal drugs in "ancient" times. Galen (130–200 A.D.), who practiced and taught pharmacy and medicine in Rome and published no fewer than 30 books on these subjects, is well known for his complex prescriptions and formulas used in compounding drugs, sometimes containing dozens of ingredients ("galenicals"). During the Dark and Middle Ages (fifth to twelfth centuries), the monasteries in countries such as England, Ireland, France, and Germany preserved the remnants of this Western knowledge, but it was the Arabs who were responsible for the preservation of much of the Greco-Roman expertise and for expanding it to include the use of their own resources, together with Chinese and Indian herbs unknown to the Greco-Roman world. The Arabs were the first to establish privately owned drug stores in the eighth century, and the Persian pharmacist, physician, philosopher, and poet Avicenna contributed much to the sciences of pharmacy and medicine through works such as *Canon Medicinae*, regarded as "the final codification of all Greco-Roman medicine." Information on this and other Arabic works may be found on the website of the National Library of Medicine (NLM), U.S. National Institutes of Health (NIH) at www.nlm.nih.gov/hmd/medieval/arabic.html. A comprehensive review of the history of medicine may be found on the NLM History of Medicine homepage at www.nlm.nih.gov/hmd/hmd.html.

Traditional Medicine and the Role of Plants in Drug Discovery

As mentioned above, plants have formed the basis for traditional medicine systems, which have been used for thousands of years in countries such as China[4] and India.[2] The use of plants in the traditional medicine systems of many other cultures has been extensively documented.[5–10] These plant-based systems continue to play an essential role in health care, and it has been estimated by the World Health Organization that approximately 80% of the world's inhabitants rely mainly on traditional medicines for their primary health care.[11] Plant products also play an important role in the health-care systems of the remaining 20% of the population, who mainly reside in developed countries. Analysis of data on prescriptions dispensed from community pharmacies in the United States from 1959 to 1980 indicates that about 25% contained plant extracts or active principles derived from higher plants, and at least 119 chemical substances, derived from 90 plant species, can be considered important drugs currently in use in one or more countries. Of these 119 drugs, 74% were discovered as a result of chemical studies directed at the isolation of the active substances from plants used in traditional medicine.[11]

The isolation of the antimalarial drug quinine from the bark of *Cinchona* species (e.g. *C. officinalis*) was reported in 1820 by the French pharmacists Caventou and Pelletier.[1,12] The bark had long been used by indigenous groups in the Amazon region for the treatment of fevers and was first introduced into Europe in the early 1600s for the treatment of malaria (for further details see www.bell.lib.umn.edu/products/cinch.html). Quinine formed the basis for the synthesis of the commonly used antimalarial drugs chloroquine and mefloquine. With the emergence of resis-

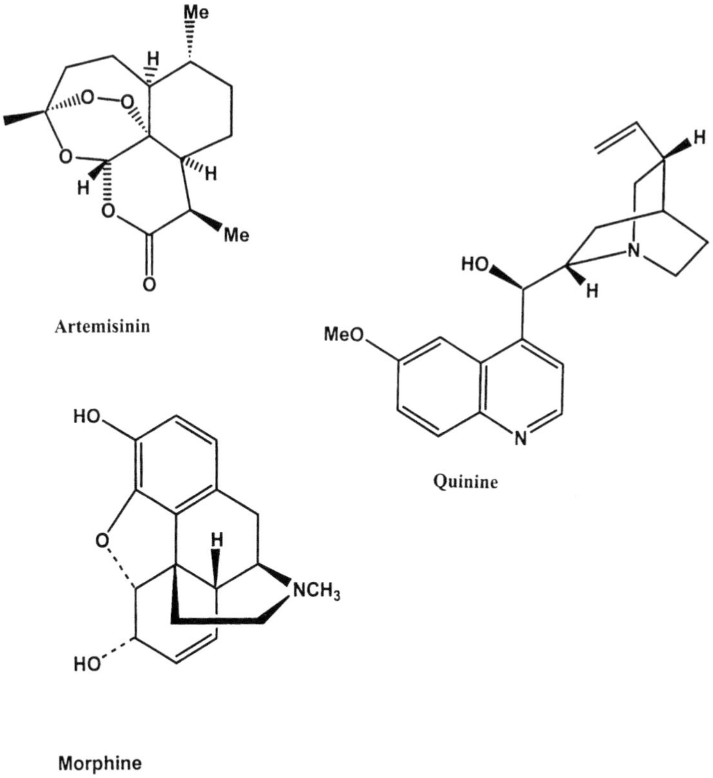

FIGURE 1. Morphine, artemisinin, and quinine.

tance to these drugs in many tropical regions, another plant long used in the treatment of fevers in traditional Chinese medicine, *Artemisia annua* (Quinhaosu), has yielded the agents artemisinin (FIG.1) and its derivatives, artemether and artether, effective against resistant strains.[12] The analgesic morphine (FIG. 1), isolated in 1816 by the German pharmacist Serturner from the opium poppy (*Papaver somniferum*) used in ancient Mesopotamia (*vide infra*), laid the basis for alkaloid chemistry, and the development of a range of highly effective analgesic agents such as codeine and buprenorphine.[1,12] In 1785, the English physician Withering published his observations on the use of the foxglove *Digitalis purpurea* for the treatment of dropsy,[13] and this eventually led to the isolation of the cardiotonic agent, digoxin.[14]

Plants have a long history of use in the treatment of cancer,[15] though many of the claims for the efficacy of such treatments should be viewed with some skepticism

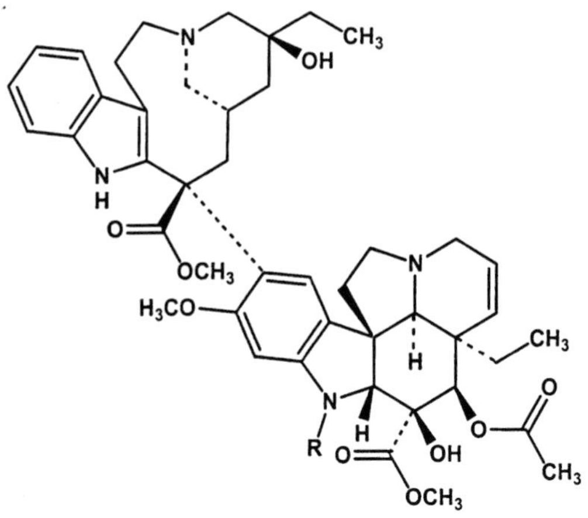

Vinblastine; R = CH₃
Vincristine; R = CHO

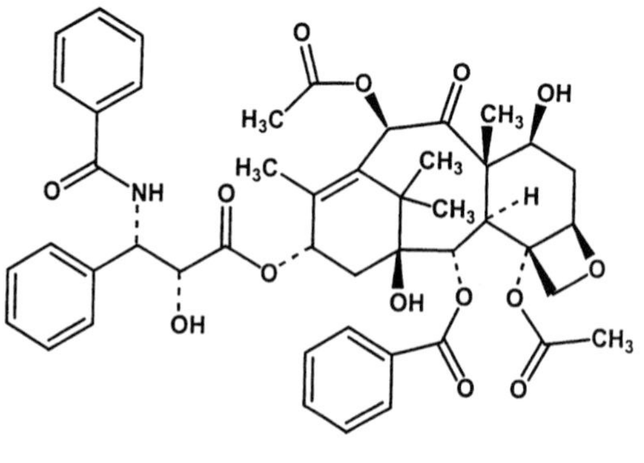

Taxol®

FIGURE 2. Vinblastine/vincristine and taxol.

because cancer, as a specific disease entity, is likely to be poorly defined in terms of folklore and traditional medicine.[16] Of the plant-derived anticancer drugs in clinical use, the best known are the so-called vinca alkaloids vinblastine and vincristine (FIG. 2), isolated from the Madagascar periwinkle *Catharanthus roseus. C. roseus* was used by various cultures for the treatment of diabetes, and vinblastine and vincristine were first discovered during an investigation of the plant as a source of potential oral hypoglycemic agents. Therefore, their discovery may be indirectly attributed to the observation of an unrelated medicinal use of the source plant. The two clinically active agents, etoposide and teniposide, which are semisynthetic derivatives of the natural product epipodophyllotoxin, may be considered to be more closely linked to a plant originally used for the treatment of cancer. Epipodophyllotoxin is an isomer of podophyllotoxin, which was isolated as the active antitumor agent from the roots of various species of the genus *Podophyllum*. These plants possess a long history of medicinal use by early American and Asian cultures, including the treatment of skin cancers and warts.[16]

More recent additions to the armamentarium of naturally derived chemotherapeutic agents are the taxanes and camptothecins. Paclitaxel (Taxol®; FIG. 2) initially was isolated from the bark of *Taxus brevifolia*, collected in Washington State as part of a random collection program by the U.S. Department of Agriculture for the National Cancer Institute (NCI).[17] The use of various parts of *T. brevifolia* and other *Taxus* species (e.g., canadensis, baccata) by several Native American tribes for the treatment of some noncancerous conditions has been reported,[16] whereas the leaves of *T. baccata* are used in the traditional Asiatic Indian (Ayurvedic) medicine system,[2] with one reported use in the treatment of cancer.[15] Paclitaxel, along with several key precursors (the baccatins), occurs in the leaves of various *Taxus* species, and the ready semisynthetic conversion of the relatively abundant baccatins to paclitaxel as well as active paclitaxel analogues, such as docetaxel,[18] has provided a major, renewable natural source of this important class of drugs. Likewise, the clinically active agents topotecan (hycamptamine), irinotecan (CPT-11), and 9-amino- and 9-nitro-camptothecin, are semisynthetically derived from camptothecin, isolated from the Chinese ornamental tree *Camptotheca acuminata*.[19] Camptothecin (as its sodium salt) was advanced to clinical trials by the NCI in the 1970s, but was dropped because of severe bladder toxicity.

Other significant drugs developed from traditional medicinal plants include the following: the antihypertensive agent reserpine isolated from *Rauwolfia serpentina* used in Ayurvedic medicine for the treatment of snakebite and other ailments[2]; ephedrine (often reported to have been originally isolated in 1923 by Chen in Beijing, but first reported in 1897 by Nagai in Tokyo[20]), from *Ephedra sinica* (Ma Huang), a plant long used in traditional Chinese medicine and the basis for the synthesis of the anti-asthma agents (beta agonists) salbutamol and salmetrol; and the muscle relaxant tubocurarine, isolated from *Chondrodendron* and *Curarea* species used by indigenous groups in the Amazon as the basis for the arrow poison curare.[12]

The Herbal Boom

Although herbal drugs (often referred to as phytomedicines) are used extensively in Europe, China, India, and much of the developing world,[21] it is only recently that there has been a resurgence in their popularity in the United States. Products such as ginseng (e.g., *Panax ginseng* and related species), ginkgo (*Ginkgo biloba*), and St. John's wort (*Hypericum perforatum*) can be traced back to the ancient traditional systems; whereas others, such as echinacea (*Echinacea angustifolia* and related species) and saw palmetto (*Serenoa repens*), are of more recent vintage. Excellent books are available to guide consumers in their choice and use of the multiplicity of products available in so-called health-food stores.[22,23] A major concern, however, is the control of the quality and standardization of the products,[24] and these issues have been addressed, particularly in Europe,[25] and the adverse effects of some of the products have also been discussed.[26] The National Center for Complementary and Alternative Medicine (NCCAM) and the Office of Dietary Supplements (http://dietary-supplements.nih.gov) of the National Institutes of Health are working with other institutes, such as the National Cancer Institute, in the standardization and testing of clinical efficacy of some of the more commonly used products. As the Director of NCCAM, Dr. Stephen Strauss, noted in his testimony to the U.S. Congress in March 2000, "As a result of rigorous scientific investigation, several therapeutic and preventative modalities currently deemed complementary and alternative will prove effective in future years. The term complementary and alternative medicine will be superceded by the concept of integrative medicine."

The Golden Age of Antibiotics

The serendipitous discovery of penicillin from the filamentous fungus *Penicillium notatum* by Fleming in 1929 and the observation of the broad therapeutic use of

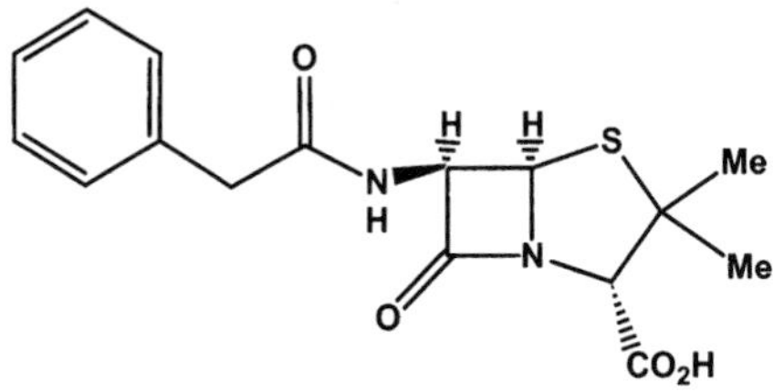

Penicillin G

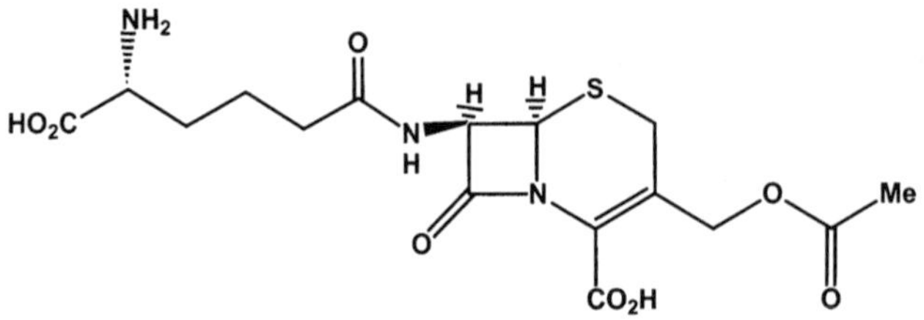

Cephalosporin C

FIGURE 3. Penicillin G and cephalosporin C.

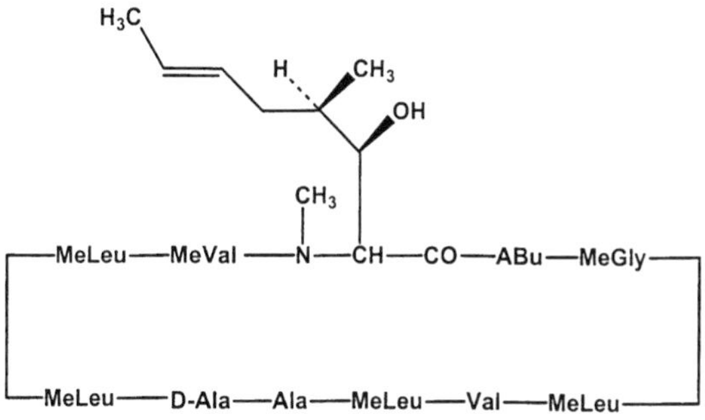

Cyclosporin A

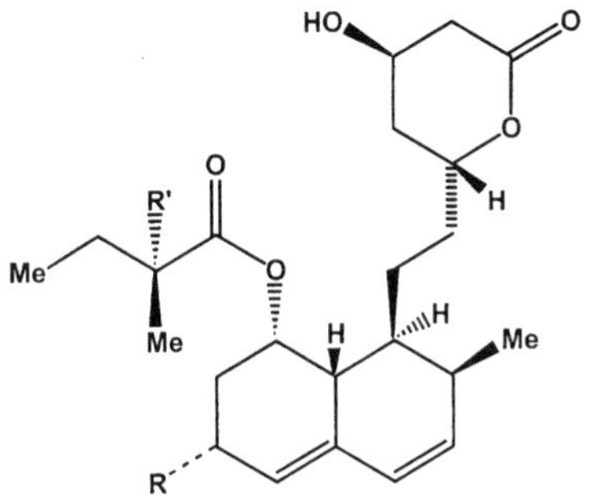

Compactin;   R, R' = H
Mevinolin;   R = CH₃, R' = H
Simvastin;   R, R' = CH₃

FIGURE 4. Cyclosporin A and some statins.

this agent in the 1940s ushered in a new era in medicine, "the Golden Age of Anti-biotics" and promoted the intensive investigation of nature as a source of novel bio-active agents.[20] Microorganisms are a prolific source of structurally diverse bioactive metabolites and have yielded some of the most important products of the pharmaceutical industry. These include antibacterial agents, such as the penicillins (from *Penicillium* species); cephalosporins (from *Cephalosporium acremonium,* FIG. 3); aminoglycosides; tetracyclines and other polyketides of many structural types (from the *Actinomycetales*); immunosuppressive agents, such as the cyclospor-ins (from *Trichoderma* and *Tolypocladium* species, FIG. 4) and rapamycin (from *Streptomyces* species); cholesterol-lowering agents, such as mevastatin (compactin, from *Penicillium* species) and lovastatin (from *Aspergillus* species) (FIG. 4); and an-thelmintics and antiparasitic drugs, such as the ivermectins (from *Streptomyces* spe-cies).[12] A recent publication reports the isolation of a potential antidiabetic agent from a *Pseudomassaria* fungal species found in the rainforests of the Congo.[27]

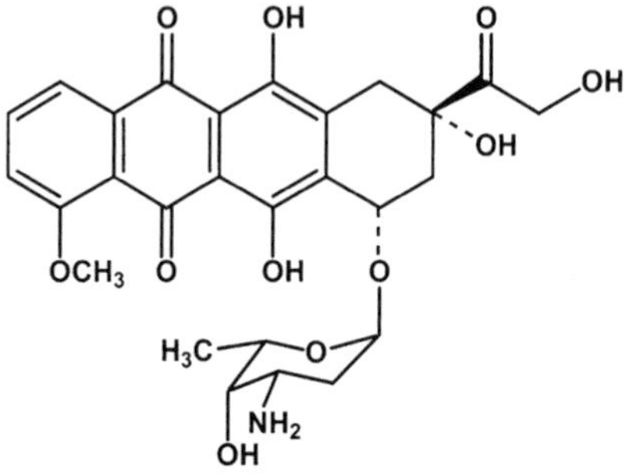

Doxorubicin (Adriamycin)

FIGURE 5. Doxorubicin.

Antitumor antibiotics, which include members of the anthracycline, bleomycin, actinomycin, mitomycin, and aureolic acid families, are among the most important of the cancer chemotherapeutic agents.[28] Clinically useful agents from these families are the daunomycin-related agents, daunomycin itself, doxorubicin (FIG. 5), idarubicin and epirubicin; the glycopeptidic bleomycins A_2 and B_2 (blenoxane®); the peptolides, exemplified by *d*-actinomycin; the mitosanes such as mitomycin C; and the glycosylated anthracenone mithramycin. All were isolated from various *Streptomyces* species, as were two other clinically active agents, streptozocin and deoxycoformycin.

Marine Sources

Although marine organisms do not have a significant history of use in traditional medicine, the ancient Phoenicians employed a chemical secretion from marine molluscs to produce purple dyes for woolen cloth, and seaweeds have long been used to fertilize the soil. The world's oceans, covering more than 70% of the earth's surface, represent an enormous resource for the discovery of potential chemotherapeutic agents. Of the 33 animal phyla listed by Margulis and Schwartz,[29] 32 are represented in aquatic environments, with 15 being exclusively marine, 17 in marine and nonmarine (with five of these having more than 95% of their species only in marine environments), and only one, *Onychophora*, being exclusively nonmarine. Before the development of reliable scuba-diving techniques some 40 years ago, the collection of marine organisms was limited to those obtainable by skin diving. Subsequently, depths from approximately 10 feet to 120 feet became routinely attainable, and the marine environment has been increasingly explored as a source of novel bioactive agents. Deep water collections can be made by dredging or trawling, but these methods suffer from disadvantages, such as environmental damage and nonselective sampling. These disadvantages can be partially overcome by use of manned submersibles or remotely operated vehicles (ROVs); however, the high cost of these forms of collecting precludes their extensive use in routine collection operations.

The first notable discovery of biologically active compounds from marine sources was the serendipitous isolation of the nonribose/deoxyribose nucleosides spongouridine and spongothymidine from the Caribbean sponge *Cryptotheca crypta* in the early 1950s. These compounds were found to possess antiviral activity, and

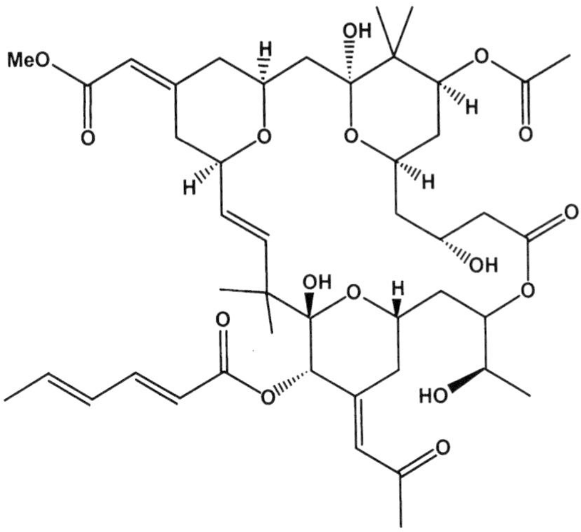

FIGURE 6. Bryostatin 1.

synthetic analogue studies eventually led to the development of cytosine arabinoside (Ara-C) as a clinically useful anticancer agent approximately 15 years later,[30] together with Ara-A as an antiviral agent. The systematic investigation of marine environments as sources of novel biologically active agents only began in earnest in the mid-1970s. During the decade from 1977 to 1987, about 2,500 new metabolites were reported from a variety of marine organisms and, to keep this in perspective, the recent review article by Faulkner,[31] covering just 1998, has over 840 novel sturctures described. These studies have clearly demonstrated that the marine environment is a rich source of bioactive compounds, many of which belong to totally novel chemical classes not found in terrestrial sources.[32]

As yet, no compound isolated from a marine source has advanced to commercial use as a chemotherapeutic agent, though several are in various phases of clinical development as potential anticancer agents. The most prominent of these is bryostatin 1 (FIG. 6), isolated from the bryozoan *Bugula neritina*.[33] This agent exerts a range of biological effects, thought to occur through modulation of protein kinase C, and has shown some promising activity against melanoma in Phase I studies.[34] The sea hare *Dolabella auricularia*, from the Indian Ocean, is the putative source of more than 15 cytotoxic cyclic and linear peptides, the dolastatins. The most active of these is the linear tetrapeptide dolastatin 10, which has been chemically synthesized and is currently in Phase I clinical trials[32]; the true source of these compounds has recently been shown to be the cyanophyte that the nudibranch grazes on.[35] Sponges are traditionally a rich source of bioactive compounds in a variety of pharmacological screens,[32] and, in the cancer area, halichondrin B, a macrocyclic polyether initially isolated from the sponge *Halichondria okadai* in 1985, was accepted for preclinical development by the NCI in 1992. Halichondrin B and related compounds have been isolated from several sponge genera, and the present source, a *Lissoden-*

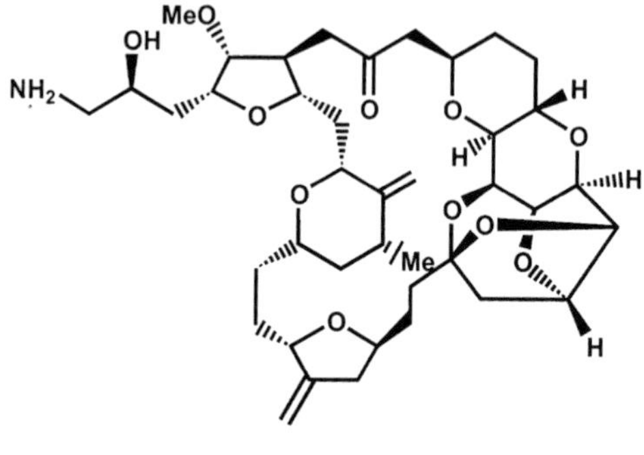

NSC707389, Eisai B1939

FIGURE 7. Halichondrin B analogue, Eisai B1939.

doryx species, is being successfully grown by in-sea aquaculture in New Zealand territorial waters.[36] Analogues derived from the total synthesis[37] of halichondrin B have shown activity superior to the natural product,[38] and one of these (FIG. 7) has now been advanced to clinical development by the NCI in collaboration with Eisai Research Institute. The mechanisms of action of discodermolide (FIG. 8),[39] isolated from the Caribbean sponge, *Discodermia* sp., and eleutherobin (FIG. 8),[40] isolated from a Western Australian soft coral, *Eleutherobia* sp., are similar to that of paclitaxel, with the former now in clinical development with Novartis.

The pseudopterosins, isolated from the Carribbean gorgonian *Pseudopterogorgia elisabethae* possess significant analgesic and antiinflammatory activity, and defined fractions obtained from extracts of the gorgonian are used topically in skin lotions. Another marine product showing potent antiinflammatory activity, manoalide, isolated from the sponge *Luffarriella variabilis*,[30] has led to a family of similar compounds via synthesis, some of which have reached clinical trial status. The extremely potent venoms (conatoxins) of predatory cone snails (*Conus* species) have yielded complex mixtures of small peptides (6–40 amino acids) that have provided models for the synthesis of novel painkillers (e.g., Ziconotide®), which is awaiting approval by the FDA at this moment.[41]

Other Sources

Teprotide, isolated from the venom of the pit viper *Bothrops jaracaca*, led to the design and synthesis of the ACE inhibitors captopril and enalapril,[12] used in the treatment of cardiovascular disease; whereas epibatidine, isolated from the skin of the poisonous frog *Epipedobates tricolor*, has led to the development of a novel class of painkillers.[42]

This interest in nature as a source of potential chemotherapeutic agents continues,[43] and an analysis of the number and sources of anticancer and antiinfective agents, reported mainly in the *Annual Reports of Medicinal Chemistry* from 1984 to 1995 and covering the years 1983 to 1994, indicates that over 60% of the approved

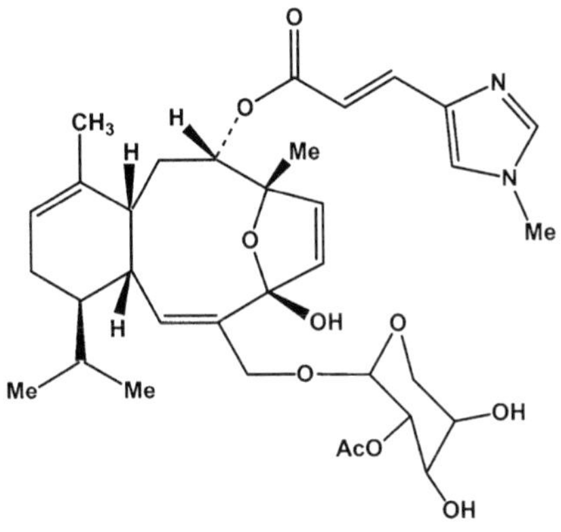

Eleutherobin [*Eleutherobia sp.*]

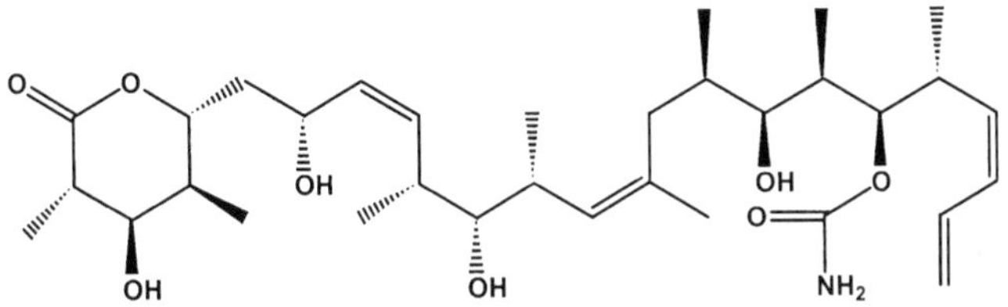

Discodermolide

FIGURE 8. Eleutherobin and discodermolide.

drugs developed in these disease areas can trace their lineage back to a natural product structure.[44]

CONTINUED GENERATION OF MOLECULAR DIVERSITY

Exploration of New Environments

The potential of the marine environment as a source of novel drugs has already
been discussed. Exciting untapped resources are the deep-sea vents occurring along
ocean ridges, such as the East Pacific Rise and the Galapagos Rift. Exploration of
these regions is being performed by several organizations, including the Center for
Deep-Sea Ecology and Biotechnology of the Institute of Marine and Coastal Sciences at Rutgers University, using deep-sea submersibles (such as Alvin); and their
rich biological resources of macro- and microorganisms are being catalogued.[45,46]

Deep-sea submersibles are being used extensively to explore the deep ocean floor and deep sea hot springs (geothermal vents) by organizations such as Woods Hole Oceanographic Institution, and further details of this research may be found on relevant websites (www.marine.whoi.edu/ships/alvin/alvin.html and pubs.usgs.gov/publications/text/exploring.html). Samples collected by the Rutgers Center are being evaluated by the NCI in collaboration with chemists at Research Triangle Institute, an institute based in Research Triangle Park, North Carolina, and involved in innovative multidisciplinary research and development programs (www.rti.org).

Despite the more intensive investigation of terrestrial flora, it is estimated that only 5–15% of the approximately 250,000 species of higher plants have been systematically investigated, chemically and pharmacologically.[47] The potential of large areas of tropical rainforests remains virtually untapped and may be studied through collaborative programs with source country organizations such as those established by the NCI.

Another vast untapped resource is that of the insect world, and organizations such as the Instituto Nacional de Biodiversidad (INBio) in Costa Rica (www.inbio.ac.cr) are investigating the potential of this resource, in collaboration with some pharmaceutical companies and the NCI.

The continuing threat to biodiversity through the destruction of terrestrial and marine ecosystems lends urgency to the need to expand the exploration of these resources as a source of novel bioactive agents.

The Unexplored Potential of Microbial Diversity

Until recently, microbiologists were greatly limited in their study of natural microbial ecosystems because of an inability to cultivate most naturally occurring microorganisms. In a report recently released by the American Academy of Microbiology entitled "The Microbial World: Foundation of the Biosphere," it is estimated that "less than 1% of bacterial species and less than 5% of fungal species are currently known," and recent evidence indicates that millions of microbial species remain undiscovered.[48]

The recent development of procedures for cultivating and identifying microorganisms will aid microbiologists in their assessment of the earth's full range of microbial diversity. In addition, procedures based on the extraction of nucleic acids from environmental samples will permit the identification of microorganisms through the isolation and sequencing of ribosomal RNA or rDNA (genes encoding for rRNA); samples from soils are currently being investigated, and the methods may be applied to other habitats, such as the microflora of insects and marine animals.[49] Valuable products and information are certain to result from the cloning and understanding of the novel genes that will be discovered through these processes.

Extreme habitats harbor a host of extremophilic microbes (extremophiles), such as acidophiles (acidic, sulfurous hot springs), alkalophiles (alkaline lakes), halophiles (salt lakes), baro- and thermophiles (deep-sea vents),[50] and psychrophiles (arctic and antarctic waters, alpine lakes).[51] While investigations thus far have focused on the isolation of thermophilic and hyperthermophilic enzymes,[52] there are reports of useful enzymes being isolated from other extreme habitats by companies such as Diversa Corporation (www.diversa.com). These extreme environments will also undoubtedly yield novel bioactive chemotypes.

Rita Colwell, Director of the United States National Science Foundation, commenting on the importance of exploration and conservation of microbial diversity, stated: "Hiding within the as-yet undiscovered microorganisms are cures for diseases, means to clean polluted environments, new food sources, and better ways to manufacture products used daily in modern society."[53]

Combinatorial Biosynthesis

Advances in the understanding of bacterial aromatic polyketide biosynthesis have led to the identification of multifunctional polyketide synthase enzymes (PKSs) responsible for the construction of polyketide backbones of defined chain lengths, the degree and regiospecificity of ketoreduction, and the regiospecificity of cyclizations and aromatizations, together with the genes encoding for the enzymes.[54-56] Because polyketides constitute a large number of structurally diverse natural products exhibiting a broad range of biological activities (e.g., tetracyclines, doxorubicin, and avermectin), the potential for generating novel molecules with enhanced known bioactivities, or even novel bioactivities, appears to be high.[57]

A recent example of the power of this technique when applied to natural products is the work recently published on the potential antitumor agents, the epothilones (FIG.9), isolated from the myxobacterium *Sorangium cellulosum*. The most active compound from this series so far reported is the des-epoxy precursor of epothilone B, epothilone D. In 2000, two groups reported on the successful isolation and sequencing of the polyketide gene cluster from two *Sorangium cellulosum* strains. The first group used the original German strain, So ce90,[58] and the second used the SMP 44 strain used by the Merck Research Laboratories group in their contemporaneous work with these agents.[59] While both groups identified the presence of the putative epoxidizing P450 enzyme, the latter reported the expression of the cytochrome P450 encoded by *epoK*, the last gene in the cluster, and demonstrated its role in epoxidizing epothilone D to epothilone B by *in vitro* conversion, using epothilone D and the expressed enzyme. Workers from KOSAN Biosciences have subsequently reported the large-scale production of crystalline epothilone D following transformation of *Myxococcus xanthus* with the gene cluster minus the *epoK* gene.[60,61]

Total Synthesis of Natural Products

The total synthesis of complex natural products has long posed challenges to the top synthetic chemistry groups worldwide and has led to the discovery of many novel reactions and to developments in chiral catalytic reactions.[62] More recently, the efforts of some groups have been focused on the synthesis and modification of drugs that are difficult to isolate in sufficient quantities for development. In the process of total synthesis, it is often possible to determine the essential features of the molecule necessary for activity (the pharmacophore); and, in some instances, this has led to the synthesis of simpler analogues having similar or better activity. Notable examples in the anticancer drug area are the synthesis of synthetic analogues of the marine organism metabolites bryostatin 1 (FIG. 6)[63] and ecteinascidin 743 (FIG. 10).[64]

The synthesis of the epothilones (FIG. 9) by several groups has permitted the preparation of a large number of designed analogues and detailed structure–activity studies, which have been reviewed.[65] These studies have identified desirable modi-

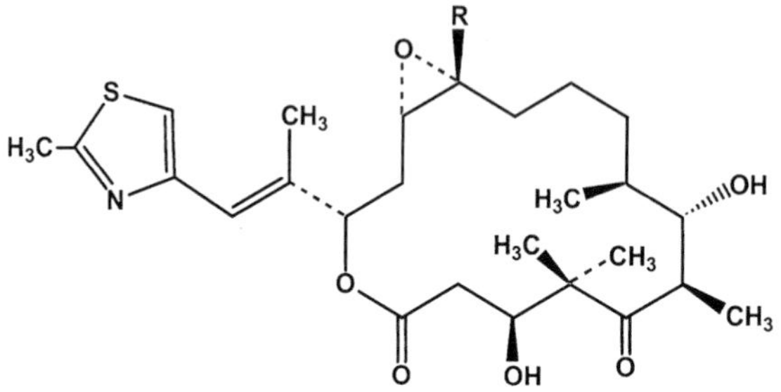

Epothilone A; R = H
Epothilone B; R = CH$_3$

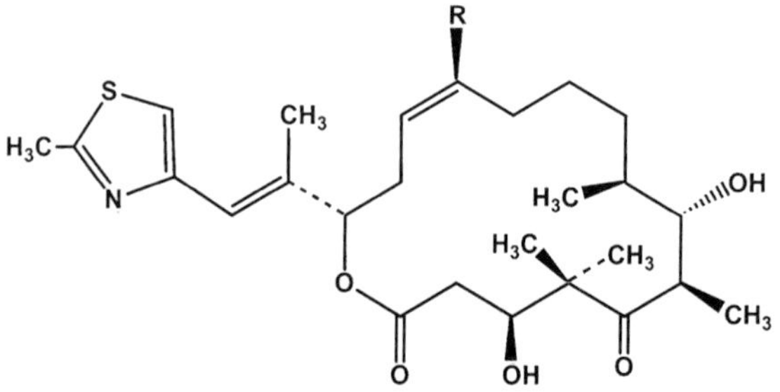

Epothilone C; R = H
Epothilone D; R = CH$_3$

FIGURE 9. Epothilones.

fications, which might eventually lead to more suitable candidates for drug development, but thus far none of the analogues has been reported to surpass epothilone B in its potency against tumor cells. Recently, however, a number of groups have reported synthetic schemes that involve *de novo* or precursor syntheses that may well lead to quite novel modifications. Thus, Bristol-Myers Squibb (BMS) recently advanced the 15-desoxy-15-aza analogue of epothilone B, in which the macrolide lactone was converted to the corresponding lactam,[66,67] to clinical trials. Danishefsky *et al.*, referring to the BMS synthesis of the 15-aza analogue, noted that production of a new compound by direct modification of a natural product can be limiting in terms of access to, and modification of, other functionalities[68]; they have reported *de novo* syntheses of lactam derivatives of both the natural epothilone B (epoxy-containing) and epothilone D (the des-epoxy precursor), which permit the synthesis of both (R) and (S) epimeric analogues at the position adjacent to the lactam.[68]

The similarity in the mechanisms of action of paclitaxel (FIG. 2), the epothilones (FIG. 9), discodermolide, and eleutherobin (FIG. 8) has led to proposals that these structurally dissimilar substances possess common pharmacophores that could lead

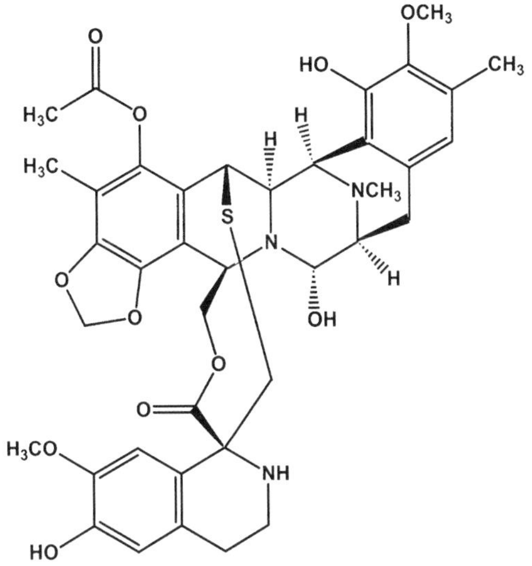

Ecteinascidin 743 [*E. turbinata*]

FIGURE 10. Ecteinascidin 743.

to the design and synthesis of analogues having substantially different structures and superior activities; different common pharmacophores have, however, been postulated by various groups.[69–71]

Combinatorial Chemistry and Natural Products

Combinatorial chemistry is a technique originally developed in the 1980s, mainly as a means to provide large numbers of chemical agents for use in assays that were then coming into existence as a result of the breakthroughs in genetic techniques and in data-processing. The genetic techniques enabled the identification of potential protein targets in a range of organisms, and, through cloning of the encoding genes in simpler host organisms, enabled the production of these targets on scales not possible through direct isolation from the original organism. When coupled to computer-controlled robotic systems, the development of high-throughput screens became possible. The capacities of such screens in industry have thus advanced from approximately 5,000 assay points per week in the early 1980s to the current rate of 30–50,000 data points per day, and, therefore, very large numbers of compounds are required to keep the screens running.

In the early days of combinatorial chemistry, large numbers of similar reactions were performed on a chemical skeleton with the aim of producing large numbers of chemically distinct, but structurally related, compounds. In some of the earliest cases, known pharmacologically active agents were used as the skeleton (e.g. the benzdiazepines), thereby providing a relatively rapid route for analogue development and lead optimization, as opposed to the traditional medicinal chemistry approach.

In some cases, the syntheses are conducted in parallel so that reasonable numbers (about 100) of relatively pure compounds are obtained; in others, however, large pools of similar materials are made without any significant purification, and, only after active pool(s) are identified, are the active constituents isolated ("deconvoluted"). The latter system functionally resembles working with an active natural product extract, in that the active principle has to be isolated and identified. Recently, however, methods used have included techniques for tagging reaction mixtures so that the "deconvolution" process is much simpler; these techniques also permit the sequential use of both solution-phase (all reactants are soluble) and solid-phase (where the initial skeleton is linked to an insoluble carrier) reactions.[72]

Over the last few years, detailed analyses of active natural product skeletons have led to the identification of relatively simple key precursor molecules that form the building blocks for use in combinatorial synthetic schemes that have produced numbers of potent molecules, thereby enabling structure–activity relationships to be probed. Thus, in the study of the structure–activity relationships of the epothilones (Fig. 9), solid-phase synthesis of combinatorial libraries was used to probe regions of the molecule important to retention or improvement of activity.[65] The combinatorial approach, using an active natural product as the central scaffold, can also be applied to the generation of large numbers of analogues for structure–activity studies, the so-called parallel synthetic approach.[73]

The importance of natural products as leads for combinatorial synthetic approaches is embodied in the concept of "privileged structures" advanced by Nicolaou et al.,[74-76] and stated as follows: "We were particularly intrigued by the possibility that using scaffolds of natural origin, which presumably have undergone evolutionary selection over time, might confer favorable bioactivities and bioavailabilities to library members." A search of the literature yielded nearly four thousand 2,2-dimethyl-2H-benzopyran moieties (Fig. 11), with another 8,000 structures identified through the inclusion of a slight modification of the search (see Fig. 2 in reference 74). Nicolaou's group then proceeded to develop the necessary solid-phase synthetic methods by modifying a reagent that they had reported in the literature a couple of years earlier, a polystyrene-based selenenyl bromide resin.[77] Application of this method has led to the identification and subsequent optimization of benzopyrans with a cyanostilbene substitution that are effective against vancomycin-resistance bacteria (Fig. 11).[78] It will be interesting to see whether these libraries provide drug lead candidates with activities in other pharmacological areas.

Chemical Genetics

The approach of probing complex biological processes by altering the function of proteins through binding with small molecules has been called chemical genetics.[79] As an example, Schreiber, using a split and pool solid-phase synthetic approach, assembled a library of over 2 million natural-product-like compounds from 18 chiral tetracyclic scaffolds, 30 terminal alkynes, 62 primary amines, and 62 carboxylic acids, using a six-step reaction sequence.[80] This library will be used to probe complex biological processes, including protein–protein interactions, for which no ligands have, as yet, been identified.

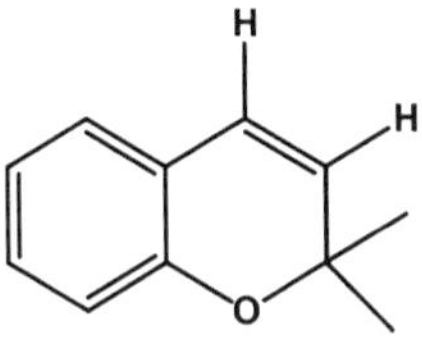

2,2-dimethyl-2*H*-benzopyran 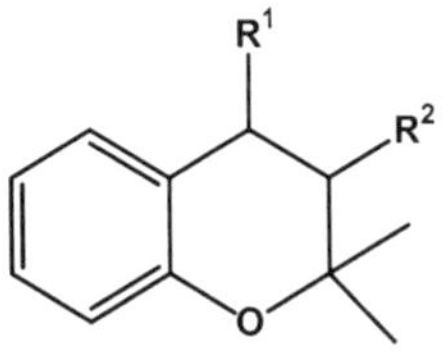   Modified double bond structures

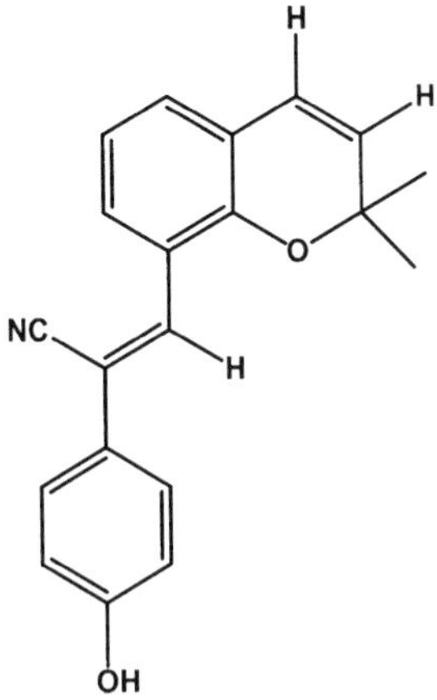

Antibacterial Product 1
Nicolaou *et al* (2001)

Privileged Structures: Benzopyrans

FIGURE 11. Benzopyrans.

In an elegant modification of this technique, Shair's group at Harvard University recently reported on the modification of the natural product galanthamine (FIG. 12),[81] using combinatorial techniques and then assaying the products using a novel screen that looked for inhibition of protein trafficking in the Golgi apparatus. They identified a modified nucleus derived from galanthamine, which they named secramine (FIG. 12), that inhibited this process. The only other known agents to do this were based on the microbial product, brefeldin, an entirely different structure in a formal sense.

Targeting Natural Products

A recurring liability of natural products, at least in the area of cancer chemother-apy, is that although many are generally very potent, they have limited solubility in

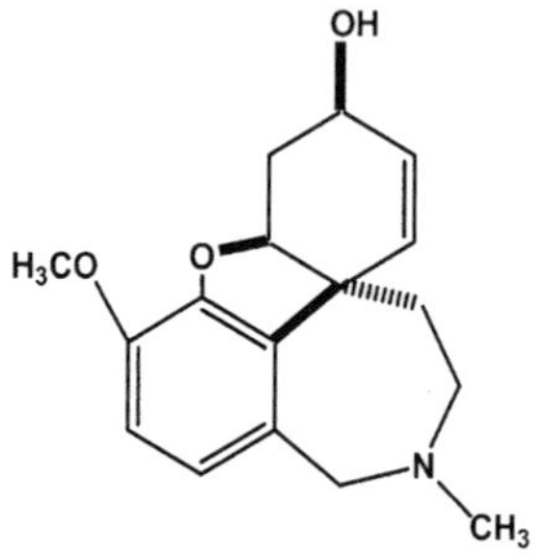

Galanthamine

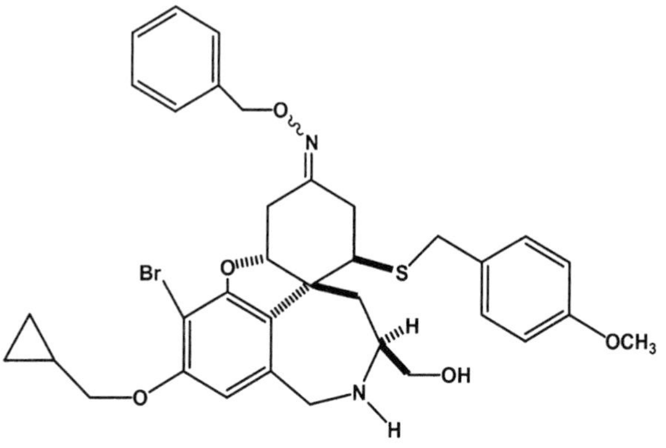

Secramine

FIGURE 12. Galanthamine and secramine.

aqueous solvents and exhibit narrow therapeutic indices. These factors have resulted in the demise of a number of pure natural products, such as bruceantin and maytansine, as promising leads.

An alternative approach to using such agents is to investigate their potential as warheads attached to monoclonal antibodies specifically targeted to epitopes on tumors of interest.[82] The first FDA-approved (middle of 2000) "defined" natural product-based molecule (Mylotarg®) has been developed by Wyeth-Ayerst Laboratories and the U.K. company Celltech Chiroscience. They developed a conjugate linking the enediyne calicheamicin and a humanized recombinant antibody with specificity for the CD33 antigen, a protein commonly expressed by myeloid leukemic cells.[83] Another conjugate, huN901-DM1, produced by the coupling of DM1, a cytotoxic agent derived from maytansine, with a monoclonal antibody targeting small-cell lung cancer cells, is being developed by the U.S. company ImmunoGen, Inc. and

British Biotech for the treatment of small-cell lung cancer.[84,85] Glaxo-SmithKline have the same maytansinoid derivative linked to a different antibody directed against the *muc*1 epitope in gastric cancers. This conjugate, known as SB408075, is currently in Phase I clinical trials in the United States.[86] At least two more natural-product conjugates are in clinical trials: genistein linked to a Mab-B43 in Phase I with the University of Minnesota and a doxorubicin-linked Mab in Phase II with Bristol-Myers Squibb.

Over the last few years, another novel strategy for delivery of anticancer drugs to the tumor site has been proven clinically; this involves the coupling of cytotoxins to water-soluble copolymers. A research group from the University of London's School of Pharmacy, working in conjunction with a polymer group at Prague and later with Farmitalia (now part of Pharmacia-Upjohn), successfully coupled doxorubicin to an *N*-(2-hydroxypropyl)-methacrylamide (HPMA) copolymer to produce the construct known as PK1, which is now in Phase II trials in the United Kingdom.[87] Later work from the same laboratory improved the targeting by adding a sugar to the polymer that was specific for the hepatocyte. This construct was named PK2 and is currently in Phase I trials in the U.K.[88]

Another strategy of interest is the use of antibodies as vectors for enzymes capable of activating a nontoxic drug precursor (prodrug) to a potent cytotoxic moiety. After injection and localization of an antibody–enzyme conjugate at the tumor, a nontoxic prodrug is administered, and, while remaining innocuous to the normal tissues, it is converted to the cytotoxin by the enzyme localized at the tumor. This approach, called "antibody-directed enzyme prodrug therapy" (ADEPT), provides further potential for the application of potent natural products to cancer treatment.[89]

CONCLUSION

As illustrated in the foregoing discussion, nature is an abundant source of novel chemotypes and pharmacophores. Nevertheless, it has been estimated that only 5 to 15% of the approximately 250,000 species of higher plants have been systematically investigated for the presence of bioactive compounds,[47] while the potential of the marine environment has barely been tapped.[30,43] The *Actinomycetales* have been extensively investigated and have been, and remain, a major source of novel microbial metabolites[90]; however, less than 1% of bacterial and less than 5% of fungal species are currently known, and the potential of novel microbial sources, particularly those found in extreme environments, seems unbounded. To these natural sources can be added the potential to investigate the rational design of novel structure types within certain classes of microbial metabolites through genetic engineering, as has been elegantly demonstrated with bacterial polyketides. The proven natural product drug discovery track record, coupled with the continuing threat to biodiversity through the destruction of terrestrial and marine ecosystems, provides a compelling argument in favor of expanded exploration of nature as a source of novel leads for the development of drugs and other valuable bioactive agents. It is apparent that nature can provide the novel chemical scaffolds for elaboration by combinatorial approaches (chemical and biochemical), thus leading to agents that have been optimized on the basis of their biological activities.

REFERENCES

1. ANONYMOUS. 1998. A Pictorial History of Herbs in Medicine and Pharmacy. Herbalgram: 33–47.
2. KAPOOR, L.D. 1990. CRC Handbook of Ayurvedic Medicinal Plants. CRC Press. Boca Raton, FL.
3. FALLARINO, M. 1994. Herbalgram **31:** 38–44.
4. CHANG, H.-M. & P.P.-H. BUT. 1986. Pharmacology and Applications of Chinese Materia Medica. World Scientific Publishing. Singapore.
5. IWU, M.M. 1993. Handbook of African Medicinal Plants. CRC Press. Boca Raton, FL.
6. JAIN, S.K. 1991. Medicinal Plants of India. Reference Publications. Algonac, MI.
7. ARVIGO, R. & M. BALICK. 1993. Rainforest Remedies. Lotus Press. Twin Lakes, WI.
8. AYENSU, E.S. 1981. Medicinal Plants of the West Indies. Reference Publications. Algonac, MI.
9. GUPTA, M.P. 1995. 270 Plantas Medicinales Iberoamericanas. CYTED. Bogota, Colombia.
10. SCHULTES, R.E. & R.F. RAFFAUF. 1990. The Healing Forest. Dioscorides Press. Portland, OR.
11. FARNSWORTH, N.R., O. AKERELE, A.S. BINGEL, et al. 1985. Medicinal plants in therapy. Bull. WHO **63:** 965–981.
12. BUSS, A.D. & R.D. WAIGH. 1995. Natural products as leads for new pharmaceuticals. In Burgers Medicinal Chemistry and Drug Discovery, fifth ed. Vol. 1. M.E. Wolff, Ed.: 983–1033. John Wiley. New York.
13. MANN, J. 1994. In Murder, Magic, and Medicine. Oxford University Press. Oxford, U.K. pp. 164–170.
14. MUSSER, J.H., P. FUGEDI & M.B. ANDERSON. 1995. Carbohydrate-based therapeutics. In Burgers Medicinal Chemistry and Drug Discovery. Vol. 1, 5th ed. M.E. Wolff, Ed.: 901–947. John Wiley & Sons. New York.
15. HARTWELL, J.L. 1982. Plants Used Against Cancer. Quarterman. Lawrence, MA.
16. CRAGG, G.M., M.R. BOYD, J.H. CARDELLINA, et al. 1994. Ethnobotany and the Search for New Drugs. In Ciba Foundation Symposium. Vol. 185. D.J. Chadwick & J. Marsh, Eds.: 178–196. Wiley & Sons. Chichester, UK.
17. CRAGG, G.M., S.A. SCHEPARTZ, M. SUFFNESS, et al. 1993. The taxol supply crisis. New NCI policies for handling the large-scale production of novel natural product anticancer and anti-HIV agents. J. Nat. Prod. **56:** 1657–1668.
18. CORTES, J.E. & R. PAZDUR. 1995. Docetaxel. J. Clin. Oncol. **13:** 2643–2655.
19. POTMEISEL, M. & H. PINEDO. 1995. Camptothecins: New Anticancer Agents. CRC Press. Boca Raton, FL.
20. SCRIABINE, A. 1999. Discovery and development of major drugs currently in use. In Pharmaceutical Innovation. R. Landau, B. Achilladelis & A. Scriabine, Eds.: 148–270. Chemical Heritage Press.
21. DE SMET, P.A.G.M. 1997. The role of plant-derived drugs and herbal medicine in healthcare. Drugs **54:** 801–840.
22. TYLER, V.E. 1993. The Honest Herbal. Haworth Press. New York.
23. TYLER, V.E. 1994. Herbs of Choice. Haworth Press. New York.
24. MATTHEWS, H.B., G.W. LUCIER & K.D. FISHER, 1999. Medicinal Herbs in the United States. Environ. Health Perspec. **107:** 773–778.
25. WICHTL, M. 1994. Herbal Drugs and Phytopharmaceuticals. Medpharm Scientific Publishers. Stuttgart, Germany.
26. DE SMET, P.A.G.M. 1992. Adverse Effects of Herbal Drugs. Springer-Verlag. Berlin.
27. ZHANG, B., G. SALITURO, D. SZALKOWSKI, et al. 1999. Discovery of a small molecule insulin mimetic with anti-diabetic activity in mice. Science **284:** 974–976.
28. FOYE, W.O. 1995. Cancer Chemotherapeutic Agents. American Chemical Society. Washington, DC.
29. MARGULIS, L. & K.V. SCHWARTZ. 1988. Five Kingdoms: An Illustrated Guide to the Phyla of Life on Earth. 2nd ed. W. H. Freeman & Co. New York.
30. MCCONNELL, O., R.E. LONGLEY & F.E. KOEHN. 1994. The discovery of marine natural products with therapeutic potential. In The Discovery of Natural Products with Therapeutic Potential. V.P. Gullo, Ed.: 109–174. Butterworth-Heinemann. Boston.

31. FAULKNER, D.J. 2000. Marine natural products. Nat. Prod. Reps. **17:** 7–55.
32. CARTE, B.K. 1996. Biomedical potential of marine natural products. Bio-Science **46:** 271–286.
33. NEWMAN, D.J. 1996. Bryostatin—from bryozoan to cancer drug. *In* 10th International Bryozoology Conference. D. P. Gordon, A.M. Smith & J.A. Grant-Mackie, Eds.: 9–17. National Institute of Water & Atmospheric Research. Wellington, N.Z.
34. PHILIP, P.A., D. REA, P. THAVASU, *et al.* 1993. Phase I study of bryostatin 1: assessment of interleukin 6 and tumor necrosis factor alpha induction in vivo. The Cancer Research Campaign Phase I Committee. J. Natl. Cancer Inst. **85:** 1812–1818.
35. LUESCH, H., R.E. MOORE, V.J. PAUL, *et al.* 2001. Isolation of dolastatin 10 from the marine cyanobacterium *Symploca* species VP642 and total stereochemistry and biological evaluation of its analogue symplostatin 1. J. Nat. Prod. **64:** 907–910.
36. MUNRO, M.H.G., J.W. BLUNT, E.J. DUMDEI, *et al.* 1999. The discovery and development of marine compounds with pharmaceutical potential. J. Biotechnol. **70:** 15–25.
37. ZHENG, W., B.M. SELETSKY, M.H. PALME, *et al.* 2000. Synthetic macrocyclic ketone analogs of halichondrin B: structure–activity relationships. Proc. Am. Soc. Cancer Res. Abstr. 1915. 91st Annual Meeting of the American Association of Cancer REseaarch, April 1–5, 2000, San Francisco.
38. TOWLE, M.J., K.A. SALVATO, J. BUDROW, *et al.* 2000. Highly potent *in vitro* and *in vivo* anticancer activities of synthetic macrocyclic ketone analogs of halichondrin B. Proc. Am. Soc. Cancer Res. Abstr. 1370. 91st Annual Meeting of the American Association of Cancer REseaarch, April 1–5, 2000, San Francisco.
39. HAAR, E., R.J. KOWALSKI, C.M. LIN, *et al.* 1996. Discodermolide, a cytotoxic marine agent that stabilizes microtubules more potently than taxol. Biochemistry **35:** 243–250.
40. LONG, B.H., J.M. CARBONI, A.J. WASSERMAN, *et al.* 1998. Eleutherobin, a novel cytotoxic agent that induces tubulin polymerization, is similar to paclitxel. Cancer Res. **58:** 1111–1115.
41. OLIVERA, B.M., C. WALKER, G.E. CARTIER, *et al.* 1999. Speciation of cone snails and interspecific hyperdivergence of their venom peptides. Potential evolutionary significance of introns. Ann. N.Y. Acad. Sci. **870:** 223–237.
42. DALY, J.W. 1998. Thirty years of discovering arthropod alkaloids in amphibian skin. J. Nat. Prod. **61:** 162–172.
43. NEWMAN, D.J., G.M. CRAGG & K.M. SNADER. 2000. The influence of natural products on drug discovery. Nat. Prod. Rep. **17:** 215–234.
44. CRAGG, G.M., D.J. NEWMAN & K.M. SNADER, 1997. Natural Products in Drug Discovery and Development. J. Nat. Prod. **60:** 52–60.
45. LUTZ, R.A. & M.J. KENNISH. 1993. Ecology of deep-sea hydrothermal vent communities: a review. Rev. Geophys. **31:** 211–242.
46. LUTZ, R.A., T.M. SHANK & D.J. FORNARI. 1994. Rapid growth at deep sea vents. Nature **371:** 663–664.
47. BALANDRIN, M.F., A.D. KINGHORN & N.R. FARNSWORTH. 1993. Plant-derived natural products in drug discovery and development: an overview. *In* Human Medicinal Agents from Plants, American Chemical Society Symposium Series, No. 534. A.D. Kinghorn & M.F. Balandrin, Eds.: 2–12. American Chemical Society. Washington, DC.
48. YOUNG, P. 1997. Major microbial diversity initiative recommended. ASM News **63:** 417–421.
49. HANDELSMAN, J., M.R. RONDON, S.F. BRADY, *et al.* 1998. Molecular biological access to the chemistry of unknown soil microbes: a new frontier for natural products. Chem. Biol. **5:** R245–R249.
50. PERSIDIS, A. 1998. Extremophiles. Nature Biotechnol. **16:** 593–594.
51. PSENNER, R. & B. SATTLER. 1998. Life at the freezing point. Science **280:** 2073–2074.
52. ADAMS, M.W. & R.M. KELLY. 1998. Finding and using hyperthermophilic enzymes. Trends Biotechnol. **16:** 329–332.
53. COLWELL, R.R. 1997. Microbial diversity: the importance of exploration and conservation. J. Ind. Microbiol. Biotechnol. **18:** 302–307.

54. HUTCHINSON, C.R. 1999. Microbial polyketide synthases: more and more prolific. Proc. Natl. Acad. Sci. USA **96:** 3336–3338.
55. KHOSLA, C. 2000. Natural product biosynthesis: a new interface between enzymology and medicine. J. Org. Chem. **65:** 8127–8133.
56. STAUNTON, J. & K.J. WEISSMAN. 2001. Polyketide biosynthesis: a millenium review. Nat. Prod. Rep. **18:** 380–416.
57. GOKHALE, R.S., S.Y. TSUJI, D.E. CANE, et al. 1999. Dissecting and exploiting intermodular communication in polyketide synthases. Science **284:** 482–485.
58. MOLNAR, I., T. SCHUPP, M. ONO, et al. 2000. The biosynthetic gene cluster for the microtubule-stabilizing agents spothilones A and B from *Sorangium cellulosum* So ce90. Chem. Biol. **7:** 97–109.
59. JULIEN, B., S. SHAH, R. ZIERMANN, et al. 2000. Isolation and characterization of the epothilone biosynthetic gene cluster from *Sorangium cellulosum*. Gene **249:** 153–160.
60. METCALF, B. 2001. The genetic manipulation of polyketide gene clusters as an approach to drug discovery. Presentation at the Asian Federation of Medicinal Chemistry 01, Brisbane, Australia.
61. FRYKMAN, S., R. REGENTIN, J. LAU, et al. 2001. Development of a scalable epothilone D fermentation process using a heterologous host. Presenttion at the Society for Industrial Microbiology, Annual Meeting, St. Louis, MO.
62. SERVICE, R.F. 1999. Drug industry looks to the lab instead of rainforest and reef. Science **285:** 186.
63. WENDER, P.A., C.M. CRIBBS, K.F. KOEHLER, et al. 1988. The design, computer modeling solution structure, and biological evaluation of synthetic analogs of bryostatin 1. Proc. Natl. Acad. Sci. USA **85:** 7197–7201.
64. MARTINEZ, E.J., T. OWA, S.L. SCHREIBER, et al. 1999. Phthalascidin, a synthetic antitumor agent with potency and mode of action comparable to ecteinascidin 743. Proc. Natl. Acad. Sci. USA **96:** 3496–3501.
65. NICOLAOU, K.C., F. ROSCHANGAR & D. VOURLOUMIS. 1998. Chemical biology of the epothilones. Angew. Chem. Int. Ed. **37:** 2014–2045.
66. VITE, G.D., R.M. BORZILLERI, S-H. KIM & J.A. JOHNSON. 1999. U.S. Patent WO99/02514; PCT/US98/12550.
67. BORZILLERI, R.M., X. ZHENG, R.J. SCHMIDT, et al. 2000. A novel application of a Pd(0)-catalyzed nucelophilic substitution reaction to the regio- and stereoselective synthesis of lactam analogues of the epithilone natural products. J. Am. Chem. Soc. **122:** 8890–8897.
68. STACHEL S.W., C.B. LEE, M. SPASSOVA, et al. 2001. On the interactivity of complex synthesis and tumor pharmacology in the drug discovery process: total synthesis and comparative in vivo evaluations of the 15-aza_epothilones. J. Am. Chem. Soc. **66:** 4369–4378.
69. OJIMA, I., S. CHAKRAVARTY, T. INOUE, et al. 1999. A common pharmacophore for cytotoxic natural products that stabilize microtubules. Proc. Natl. Acad. Sci. USA **96:** 4256–4261.
70. GIANNAKAKOU, P., R. GUSSIO, E. NOGALES, et al. 2000. A common pharmacophore for epithilone and taxanes: molecular basis for drug resistance conferred by tubulin mutations in human cancer cells. Proc. Natl. Acad. Sci. USA **97:** 2904–2909.
71. NICOLAOU, K.C., K. NAMOTO, J. LI, A. RITZEN, et al. 2001. Synthesis and biological evaluation of 12,13-cyclopropyl and 12,13 cyclobutyl epothilones. Chembiochem **1:** 69–75.
72. BORMAN, S. 2001. Combinatorial chemistry. C&EN August 27, 2001: 49–58.
73. NICOLAOU, K.C., S. KIM, J. PFEFFERKORN, et al. 1998. Synthesis and biological activity of sarcodictyins. Angew Chem. Int. Ed. **37:** 1418–1421.
74. NICOLAOU, K.C., J.A. PFEFFERKORN, S. BARLUENGA, et al. 2000. Natural product-like combinatorial libraries based on privileged structures. 3. The "libaries from libraries" principle for diversity enhancement of benzopyran libraries. J. Am. Chem. Soc. **122:** 9968–9976.
75. NICOLAOU, K.C., J.A. PFEFFERKORN, H.J. MITCHELL, et al. 2000. Natural product-like combinatorial libraries based on privileged structures. 2. Construction of a 10,000-

membered benzopyran library by directed split-and-pool chemistry using Nano-Kans and optical encoding. J. Am. Chem. Soc. **122:** 9054–9967.

76. NICOLAOU, K.C., J.A. PFEFFERKORN, A.J. ROECKER, *et al.* 2000. Natural product-like combinatorial libraries based on privileged structures. 1. General prinicples and solid-phase synthesis of benzopyrans. J. Am. Chem. Soc. **122:** 9939–9953.

77. NICOLAOU, K.C., J. PASTOR, S. BARLUENGA & N. WINSSINGER. 1998. Polymer-supported selenium reagents for organic synthesis. Chem. Commun. **1998:** 1947–1948.

78. NICOLAOU, K.C., S.Y. CHO, R. HUGHES, *et al.* 2001. Solid and solution-phase synthesis of vancomycin and vancomycin analogues with activity against vancomycin-resistant bacteria. Chem. Eur. J. **7:** 3798–3823.

79. SCHREIBER, S.L. 1998. Chemical genetics resulting from a passion for synthetic organic chemistry. Bioorg. Med. Chem. **6:** 1127–1152.

80. SCHREIBER, S.L., D.S. TAN, M.A. FOLEY, *et al.* 1998. Stereoselective synthesis of over two million compounds having structural features both eminiscent of natural products and compatible with miniaturized cell-based assays. J. Am. Chem. Soc. **120:** 8565–8566.

81. PELISH, H.E., N.J. WESTWOOD, Y. FENG, *et al.* 2001. Use of biomimetic-oriented synthesis to discover galanthamine-like molecules with biological properties beyond those of the natural product. J. Am. Chem. Soc. **123:** 6740–6741.

82. SAUSVILLE, E.A. 1997. Targeted toxins. *In* Encyclopedia of Cancer. Vol. III. J. Bertino, Ed.: 1703–1714. Academic Press. San Diego.

83. BORMAN, S. 2000. Enediyne research continues apace. Chem. Eng. News **13:** 47–49.

84. ANONYMOUS. 2000. Cancer Lett. Bus. Reg. Rep. **15:** 7.

85. LIU, C., B.M. TADAYONI, L.A. BOURRET, *et al.* 1996. Eradication of large colon tumor xenografts by targeted delivery of maytansanoids. Proc. Natl. Acad. Sci. USA **93:** 8618–8623.

86. JOHNSON, R. 2000. Personal communication with Dr. Randall Johnson, SKB Pharmaceutical R & D. Sept. 1, 2000.

87. VASEY, P.A., S.B. KAYE, R. MORRISON, *et al.* 1999. Phase I clinical and pharmacokinetic study of PK1 [*N*-(2-hydroxypropyl)methacrylamide copolymer doxorubicin]: first member of a new class of chemotherapeutic agents—drug–polymer conjugates. Cancer Research Campaign Phase I/II Committee. Clin. Cancer Res. **5:** 83–94.

88. JULYAN, P.J., L.W. SEYMOUR, D.R. FERRY, *et al.* 1999. Preliminary clinical study of the distribution of HPMA copolymers bearing doxorubicin and galactosamine. J. Con. Rel. **57:** 281–290.

89. MELTON, R.G. & R.F. SHERWOOD. 1996. Antibody–enzyme conjugates for cancer therapy. J. Natl. Can. Inst. **88:** 153–165.

90. HORAN, A.C. 1994. Actinomycetes. *In* The Discovery of Natural Products with Therapeutic Potential. V.P. Gullo, Ed.: 3–30. Butterworth-Heinemann. Boston.

Gene Therapy

A Brief Overview of the Past, Present, and Future

ROLAND SCOLLAY

Genteric, Alameda, California 94501, USA

ABSTRACT: Gene therapy has only recently begun to make serious progress, beginning with two approved gene therapy trials in the United States in late 1990. The death of an 18-year-old man participating in a gene therapy trial delivered a major setback in terms of public concerns, but the resulting improvements in scrutiny of trial design and ethical standards will benefit the field in the long run. The three main issues for the coming decade will be public perceptions, scale-up and manufacturing, and commercial considerations. Focusing on single-gene applications, which tend to be rarer diseases, will produce successful results sooner than the current focus on the commoner, yet more complex, cancer and heart disease.

KEYWORDS: gene therapy; clinical trials; trial design; cancer; cardiovascular disease; hemophilia

Gene therapy has had rather a bad decade. In fact, it got off to a shaky start long before the 1990s began with two unapproved trials in the early 70s and early 80s. In the first, an attempt was made to treat two young girls with arginase deficiency syndrome using *in vivo* gene therapy with wild-type Shope papilloma virus, in the hope that the viral arginase would replace the missing enzyme in the patients. The second was *ex vivo* gene therapy for β-thalassemia, a bone marrow transplant using marrow cells treated with a β-globin-containing plasmid, again in two patients. In neither case was any real follow-up reported, since both trials were stopped, but apparently neither good nor harm resulted for the patients, although the investigators did not fare so well (for discussion of the early history of gene therapy, see Wolff and Lederberg[1]).

The first serious, approved gene therapy trials happened in the United States in late 1990, when two *ex vivo* trials began. One trial employed enzyme-transduced T cells for an enzyme deficiency that causes severe combined immunodeficiency (SCID)[2]; the other used cytokine (TNF)-transduced lymphocytes that had been extracted from tumors as immunotherapy for melanoma.[3] Both trials relied on retroviruses to transfect the cells. Neither was successful, for reasons we now understand. During the rest of the 90s, the pace accelerated, and in 1999 alone 84 new trials were approved by NIH/RAC.[4] In all, as of mid-2000, almost 4000 patients have been

Address for correspondence: Roland Scollay, Ph.D., Chief Scientific Officer, Genteric, 2061 Challenger Drive, Alameda, CA 94501. Voice: 510 749 6063.

rscollay@genteric.com

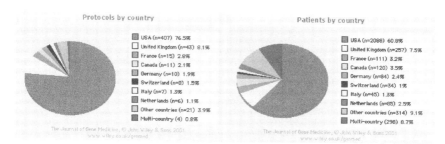

FIGURE 1. Geographic distribution of gene therapy clinical trials. Reproduced from the John Wiley and Sons, Ltd. website[5] with permission.

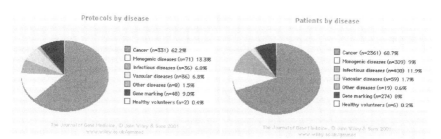

FIGURE 2. Diseases being treated in gene therapy clinical trials. Reproduced from the John Wiley and Sons, Ltd. website[5] with permission.

treated with gene therapy in more than 500 trials. A Medline search for "gene therapy" publications will find a handful in 1985, a few hundred in 1990, and more than 2000 by 1999. According to the Wiley website (Ref. 5, a good source of information on clinical trials) 77% of these protocols were in the United States, and in 69% of patients, the target disease was cancer (FIGS. 1 and 2). Only 1% of protocols reached phase three, and none have gone beyond.

The decade of the 90s was discouraging: all those trials and almost no success. And it finished badly in September 1999 with the widely publicized death of an eighteen-year-old man undergoing gene therapy for a liver disease at the University of Pennsylvania, an event that brought the scrutiny of the press onto the world of gene therapy. This was the first death directly attributable to gene therapy, and the ensuing publicity and investigations not only bought to light a number of clinical trials in which trial design or ethical standards were not satisfactory, but also unfairly cast a shadow over the whole field of gene therapy. The improved control and scrutiny resulting from these events can only be good for the future of the field, but the lingering concerns will take time to dispel.

Then, at the turn of the millennium, through the year 2000, anecdotal reports of the first apparent successes began to be heard, hopeful hints that real success may be just around the corner: factor IX for hemophilia,[6] transduced stem cells for X-linked SCID,[7] and oncolytic vectors.[8] In some cases, the progress came from improvements in our understanding of the vectors (e.g., hemophilia and improved adeno-associated virus vectors); in others, the vectors have changed little, but our understanding of the genes and of the biology of the transduced cells made all the difference (e.g., treatment of SCID patients by transduction of stem cells with the common gamma chain of the interleukin receptor). Indeed, the field is learning from its mistakes, and many of the problems are now better understood. Scale-up and manufacturing issues, as well as those of quality control and safety, are being intensely studied. Well-founded skepticism has forced the field to be more rigorous, leading to a higher likelihood of success. Ten years of hard times has weeded out many approaches and put the focus on realistic and achievable technologies.

In fact this ten-year cycle is rather similar to the one that monoclonal antibodies followed: a lot of noise and high expectations based on preclinical science; ten years of failed clinical trials as the problems became apparent; then, a much more realistic approach and solutions to many of the problems; and now major clinical and commercial successes. I believe that gene therapy will follow a similar pattern and that the recent successes herald the beginnings of a decade of real progress, leading to gene therapies that will have a major impact on the practice of medicine.

What, then, are the main issues (apart from just getting it to work in the clinic) going forward over the next 10 years? They can be broadly divided into three categories:

- public perceptions
- scale-up and manufacturing
- commercial considerations

Public perceptions have indeed been influenced by the gene therapy–related death mentioned above. Furthermore, there is a general public concern about genetic engineering and genetically modified organisms, concern that has lead to demonstrations and legal challenges in Europe. The public often has a limited ability to discriminate between different forms of "genetic manipulation" and will lump even the simplest clinical gene therapy together with gene-modified crops, transgenic farm animals, and Dolly the cloned sheep, generating public resistance to all. Many people can discriminate among these issues, however, and do realize that some setbacks are inevitable with cutting-edge therapies. It will be crucial in the future that gene therapy trials are well planned and in accordance with all relevant guidelines. Then a few real successes in the clinic will soon regain popular support. The addition of a growing number of safety features into vectors should also allay fears as we move forward.

Scale-up and manufacture have long been significant obstacles for many of the best vector systems; and, even now, producing enough vector for large clinical trials is still problematic. It remains a challenge to produce vectors at commercial scale and to control production runs for mutated or recombined viruses. Nevertheless, tangible progress is being made, and it is likely that adequate systems will be available for the manufacture of many vectors by the time clinical efficacy is established in Phase III clinical trials.

Commercial considerations have heavily influenced the direction of gene therapy development. The fact that many gene therapy trials and much gene therapy research is being done within companies or sponsored by companies, with the ultimate aim of developing these therapies commercially as "drugs," has put pressure on researchers and companies to develop therapies for large-market indications. This means that rarer diseases, such as some of the single-gene-mutation, inherited diseases, get less attention, while major diseases, such as cardiovascular disease and cancer, are greatly emphasized. This is a pity for two reasons. First, rare diseases that could potentially be treated quite soon using gene therapy are getting little attention. Second, these same "rare" diseases are, in fact, often much easier targets for gene therapy, with well-defined, well-understood target genes for delivery. Factors VIII and IX for the treatment of hemophilia are good examples of well-understood drugs with very accessible clinical targets. They have received some attention from smaller biotechnology companies, but many other diseases remain untouched. The pressure to treat larger indications like cancer has lead to a predominance of trials for these diseases (approximately 70% of all gene therapy trials to date have been in cancer), and this has been one of the reasons there have been so many unsuccessful clinical trials in the last 10 years. In most cases it has not been clear which genes to use in the treatment of these complex diseases, and many trials have been tests for the efficacy of the genes being investigated, rather than tests of a gene delivery technology using genes that we know will work if delivered at adequate levels. In other words, many of these trials have involved two very serious unknowns, the ability to deliver the gene and the efficacy of the gene, once delivered. Furthermore, it has not always been clear which of the two failed.

The second major commercial issue relates to intellectual property. Most gene therapies involve complex treatments upon which multiple patents impinge. Patents or licenses for vector systems or their individual components, promoters, regulatory elements, targeting elements, the therapeutic gene, the manufacturing process, and so forth are all required for a single therapy. Few, if any, companies can gather together all they need for the optimal treatment, because other companies that control key components often have unrealistically high ideas of their value, and the additive effect of the royalties on the many components involved (royalty stacking) becomes seriously limiting. This means that therapies going to the clinic are not always the very best available; rather, they are those for which the licenses are held, another factor contributing to the high failure rate of gene therapy trials to date. This is quite distinct from the world of small molecular drugs, where each competing company fully controls a single drug entity, and the public process of clinical trials can select the best among them.

Because the field of gene therapy urgently needs some additional successes in order to continue to attract public support as well as research funds and investments, it would perhaps be wise to focus on achieving success in the short term with the easier, but less profitable diseases, rather than failing with the big-market indications. Furthermore, it may be in everyone's best interest if there were many more cooperative arrangements between diverse interests (collaborations, joint ventures, consortia, etc.) in order to bring the very best combinations of technology to bear on the clinical problems being addressed. This will require a cooperative, rather than a competitive, spirit. Commercially, this may mean waiting for success to bring recognition or profit, rather than demanding short-term gain in the form of large upfront licenses and fees. There has been some evidence of such positive interactions in recent months, but a lot more cooperation will be needed if the new field of gene therapy is to reach its potential in the near future. I am optimistic that both the cooperation and the success will happen in the coming decade.

NOTES AND REFERENCES

1. WOLFF, J.A. & J. LEDERBERG. 1994. An early history of gene transfer and therapy. Hum. Gene Ther. **5:** 469–480.
2. BLAESE, R.M., K.W. CULVER, A.D. MILLER, et al. 1995. T-lymphocyte-directed gene therapy for ADA-SCID: initial trial results after 4 years. Science **270(5235):** 475–480.
3. ROSENBERG, S.A., et al. 1992. Immunization of cancer patients using autologous cancer cells modified by insertion of the gene for tumor necrosis factor. Hum. Gene Ther. **3:** 57–73.
4. More information on U.S. clinical trials can be obtained from the NIH site (http://www4.od.nih.gov/oba/clinicaltrial.htm).
5. John Wiley website: http://www.wiley.co.uk/wileychi/genmed/clinical/.
6. KAY, M.A., C.S. MANNO, M.V. RAGNI, et al. 2000. Evidence for gene transfer and expression of factor IX in hemophilia patients treated with an AAV vector. Nat. Genet. **24:** 257–261.
7. CAVAZZANA-CALVO, M., S. HACEIN-BEY, G. DE SAINT BASILLE, et al. 2000. Gene therapy of severe combined immunodeficiency (SCID)-X1 disease. Science **288:** 669–672.
8. KHURI, F.R., J. NEMUNAITIS, I. GANLY, et al. 2000. A controlled trial of intratumoral ONYX-015, a selectively-replicating adenovirus, in combination with cisplatin and 5-fluorouracil in patients with recurrent head and neck cancer. Nature Med. **8:** 879–885.

Gene Therapy for Cardiovascular Disorders

Is There a Future?

BEVERLY L. METCALFE,[a] KATHLEEN W. SELLERS,[a]
MICHAEL JING-REN JENG,[a] MATTHEW J. HUENTELMAN,[a]
MICHAEL J. KATOVICH,[b] AND MOHAN K. RAIZADA[a]

[a]*Department of Physiology and Functional Genomics, College of Medicine,*
[b]*Department of Pharmacodynamics, College of Pharmacy,*
Evelyn F. and William L. McKnight Brain Institute, University of Florida,
Gainesville, Florida 32610, USA

ABSTRACT: Incidence of cardiovascular disease has reached epidemic proportions in spite of recent advances in improving the efficacy of pharmacotherapeutics. This has led many to conclude that drug therapy has reached a plateau in its effectiveness. As a result, our efforts have been diverted to explore the use of gene transfer approaches for long-term control of these pathophysiological conditions. The purpose of this review is to present various approaches that are being undertaken to provide "proof of principle" for gene therapy for cardiovascular diseases. Finally, we will discuss the future of gene therapy and other new technologies that may further advance this field of therapeutics.

KEYWORDS: gene therapy; cardiovascular disorders; viral vectors; restenosis; thrombosis; hypertension; ischemia; heart failure

INTRODUCTION

The cardiovascular (CV) system is a complex physiological organization with regulators ranging from the heart to the adrenals to the kidney and the brain. While recent advances have significantly improved the beneficial outcome, CV diseases, including hypertension, remain the leading cause of mortality and morbidity in industrialized nations.[1]

In spite of effective pharmacotherapies, patient incompliance due to the strict daily regime has disabled our ability to control hypertension. Other diseases such as atherosclerosis demand a fast and targeted preventative measure that available drugs cannot provide. Given these limitations in traditional pharmacotherapies, many researchers have turned their attention to investigate a genetic-based therapy that could be the next step forward to combat or prevent CV disorders. Gene therapy is an emerging field that offers targeted and time-controlled parameters especially relevant to CV diseases ranging from hypertension to ischemia to restenosis.

Address for correspondence: Mohan K. Raizada, Department of Physiology and Functional Genomics, University of Florida, College of Medicine, P.O. Box 100274, Gainesville, FL 32610. Voice: 352-392-9299; fax: 352-294-0191.

mraizada@phys.med.ufl.edu

Principally, gene therapy is a strategy in which a vector is used to deliver beneficial gene(s), either systemically or directly into the tissue. Successful delivery thereby changes the expression levels of that gene to correct the altered expression in the pathophysiological state. Gene therapy is being explored in a multitude of diseases due to its diversity in vector types and delivery methods. CV research is no exception. In accordance with the variety of CV diseases, a number of different gene therapy strategies have been implemented. In hypertension research, where reversal and prevention are key, long-term gene regulation is necessary. In terms of disorders such as ischemia and restenosis, short-term gene control would serve to prevent such incidences. Different gene therapy vectors are therefore effective against specific CV diseases.

In this review, we will summarize our current understandings of gene therapy for CV diseases, describe various vehicles to deliver therapeutic genes, and present many approaches that are being taken to provide "proof of concept" from animal and human experimentation. Then, we will summarize our studies on the use of antisense gene therapy for long-term control of hypertension and finally discuss novel technologies that may provide additional advances in the gene therapy field.

GENE DELIVERY VEHICLES: NONVIRAL AND VIRAL VECTORS

Several methods have been used to deliver exogenous genes related to various CV diseases. Each method has its own advantages and disadvantages that determine its use for a particular subset of CV diseases.

The simplest way to deliver exogenous genes is by directly injecting "naked" plasmid DNA. This method is effective for localized delivery into a particular tissue such as skeletal muscle.[2] "Naked" DNA delivery is effective for approximately one month, it has little or no toxic or adverse side effects, and repeated injection is effective.[3] Disadvantages of this technique include inefficient delivery, limited time for transgene expression, high levels of vector breakdown in circulation, and lack of chromosomal integration.[4] Liposomes and hemagglutinating virus of Japan (HVJ-liposomes) have been developed to deliver "naked" DNA in an attempt to overcome some of these disadvantages. Both of these methods increase infection efficiency over "naked" DNA delivery, minimize immunogenicity, and prevent DNA degradation in circulation. This makes "naked" DNA delivery an ideal choice for short-term transgene expression. Consequently, it has been used to deliver transgenes relevant in the inhibition of cell proliferation during restenosis.[5] However, these methods of delivery still do not elicit target specificity and do not allow the DNA to integrate into the recipients' genome. Thus, it is of less therapeutic significance in situations where long-term transgene expression is required.[6,7]

Viral-mediated gene delivery is emerging as the preferred choice of gene delivery vehicles. Viral vectors are designed to be replication-defective, while retaining their ability to infect target cells and transduce genetic material.[8] Several types of these viral-mediated systems exist, each having its own unique qualities. The major classes of viral vectors include the adenovirus, adeno-associated virus (AAV), herpes simplex virus (HSV), and a family of retroviruses including the murine leukemia virus (MLV) and lenti-based HIV-1 viral vectors.

Adenovirus is one of the most widely used viral vectors for gene therapy for CV diseases. Advantages of using the adenovirus as a gene therapy vector include ease of manipulation, generation of high titers, large insert capacity, infection of a wide variety of dividing and nondividing cells and tissue types, and extensive characterization.[9] While adenovirus has been readily used for studying various CV diseases, this vector system has some drawbacks that may prevent its use in the future. First, it does not integrate into the host genome, thus allowing only transient expression of the desired transgene. Adenovirus can also cause acute and chronic toxicity and immune response. Finally, this viral vector will not be an effective transducing agent if test animals and patients have existing acquired immune response to adenovirus. Such an immune response reduces the efficiency of readministration of adenovirus to increase the transgene expression.[10]

Adeno-associated virus (AAV) is increasingly gaining popularity as a gene therapy vector because of its ability to infect a large number of both dividing and nondividing cell types. The wild-type AAV has a known integration site into chromosome 19 and is nonpathogenic. In spite of these positive qualities, many drawbacks must be overcome before this vector system can be an ideal vector for gene therapy. These include (i) increasing the genomic capacity to include various regulators and promoters for a transgene, (ii) technical advances to allow production of large-scale quantities of virus, and (iii) identifying the chromosomal integration site of the recombinant AAV.[11]

Several groups have used the herpes simplex virus (HSV) as a gene therapy vector as well. The advantages of this vector system are its natural infection of nondividing neurons, its production of latent infections without damaging the neuronal cells, its large transgene capacity, and its capability to be made with high titers. The major disadvantage of using HSV as a gene therapy vector is that, when the virus is in its latent phase, none of its genes are expressed and studies must be made to disable wild-type HSV since it can cause damaging effects.[12]

The retrovirus was the first family of viruses to be used for gene therapy; thus, it is the most used viral vector in clinical trials. There are many different types of viruses in this family, but this review will focus on the Moloney murine leukemia virus (MLV) and lentivirus. The majority of retroviruses used for gene therapy are derived from the MLV. The advantages of using MLV for gene therapy are that it can infect a variety of cells and tissues, large genes can be inserted into the vector, it is easy to manipulate *in vitro*, and it can be made with high titers. There is no pathogenicity associated with the MLV because the viral system is designed to not transfer any of the viral genes, and it stably integrates into the host genome, allowing for long-term expression of the transgene. This type of virus, however, has limitations because its random insertions can cause mutations, and it can only infect dividing cells. MLV requires the cell cycle to integrate and express the transgene.[13,14] Because of these drawbacks of the MLV, lentivirus has become a novel and exciting new gene therapy vector. The lentivirus maintains all of the advantages of the MLV, but it can infect both nondividing and dividing cells. This virus is based on the human HIV-1 virus and, thus, one of the major drawbacks of this virus is establishing its efficacy and safety.[15]

In summary, major strides have been made in the last several years to develop both nonviral and viral vectors for gene delivery. Choice of a gene delivery method is dependent on the needs of a given pathophysiological situation. For example, an ideal vector for the control of hypertension would be the one that could be produced in large quantities, could integrate into the genome and have long-term transgene expression, and be safe and nonimmunogenic. At this time, the retroviral vector family seems to fit these criteria. On the other hand, the adenoviral vector or HVJ-based "naked" DNA delivery may serve a prominent role in which transient expression of a given transgene is needed, as for the case with restenosis or ischemia.

RESTENOSIS

Interventions such as balloon angioplasty are highly effective for the treatment of stenosis in coronary and renal arteries. However, after initial success, these arteries undergo restenosis at a rate of 30%. While various mechanical and pharmacological strategies are used to circumvent restenosis, they all have limited success. As a result, innovative gene transfer approaches are being tried to improve the success in inhibiting restenosis.

Principally, the objective has been to introduce genes that inhibit cell multiplication by either obstructing or inhibiting entry of cells into the cell cycle. Research by Dzau's group has used HVJ-liposome-mediated delivery of antisense oligonucleotides to cyclin B1 and CDC2 kinase encoding genes. They demonstrated that HVJ-liposomes increased the half-life of the oligos and transduction efficiency and that combined administration of the antisense oligos inhibited neointima formation after balloon injury.[16,17]

Several genes have been delivered after balloon injury via the adenoviral vector to prevent entry of the cell into the cell cycle. Leiden's group has paved the path for this approach by expressing a constitutively active mutant of the retinoblastoma protein, RB. This mutant forms a complex with the E2F family of transcription factors to prevent cell cycle entry.[18] Another group has fused the active sites of two cell cycle inhibitors, p27 and p16, and delivered it using an adenovirus.[19] A third approach used the adenovirus to express the HSV thymidine kinase gene that phosphorylates the pro-drug ganciclovir to inhibit DNA synthesis.[20] Recently, a group has constructed a hybrid protein of the amino-terminal fragment of urokinase-type plasminogen activator (u-PA) linked to bovine pancreas trypsin inhibitor. This hybrid binds to the u-PA receptor to inhibit plasmin activity, acting as a potent cell migration inhibitor.[21,22] All of these methods show a significant reduction in the intima-to-media ratio.

While the use of the adenoviral vector has been instrumental in establishing proof of principle for the use of gene therapy in restenosis, the concerns regarding the adverse immune response restricts its possible use for human gene therapy. As a result, our research group has investigated if the retroviral family of viral vectors can be more efficacious for the control of restenosis. Our approach has been to deliver a transgene into an artery using the lentiviral vector.

The lentiviral vector may be ideal for this delivery because, like the adenovirus, it can infect both dividing and nondividing cells. In contrast, however, it also integrates into the host genome, allowing long-term expression if desired, and it has little or no immunogenic response. The external, internal, and common carotid arteries were ligated and a balloon catheter was inflated and passed three times in the pres-

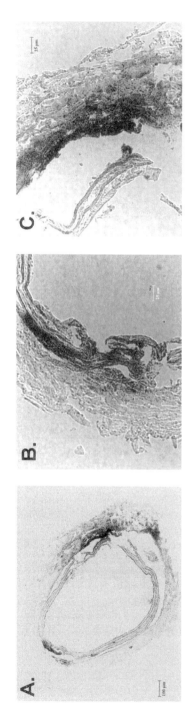

FIGURE 1. (A) Arterial cross sections demonstrating lentiviral-mediated delivery of hPLAP in a balloon-injured artery. This technique was able to transduce both vascular smooth muscle and adventitial layers. **(B, C)** Higher magnifications of the arterial cross sections.

ence of heparin (0.1 units/mg) and elastase (2×10^{-7} units). Following the injury, approximately 4.5×10^8 viral particles of lentivirus containing a human placental alkaline phosphatase gene (hPLAP) were injected and allowed to incubate in the artery for 15 minutes. Three days later, arteries were perfused, sectioned, and examined for alkaline phosphatase activity. A robust and high degree of transduction was observed (FIG. 1). It appears that the lentiviral vector was able to transduce both vascular smooth muscle and adventitial cellular layers. This observation, although preliminary, provides important evidence that the lentiviral vector seems to pass through many cell layers.

THROMBOSIS

Prevention of thrombosis is a clinically relevant problem to study, not only because it plays a pivotal role in vascular occlusion following balloon injury, but because thrombolytic therapy has also been monumental in increasing survival rate following an acute myocardial infarction or a cerebrovascular incident.

The research groups led by Drs. Woo and Shenaq have been instrumental in establishing the potential use of adenovirus for "thromboresistance" in a rabbit model. Using local delivery into the common femoral artery, they were successful in increasing the expression of both plasminogen and thrombomodulin. Tissue-type plasminogen activator is a protease that catalyzes the conversion of plasminogen to plasmin to prevent the formation of fibrin. Thrombomodulin binds to thrombin to initiate the conversion of protein C to its active form, an anticoagulant. Both methods have been proven successful in preventing thrombosis, decreasing evidence of occlusion by approximately 50%.[23,24] Recombinant tissue factor pathway inhibitor (rTFPI) has also been used to prevent thrombosis and restenosis after balloon injury. TFPI inhibits factor Xa and the coagulation initiator, factor VIIa. Adenoviral and retroviral administration encoding TFPI have been shown to decrease or prevent thrombosis following injury.[25,26]

HYPERTENSION

Essentially two approaches have been used to provide "proof of concept" for the use of gene therapy for hypertension. One consists of overexpression of vasodilatory relevant genes (sense approach) and the other is an "antisense" approach in which vasoconstrictive genes are inhibited.

Chao and associates have led the way in using the "sense" approach overexpressing the kallikrein and adrenomedullin genes using the adenoviral vector. Kallikrein hydrolyzes kininogen to kinin. Kinin binds to its receptor (bradykinin B2 receptor) and induces vasodilation. Systemic delivery of an adenovirus expressing kallikrein showed a reversal in hypertension for 20–25 days. This was associated with protection against hypertension-induced renal injury and cardiac remodeling.[27,28] Additionally, they have established that a single intramuscular injection of the same virus leads to a continuous supply of kallikrein in the circulation, thus reducing blood pressure.[29] Adrenomedullin is a potent vasodilator that plays an important role in cardiac function. Overexpression of adrenomedullin using the adenoviral vector provided protection against hypertension, cardiac hypertrophy, and renal damage in both salt-sensitive and volume-dependent hypertension.[30,31]

Our research group and Phillips' group have used an "antisense" approach to target the renin angiotensin system (RAS). In the RAS, angiotensinogen is converted to angiotensin I by the enzyme renin. Angiotensin I is then converted to angiotensin II by the angiotensin-converting enzyme (ACE). Angiotensin II is the physiologically active hormone of the RAS, causing vasoconstriction, among other effects, when bound to its receptor, the angiotensin II type 1 receptor (AT_1R). Using liposomes to deliver AT_1R antisense, Phillips and his associates were able to demonstrate a significant decrease in blood pressure in the spontaneously hypertensive rat (SHR).[3,32] While these results are impressive, the antihypertensive effects were transient and seem to be of little improvement over traditional therapy.

Our laboratory has used a retroviral vector (MLV) to determine if antihypertensive effects of AT_1R-AS could be prolonged. A single intracardiac injection in 5-day-old rats results in a significant attenuation of high blood pressure in the SHR for the life of the animal. The AT_1R-AS transductions also prevent left ventricular hypertrophy, cardiac fibrosis, and neointimal thickening in the SHR.[33–36] Proof of principle has been provided by demonstrating that the AT_1R-AS gene therapy prevents hypertension in many other animal models.[37] Similar results were seen using a retrovirus delivering antisense to the angiotensin-converting enzyme.[38,39]

ISCHEMIA

Ischemia, the reduction of oxygen to a specific area of the body, affects over 3 million Americans.[1] Ischemic heart disease leads to myocardial infarction and other cardiac complications. Cerebral ischemia is fatal and can result from subarachnoid hemorrhage (SAH). Ten days following SAH, arterial constriction known as cerebral vasospasm can lead to ischemia and death. Gene therapy, because of its potential to be targeted and rapid response to ischemia, offers a promising technology to prevent SAH.

Adenovirus is the most widely used viral vector in ischemia research. Success in the prevention of ischemia has been demonstrated in the induction of angiogenesis using the adenoviral vector. The principle behind the treatment of ischemia has been to deliver growth-promoting and vasodilatory genes to increase blood volume and oxygen availability. One such gene is the basic fibroblast growth factor (bFGF), an angiogenic factor that has effects on multiple classes of cells including neurons. Administration of the bFGF protein is effective for only a short time; therefore, it is a good target for gene therapy. Ventricular delivery of bFGF to male Wistar Kyoto (WKY) rats resulted in an increased vessel-to-area ratio in the paraventricular region.[40]

Using an adenoviral vector to deliver prepro-calcitonin gene–related peptide (CGRP), a known vasodilator, Toyoda demonstrated a decreased arterial constriction in rabbits. In addition, a similar beneficial outcome in arterial diameter was observed with prepro-CGRP gene delivery in SAH *in vivo*. These results led to the conclusion that vasospasm can be prevented following SAH.[41] In parallel experiments, Katusic demonstrated that adenoviral delivery of endothelial nitric oxide synthase (eNOS), another known vasodilator, partially restored relaxation in cerebral basilar arteries, a significant stepping stone in the prevention of vasospasm after SAH.[42] Thus, the quick response from the delivery of ischemia-related gene(s) holds promise in the prevention of this fatal disease.

Vascular endothelial growth factor (VEGF) is a promising candidate for gene therapy because it stimulates the angiogenic process at all stages. Adenovirus was used to successfully deliver VEGF to 21 patients with areas of reversible ischemia, and ischemic effects were later assessed.[43] Thirty days after myocardial injections, coronary artery filling increased and reversible ischemia decreased in patients with coronary artery disease.[44,45]

Other viral and nonviral vectors are also being developed to prevent ischemia. Using the HSV, Yenari has enhanced neuronal survival even following injury by effectively overexpressing genes essential to neuronal function.[46] Double-stranded (ds) oligo/DNA delivery of a decoy nuclear factor KB (NF-kappaB), which normally functions in elevating inflammation after SAH, resulted in a prevention of vasospasm and morphological changes in vessel walls.[47]

Finally, risk of ischemia associated with heart transplants is being addressed with a gene therapy strategy. During heart transplantation, the process of preserving the heart is countered with potential ischemia-reperfusion injury. Current methods focus on elevating cardioprotective proteins that would protect the cells against ischemia. The HVJ-liposome technique was used to deliver the heat-shock protein 70 (HSP70) via intracoronary infusion. HSP70 functions in regulating myocardial metabolism, and results show a protection in both mitochondrial and ventricular functions.[48] Gene therapy thus presents a promising route to prevent ischemia even after SAH.

HEART FAILURE

Despite pharmacological advance, incidence of heart failure has increased for the past 20 years. Gene therapy for this disease is promising for several reasons. First, the targeted demographic for heart failure focuses on the elderly, where lifelong transgene expression is within reach with current technology. Second, elderly patients are often not ideal candidates for a heart transplant because of increased surgical risk or limited availability of donor organs. Third, since biochemistry and physiology of the heart are well studied, specific genes that could be targeted for therapy can be easily identified. Finally, gene therapy aimed at targeting a specific organ rather than the entire body is more obtainable and effective.[49]

Proteins involved in heart failure include the sarcoplasmic reticulum (SR) Ca(2+)-ATPase (SERCA2a). This enzyme drives Ca(2+) reaccumulation into the SR from the cytoplasm; a defect in SERCA2a results in a decrease in contraction and thus heart failure. In a recent study, adenoviral vector was used to deliver SERCA2a via catheter to rats with established heart failure. Results showed a 63% increase in survival rate, decreased left ventricular volumes, and normalized cardiac metabolism.[50] Beta2-adrenergic receptor has also been used as a target for gene therapy in heart failure. Activation of this receptor controls catecholamine response through cAMP regulation and, thus, a decrease in beta2-adrenergic receptors causes a decrease in cardiac responses to catecholamines and leads to heart failure. The Epstein-Barr virus (EBV) vector has been used to deliver human beta2-AR gene to the left ventricular muscle of hamsters with decreased beta2-AR and failing cardiomyocytes.[51] EBV has been used based on its specificity and efficient transduction. Two days after transduction, cardiac output increased 1.6-fold and stroke volume increased 1.7-fold. Results show an increase in both cardiac output and stroke volume, indicating improved cardiac function. Therefore, cardiac function improved in hamsters with failing hearts, demonstrating how gene therapy can reverse effects of heart failure.

FUTURE DIRECTIONS AND GENE THERAPY ALTERNATIVES

While gene therapy is an exciting field and without a doubt will play a pivotal role in the treatment of many cardiovascularly related diseases, more research is needed before taking this strategy to the clinical trial level. Many of the first-generation gene therapy vectors have been useful in studying proof of principle for many genes and how they may play a role or regulate various CV diseases. However, newer second- and third-generation vectors are being developed that combine the advantages of several vectors, while eliminating some disadvantages of each. The potential of these newer generations of viral vectors must be evaluated in terms of their ability to increase transgene transduction.

Other emerging technologies may prove to be beneficial in the treatment of CV disease and thus must be explored. Recent studies have demonstrated that an amino acid sequence, Tat, has the potential to transport proteins across the cell membrane and into the intracellular compartments. With this Tat fusion, the investigators have successfully introduced their protein of interest in most major organs including the brain.[52] Davidson's group has taken advantage of this technology and combined it with a viral vector. They have designed an adenoviral vector to induce a Tat fusion protein whose expression can be demonstrated for a longer period of time.[53]

Finally, the potential for a newly discovered technique called chimeraplasty must be explored. Chimeraplasts are DNA-RNA oligomers that, by taking advantage of the cell's DNA repair machinery, can identify and correct a point mutation. Recently, this technique was used to convert the hyperlipidemia-causing variant of the apolipoprotein E (apoE2) to its anti-atherogenic form, apoE3.[54]

CONCLUSIONS

All of the existing data presented here indicate that the gene therapy approach holds immense potential for the treatment of various CV disorders. Continuing research will lead to the identification of the "ideal" genes to target for the treatment of each CV disease. With ongoing research in collaboration with virologists, molecular biologists, pharmacologists, geneticists, and physiologists, the development of new and improved viral vectors will lead us to the "perfect" viral vectors and genes to treat certain CV-related diseases.

ACKNOWLEDGMENTS

This research was supported by NIH Grant No. HL52691. M. J. Huentelman and B. L. Metcalfe are predoctoral fellows of the American Heart Association, Florida affiliate. Michael Jing-Ren Jeng was a visiting fellow from the Department of Medicine, National Defense Medical Center, Taipei, Taiwan.

REFERENCES

1. AMERICAN HEART ASSOCIATION. 2001. Heart and Stroke Statistical Update. American Heart Association. Dallas.
2. WOLFF, J.A., et al. 1990. Direct gene transfer into mouse muscle in vivo. Science 247(4949, pt. 1): 1465–1468.
3. PHILLIPS, M.I., S.M. GALLI & J.L. MEHTA. 2000. The potential role of antisense oligodeoxynucleotide therapy for cardiovascular disease. Drugs 60(2): 239–248.
4. NISHIKAWA, M. & L. HUANG. 2001. Nonviral vectors in the new millennium: delivery barriers in gene transfer. Hum. Gene Ther. 12(8): 861–870.
5. NIKOL, S., et al. 2000. Prevention of restenosis using the gene for cecropin complexed with DOCSPER liposomes under optimized conditions. Int. J. Angiol. 9(2): 87–94.
6. ROMANO, G., et al. 1998. Recent advances, prospects, and problems in designing new strategies for oligonucleotide and gene delivery in therapy. In Vivo 12(1): 59–67.
7. KANEDA, Y., Y. SAEKI & R. MORISHITA. 1999. Gene therapy using HVJ-liposomes: the best of both worlds? Mol. Med. Today 5(7): 298–303.
8. VERMA, I.M. & N. SOMIA. 1997. Gene therapy—promises, problems, and prospects. Nature 389(6648): 239–242.
9. DANTHINNE, X. & M.J. IMPERIALE. 2000. Production of first generation adenovirus vectors: a review. Gene Ther. 7(20): 1707–1714.
10. PARKS, R.J. 2000. Improvements in adenoviral vector technology: overcoming barriers for gene therapy. Clin. Genet. 58(1): 1–11.
11. MONAHAN, P.E. & R.J. SAMULSKI. 2000. Adeno-associated virus vectors for gene therapy: more pros than cons? Mol. Med. Today 6(11): 433–440.
12. LATCHMAN, D.S. 2001. Gene delivery and gene therapy with herpes simplex virus–based vectors. Gene 264(1): 1–9.
13. MILLER, A.D., et al. 1993. Use of retroviral vectors for gene transfer and expression. Methods Enzymol. 217: 581–599.
14. KIM, S.H., S. KIM & P.D. ROBBINS. 2000. Retroviral vectors. Adv. Virus Res. 55: 545–563.
15. BUCHSCHACHER, G.L., JR. & F. WONG-STAAL. 2000. Development of lentiviral vectors for gene therapy for human diseases. Blood 95(8): 2499–2504.
16. MORISHITA, R., et al. 1994. Pharmacokinetics of antisense oligodeoxyribonucleotides (cyclin B1 and CDC 2 kinase) in the vessel wall in vivo: enhanced therapeutic utility for restenosis by HVJ-liposome delivery. Gene 149(1): 13–19.
17. KANEDA, Y., R. MORISHITA & V.J. DZAU. 1997. Prevention of restenosis by gene therapy. Ann. N.Y. Acad. Sci. 811: 299–308; 308–310 (discussion).
18. CHANG, M.W., et al. 1995. Cytostatic gene therapy for vascular proliferative disorders with a constitutively active form of the retinoblastoma gene product. Science 267(5197): 518–522.
19. TSUI, L.V., et al. 2001. p27-p16 fusion gene inhibits angioplasty-induced neointimal hyperplasia and coronary artery occlusion. Circ. Res. 89(4): 323–328.
20. GUZMAN, R.J., et al. 1994. In vivo suppression of injury-induced vascular smooth muscle cell accumulation using adenovirus-mediated transfer of the herpes simplex virus thymidine kinase gene. Proc. Natl. Acad. Sci. U.S.A. 91(22): 10732–10736.
21. LAMFERS, M.L., et al. 2001. In vivo suppression of restenosis in balloon-injured rat carotid artery by adenovirus-mediated gene transfer of the cell surface–directed plasmin inhibitor ATF.BPTI. Gene Ther. 8(7): 534–541.
22. QUAX, P.H., et al. 2001. Adenoviral expression of a urokinase receptor–targeted protease inhibitor inhibits neointima formation in murine and human blood vessels. Circulation 103(4): 562–569.
23. WAUGH, J.M., et al. 1999. Gene therapy to promote thromboresistance: local over-expression of tissue plasminogen activator to prevent arterial thrombosis in an in vivo rabbit model. Proc. Natl. Acad. Sci. USA 96(3): 1065–1070.

24. WAUGH, J.M., *et al.* 1999. Local overexpression of thrombomodulin for *in vivo* prevention of arterial thrombosis in a rabbit model. Circ. Res. **84**(1): 84–92.
25. GOLINO, P., *et al.* 2001. Expression of exogenous tissue factor pathway inhibitor *in vivo* suppresses thrombus formation in injured rabbit carotid arteries. J. Am. Coll. Cardiol. **38**(2): 569–576.
26. ZOLDHELYI, P., *et al.* 2000. Thromboresistance of balloon-injured porcine carotid arteries after local gene transfer of human tissue factor pathway inhibitor. Circulation **101**(3): 289–295.
27. WOLF, W.C., *et al.* 2000. Human tissue kallikrein gene delivery attenuates hypertension, renal injury, and cardiac remodeling in chronic renal failure. Kidney Int. **58**(2): 730–739.
28. DOBRZYNSKI, E., *et al.* 1999. Adenovirus-mediated kallikrein gene delivery attenuates hypertension and protects against renal injury in deoxycorticosterone-salt rats. Immunopharmacology **44**(1–2): 57–65.
29. ZHANG, J.J., *et al.* 1999. Human tissue kallikrein attenuates hypertension and secretes into circulation and urine after intramuscular gene delivery in hypertensive rats. Clin. Exp. Hypertens. **21**(7): 1145–1160.
30. ZHANG, J.J., *et al.* 2000. Human adrenomedullin gene delivery protects against cardiac hypertrophy, fibrosis, and renal damage in hypertensive dahl salt-sensitive rats. Hum. Gene Ther. **11**(13): 1817–1827.
31. DOBRZYNSKI, E., *et al.* 2000. Adrenomedullin gene delivery attenuates hypertension, cardiac remodeling, and renal injury in deoxycorticosterone acetate–salt hypertensive rats. Hypertension **36**(6): 995–1001.
32. KAGIYAMA, S., T. KAGIYAMA & M.I. PHILLIPS. 2001. Antisense oligonucleotides strategy in the treatment of hypertension. Curr. Opin. Mol. Ther. **3**(3): 258–264.
33. IYER, S.N., *et al.* 1996. Chronic control of high blood pressure in the spontaneously hypertensive rat by delivery of angiotensin type 1 receptor antisense. Proc. Natl. Acad. Sci. USA **93**(18): 9960–9965.
34. LU, D., *et al.* 1997. Losartan versus gene therapy: chronic control of high blood pressure in spontaneously hypertensive rats. Hypertension **30**(3, pt. 1): 363–370.
35. PACHORI, A.S., *et al.* 2000. Inability to induce hypertension in normotensive rat expressing AT(1) receptor antisense. Circ. Res. **86**(11): 1167–1172.
36. MARTENS, J.R., *et al.* 1998. Prevention of renovascular and cardiac pathophysiological changes in hypertension by angiotensin II type 1 receptor antisense gene therapy. Proc. Natl. Acad. Sci. USA **95**(5): 2664–2669.
37. KATOVICH, M.J., *et al.* 2001. Gene therapy attenuates the elevated blood pressure and glucose intolerance in an insulin-resistant model of hypertension. J. Hypertens. **19**(9): 1553–1558.
38. WANG, H., *et al.* 1999. Sustained inhibition of angiotensin I–converting enzyme (ACE) expression and long-term antihypertensive action by virally mediated delivery of ACE antisense cDNA. Circ. Res. **85**(7): 614–622.
39. WANG, H., *et al.* 2000. Angiotensin I–converting enzyme antisense gene therapy causes permanent antihypertensive effects in the SHR. Hypertension **35**(1, pt. 2): 202–208.
40. YUKAWA, H., *et al.* 2000. Adenoviral gene transfer of basic fibroblast growth factor promotes angiogenesis in rat brain. Gene Ther. **7**(11): 942–949.
41. TOYODA, K., *et al.* 2000. Gene transfer of calcitonin gene–related peptide prevents vasoconstriction after subarachnoid hemorrhage. Circ. Res. **87**(9): 818–824.
42. ONOUE, H., *et al.* 1999. Expression and function of recombinant endothelial nitric oxide synthase gene in canine basilar artery after experimental subarachnoid hemorrhage. Stroke **29**(9): 1959–1965; 1965–1966 (discussion).
43. ROSENGART, T.K., *et al.* 1999. Angiogenesis gene therapy: phase I assessment of direct intramyocardial administration of an adenovirus vector expressing VEGF121 cDNA to individuals with clinically significant severe coronary artery disease. Circulation **100**(5): 468–474.
44. ROSENGART, T.K. & K. HILLEBRAND. 2001. Gene therapy for coronary artery disease. Adv. Card. Surg. **13**: 107–120.
45. TEIGER, E., *et al.* 2001. Gene therapy in heart disease. Biomed. Pharmacother. **55**(3): 148–154.

46. YENARI, M.A., *et al.* 2001. Gene therapy for treatment of cerebral ischemia using defective herpes simplex viral vectors. Ann. N.Y. Acad. Sci. **939:** 340–357.

47. ONO, S., *et al.* 1998. Decoy administration of NF-kappaB into the subarachnoid space for cerebral angiopathy. Hum. Gene Ther. **9**(7): 1003–1011.

48. JAYAKUMAR, J., *et al.* 2001. Heat shock protein 70 gene transfection protects mitochondrial and ventricular function against ischemia-reperfusion injury. Circulation **104**(12, suppl. 1): I303–I307.

49. HAJJAR, R.J., *et al.* 2000. Prospects for gene therapy for heart failure. Circ. Res. **86**(6): 616–621.

50. DEL MONTE, F., *et al.* 2001. Improvement in survival and cardiac metabolism after gene transfer of sarcoplasmic reticulum Ca(2+)-ATPase in a rat model of heart failure. Circulation **104**(12): 1424–1429.

51. TOMIYASU, K., *et al.* 2000. Direct intra-cardiomuscular transfer of beta2-adrenergic receptor gene augments cardiac output in cardiomyopathic hamsters. Gene Ther. **7**(24): 2087–2093.

52. SCHWARZE, S.R., *et al.* 1999. *In vivo* protein transduction: delivery of a biologically active protein into the mouse. Science **285**(5433): 1569–1572.

53. XIA, H., Q. MAO & B.L. DAVIDSON. 2001. The HIV Tat protein transduction domain improves the biodistribution of beta-glucuronidase expressed from recombinant viral vectors. Nat. Biotechnol. **19**(7): 640–644.

54. TAGALAKIS, A.D., *et al.* 2001. Gene correction of the apolipoprotein (Apo) E2 phenotype to wild-type ApoE3 by *in situ* chimeraplasty. J. Biol. Chem. **276**(16): 13226–13230.

Retroviral Approaches to Gene Therapy of Cystic Fibrosis

LARRY G. JOHNSON

Cystic Fibrosis Pulmonary Research and Treatment Center and the Departments of Medicine and Pharmacology, The University of North Carolina at Chapel Hill, Chapel Hill, North Carolina 27599, USA

ABSTRACT: Retroviral vectors are attractive as vectors for gene therapy of cystic fibrosis because of their ability to integrate into the host cell genome, which may lead to long-term expression and, perhaps, a cure. Nevertheless, retroviral applications for gene transfer to airway epithelia have been limited by low titers and a requirement for proliferating cells. Significant advances in pseudo-typing of retroviruses and in retroviral production have reduced some of the concerns regarding titer. The development of lentiviral vectors that transduce nondividing cells has also helped to establish that retroviral approaches for gene therapy of cystic fibrosis are feasible. However, the apical membrane of the airway epithelium remains a formidable barrier to gene transfer. In this review, I will discuss limitations of current retroviral gene transfer vectors and strategies to improve retroviral gene transfer efficiency to airway epithelia *in vivo*.

KEYWORDS: retroviral vectors; gene therapy; cystic fibrosis; gene transfer; airway epithelia

INTRODUCTION

Cystic fibrosis (CF) is a common inherited disorder affecting a variety of epithelial tissues. The disease is caused by mutations in the cystic fibrosis transmembrane conductance regulator gene (CFTR) that lead to abnormal secretions recurrent infection and inflammation, bronchiectasis, and premature death. Because lung disease is the major cause of morbidity and mortality in this disorder, gene therapy efforts to date have focused primarily on treatment of CF lung disease. A variety of gene transfer vectors have been considered for treatment of CF, including adenoviral (Ad) vectors, adeno-associated viral (AAV) vectors, cationic liposomes, and other nonviral vectors, for example, molecular conjugates. Until recently retroviruses had not been considered promising vectors for lung gene transfer because of the low rates of epithelial cell proliferation in human airways (~0.1–0.2%) combined with the relatively low titers of simple oncogenic retroviruses. Nevertheless, retroviruses remain attractive as gene transfer vectors because integration into the host genome may lead to

Address for correspondence: Larry G. Johnson, M.D., Associate Professor of Medicine and Pharmacology, Cystic Fibrosis Pulmonary Research and Treatment Center, 7123A Thurston Bowles Bldg., CB#7248, The University of North Carolina at Chapel Hill, Chapel Hill, NC 27599-7248. Voice: 919-966-7052; fax 919-966-7524.
Larry_Johnson@med.unc.edu

long-term expression and, perhaps, a cure. Advances in vector design and production including the development of human and animal lentiviruses that transduce nondividing cells have raised hopes for retroviral approaches for treatment of CF lung disease. In this article, I will review the features of retroviral and lentiviral vector design, discuss limitations of gene transfer to airway epithelia, and review strategies to overcome these limitations. The safety considerations of retroviral and lentiviral vectors will not be discussed, as overcoming inefficient gene transfer to airways is the current focus of this area of investigation.

CLASSIFICATION OF RETROVIRUSES

Retroviruses are members of a large group of viruses that infect vertebrates; they are known as the Retroviridae,[1,2] and can be subclassified into seven genera. Several members of the mammalian C-type genus, which includes a variety of oncogenic retroviruses, and the lentivirus genus, a group of viruses that are associated with slowly progressive immunodeficiency states, have been developed as gene transfer vectors. Lentiviruses are particularly attractive as gene transfer vectors because of their ability to transduce nondividing cells. The best known and perhaps most actively studied lentiviruses are the human immunodeficiency viruses (HIV-1 and 2) and the simian immunodeficiency viruses (SIV). Feline immunodeficiency virus (FIV) and equine infectious anemia virus (EIAV) are also actively being developed as gene transfer vectors for cystic fibrosis.

RETROVIRAL AND LENTIVIRAL VECTORS

Retroviruses have been extensively used in the laboratory for stable expression of foreign cDNAs. Simple retroviruses are RNA viruses whose simple genomes consist of two viral long-terminal repeats (LTRs) that are important for cellular integration, but also contain promoter elements, a packaging signal, and a series of structural genes, *gag, pol,* and *env.* These structural genes encode the capsid protein, reverse transcriptase, protease, an integrase, and the envelope glycoprotein. Deletion of *gag, pol,* and *env* creates room for insertion of therapeutic cDNAs (genes) into the retroviral genome forming a replication defective retroviral vector.[3]

The genomes of lentiviruses are more complex, encoding a variety of regulatory accessory proteins and pathogenesis factors that are not present in the genomes of simple retroviruses.[4–6] Furthermore, genes encoding proteins that utilize the cellular nuclear import machinery, for example, MA, IN, and Vpr of HIV-1, to target the preintegration complex to the nucleus are also encoded within this complex genome. Major deletions in these accessory and pathogenesis factor genes have enabled the development of lentiviral vectors for gene transfer.[4–6] Exogenous (internal) promoters have also been included within the sequences of the inserted gene cassette, since transcription from the viral LTR may constitute a safety hazard. Deletions in the LTR to prevent transcription (self-inactivating or SIN vectors) have been recently introduced as a safety feature of retroviruses based on Moloney murine leukemia virus (MLV) and human lentiviral (HIV) vectors.[7,8] Replication-defective vectors have traditionally been produced from packaging cell lines that provide the retroviral structural and replication proteins in *trans*. Transient transfection techniques that place vector, helper, and envelope functions on separate plasmids have also been developed to permit rapid production of retroviral and lentiviral vectors for testing *in vitro* and *in vivo*.[9–10]

The envelope glycoproteins of wild-type retroviruses and lentiviruses bind to cell surface receptors to facilitate entry of the virus into the cytoplasm where the viral RNA is reverse transcribed to form a cDNA, the provirus. This provirus is translocated to the nucleus where it integrates into the host cell chromosomes and, through the normal process of DNA transcription, encodes new viral proteins and new viral RNA, which are assembled at the cell surface into new viral particles. Replication-defective retroviral and lentiviral vectors infect cells by similar mechanisms, but unlike wild-type viruses, the integrated provirus from these vectors encodes the therapeutic gene, and viral particles are not produced.

BARRIERS TO RETROVIRAL AND LENTIVIRAL GENE TRANSFER

A number of barriers to retroviral and lentiviral gene transfer to human airways have been delineated. These can be grouped into nonspecific barriers arising from inflammation and the biology of the CF airway epithelium, for example, airway mucus, innate immunity, and the glycocalyx, and vector-specific barriers including a requirement for cell proliferation by simple retroviruses and a lack of receptor expression on the apical membranes of polarized human airway epithelial cells.

Nonspecific Barriers

Innate immunity has been suggested as a potential barrier to lung gene transfer.[11] Components of the innate immune system serving as potential barriers include alveolar macrophages and airway surface fluid. Alveolar macrophages have been shown to inhibit retrovirus-mediated gene transfer to airway epithelia *in vitro*.[11] McCray *et al.* demonstrated that alveolar macrophages inhibited amphotropic-enveloped retroviral vector-mediated transduction of human airway epithelial cells by 40% and that LPS-activated alveolar macrophages inhibited transduction by more than 60%.[11] Incubation of macrophages with dexamethasone (1 μM) partially reversed this inhibition of retroviral transduction. Furthermore, the rapid uptake of labeled vector into vesicles of macrophages was associated with loss of DNA within 24 hours, consistent with rapid degradation—rather than rapid transduction—of alveolar macrophages. These data suggest that macrophages may play a significant role in inhibiting *in vivo* gene transfer to lung epithelia.

Airway surface liquid may also have potential inhibitory effects on airway gene transfer. Batra and colleagues demonstrated that high concentrations of proteoglycans and glycosaminoglycans in pleural fluid from patients with malignant pleural effusions could have inhibitory effects on amphotropic, GALV, and vesicular stomatitis virus (VSV) glycoprotein (G) pseudotyped retroviral vectors *in vitro*.[12] Because human airways are lined by a glycocalyx that may contain proteoglycans and glycosaminoglycans, molecules shed from this glycocalyx into the airway surface liquid may potentially inhibit gene transfer. In an *in vitro* study, airway surface liquid from well-differentiated human epithelial cell cultures harvested in a small volume of distilled water failed to inhibit retroviral transduction to naïve airway cells *in vitro*.[11] Similarly, freshly isolated murine bronchoalveolar lavage fluid also had no effect on transduction of airway epithelial cells by VSV-G-pseudotyped retroviral vectors.[13] Although dilution of the airway surface fluid occurred during sampling, these data suggest that the soluble components of airway surface fluid do not contain significant levels of vector inhibitory substances.

Cell Proliferation and Titer

The lack of cell proliferation in well-differentiated airway epithelia *in vivo*[14] and low titers have served as major barriers to the use of retroviral vectors derived from MLV for *in vivo* airway gene transfer. The development of HIV, EIAV, and FIV vectors,[4–6,8,15,16] which can transduce nondividing airway cells, may soon overcome the requirement for cell proliferation by oncogenic retroviruses.[17] Advances in retroviral technology, including production techniques and pseudotyping of vectors to permit concentration of vector stocks, may also soon overcome the limitations of titer.[18]

Lack of Apical Membrane Receptors

Apical membrane barriers to efficient transduction of well-differentiated airway cells by retroviruses across the apical membrane also exist. Wang *et al.* have demonstrated efficient transduction of polarized, well-differentiated airway cells stimulated to proliferate with keratinocyte growth factor (KGF) when amphotropic-enveloped MLV vectors were applied to basolateral surface as compared to minimal to no gene transfer when vector was applied to the apical surface.[19] These data are consistent with localization of the amphotropic receptor, RAM-1 or Pit-2, to the basolateral surface of polarized well-differentiated airway cells. Western blot data from this study suggested that receptor levels were extremely low in the absence of KGF.[19] *In vivo* studies have also confirmed very low levels of expression of RAM-1 or Pit-2 in murine lung.[20,21]

Similar findings have been observed with retroviral vectors bearing different envelopes. Wild-type vesicular stomatitis virus (VSV) has been shown to preferentially infect polarized MDCK cells, a model for polarized airway epithelia, across the basolateral membrane.[22] Since the envelope glycoprotein of vesicular stomatitis virus has been used to pseudotype MLV [MLV (VSV-G)] and lentiviral vectors derived from HIV [HIV (VSV-G)] and EIAV [EIAV (VSV-G)], these pseudotyped vectors would be expected to preferentially transduce polarized MDCK cells from the basolateral surface. *In vitro* studies of transduction have confirmed this notion in MDCK cells and in polarized, well-differentiated airway cells.[23]

Strategies to Overcome Barriers to Airway Epithelial Gene Transfer

Strategies to overcome *in vivo* barriers to retroviral transduction must address issues of titer, cell proliferation, and receptor localization. Significant progress has been made in improving retroviral titers, and the development of lentiviral vectors that transduce nondividing cells has made retroviral approaches for CF lung disease feasible.[4–6,8,15–18] However, developing successful methods to overcome the lack of apical membrane receptors on airway cells remains a significant challenge. Two strategies have been proposed: (1) host modification with injury models and agents that permeabilize tight junctions to increase vector access to basolateral membrane receptors and basal cells,[13,15,16,19,23] which possess pleuripotential properties, and (2) targeting the apical membrane of polarized airway epithelia by pseudotyping retroviruses with envelope proteins from other viruses to increase binding and entry of vectors across the apical membrane of polarized airway epithelial cells.[24,25]

Titer

Traditionally, retroviral vectors have been produced by the generation and selection of stable cell lines, which then allow continuous production of vector over many passages. These cell lines have generally been derived from fibroblast and human embryonic kidney 293 cells stably transfected with envelope, helper, and vector. Clones producing the highest titers are selected and propagated. These titers have traditionally been in the range of 10^5–10^6 infectious units/ml, with further increases in titer limited in part by the stability of the envelope protein. The use of pseudotyping has improved the ability to produce stable vectors with altered tropisms that have higher titers after concentration. The ability to form pseudotypes is common to most retroviruses, including lentiviruses. Gibbon ape leukemia virus (GALV)-pseudotyped retroviral vectors have been found to infect primate airway epithelium *in vitro* more efficiently than murine amphotropic vectors.[26] VSV-G-pseudotyped MLV and lentiviral vectors have also been developed that can be concentrated to high titer by ultracentrifugation without significant loss of infectivity.[4–6,13,16,18] This concentration step allows the preparation of retroviral vectors with higher titers that approach titers typical of AAV and Ad vectors, thereby permitting direct *in vivo* gene transfer applications. However, the toxicity of VSV-G envelope protein and some lentiviral accessory proteins have limited the ability to develop stable packaging cells lines for vector production. Recently, regulated expression of helper and envelope components with tetracycline-inducible promoters has permitted the development of stable VSV-G-pseudotyped MLV and lentiviral vector producer lines.[27–29]

The generation of high-titer VSV-G-pseudotyped MLV vectors has permitted the correction of Cl⁻ permeability defect in dividing (subconfluent), but undifferentiated primary CF human airway epithelial cells grown on permeable collagen substrates without selection for vector.[13] The level of Cl⁻ secretion induced in the CFTR-corrected CF cells was similar to that observed with an Ad-CFTR at a multiplicity of infection of 100. Western blot analysis of these cultures demonstrated CFTR expression in CF cells transduced with the MLV (VSV-G) CFTR, but not in uninfected CF cells. Similar findings have been reported with VSV-G-pseudotyped lentiviral vectors.[16] Thus, vectors with high titer permit correction *in vitro* without having to enrich the population of cells transduced by selection.

Cell Proliferation

Oncogenic retroviral vectors based on MLV require cell proliferation for nuclear entry, integration, and subsequent transgene expression. Studies in freshly excised human airways from CF and non-CF persons suggest that the rates of airway epithelial cell proliferation in the chronically inflamed CF lung may be as high as 18% in some regions as compared to 0.1–0.2% in non-CF persons.[14] Areas of increased proliferation were patchy and perhaps more frequent in regions of severe injury. One strategy to overcome low rates of epithelial cell proliferation is to deliver gene transfer vectors *in utero*, where rates of epithelial proliferation are presumed to be higher. Pitt *et al.* demonstrated successful retroviral-mediated gene transfer to fetal lamb airways *in utero*.[30] Although the efficiency of transduction was not quantified in this particular study, it established the feasibility of retroviral gene transfer to proliferating airways *in vivo*. However, techniques that stimulate epithelial cell proliferation will likely be required for successful mediation of retroviral gene transfer to airway epithelia in the postnatal lung. Two models have been developed to stimulate epithelial cell proliferation *in vivo*: (1) oxidant gas injury models and (2) growth factors.[13,23,19,20,2]

Johnson and coworkers developed a sulfur dioxide (SO_2) inhalational injury model to stimulate airway epithelial cell proliferation *in vivo*.[13] Mice exposed to SO_2 (500 ppm for 3 hr) demonstrated an increase in the number of proliferating tracheal epithelial cells to ≥50% of cells that peaked at 24 hr after SO_2 inhalation with a rapid decline in the number of proliferating cells over the ensuing 48 hr. Importantly, no significant cell proliferation was detected in the first 12 hr after SO_2 exposure. Subsequently, vector was instilled into the tracheas of anesthetized mice through a proximal tracheostomy while the mice breathed through a distal tracheostomy, limiting vector to the region between the two ostomies for up to 2 hr. This technique produced relatively efficient gene transfer to murine tracheas (~6% of cells) with a MLV (VSV-G) *lacZ* vector construct, compared to <0.1% of cells in air-exposed tracheas, which were not different from vehicle controls. A significantly greater fraction of cells were transduced in mice aged 3–4 weeks than in mice ≥6 weeks of age.[13]

Wang *et al.* demonstrated that well-differentiated human airway epithelial cell cultures treated with keratinocyte growth factor (KGF) to stimulate epithelial cell proliferation could be transduced with amphotropic-enveloped MLV vectors following apical application of vector, but only if pretreatment or coadministration of vector with ethylene glycol bis(β-aminoethyl ether)-*N,N,N′,N′*-tetraacetic acid (EGTA) and hypotonic solutions was performed.[19] Because no significant gene transfer occurred in the absence of EGTA and hypotonic solutions, however, factors other than proliferation were limiting. Similarly, intratracheal administration of KGF *in vivo* stimulated bronchiolar and alveolar type II cell proliferation in murine lung, which increased transduction by amphotropic and 10A1-enveloped vectors in murine lung *in vivo*.[20,21] Despite the increased rate of epithelial cell proliferation, retrovirus-mediated gene transfer was inefficient. Subsequent immunohistochemical and molecular studies demonstrated minimal levels of amphotropic receptor expression (RAM-1 or Pit-2) in murine lung. Thus, retroviral vectors must not only overcome the limitations of cell proliferation, but must also circumvent the lack of apical membrane receptors to transduce airway epithelial cells *in vivo*.

Lentiviral vectors have been shown to transduce a variety of nondividing cell types *in vitro* and *in vivo* and thus offer a chance to overcome the limitation of cell proliferation typical of oncogenic retroviruses.[4–6,8,15,16,23] Goldman and colleagues demonstrated that HIV (VSV-G vectors) failed to transduce well-differentiated primary human airway epithelia cells in bronchial xenografts.[31] Subsequently, Johnson *et al.* evaluated whether HIV (VSV-G) vectors could transduce nondividing airway epithelial cells.[23] An amphotropic-enveloped vector [MLV (ampho)], an HIV (VSV-G) vector, and an MLV (VSV-G) vector each efficiently transduced growing or dividing CF tracheal epithelia cells (CFT1), whereas only the HIV (VSV-G) vector efficiently transduced aphidicolin-treated (growth-arrested) airway epithelial cells. Thus, HIV vectors can transduce nondividing airway epithelial cells. However, because luminal application of pseudotyped lentiviral vectors failed to transduce well-differentiated primary human airway epithelia in bronchial xenografts, strategies to circumvent lack of apical membrane receptors will still be required.

Lack of Apical Membrane Receptors

To evaluate the polarity of lentiviral transduction, HIV VSV-G vectors were applied to either the apical or the basolateral surfaces of polarized, well-differentiated human airway epithelial cell cultures.[23] HIV vectors efficiently transduced cells when vector was applied to the basolateral surface as compared to minimal levels of gene transfer following application of vector to the apical surface of cells. Furthermore, basolateral infection by HIV (VSV-G) vectors was 30-fold more efficient than transduction across the apical membrane. These data suggest that while HIV vectors can transduce nondividing cells, the receptors for uptake and entry of both HIV and MLV vectors are predominantly localized to the basolateral membrane.

Injury models are one method by which to increase access to basolateral receptors and pleuropotential basal cells lining the basement membrane. Johnson et al. exposed mice to SO_2 inhalation to increase vector delivery to the basolateral surface and/or basal cells of murine tracheas.[13,23] In this injury model, SO_2 not only increased airway cell proliferation, but also caused a dose-related denuding of the surface epithelium, leaving the basal cell layer intact.[13,23,32] In regions less severely injured by the SO_2, permeability is increased through the tight junctions.[13] This observation has been confirmed in murine tracheal epithelia exposed to 500 ppm SO_2 for 3 hr using the electron-dense tracer lanthanum, which permeates into the intercellular junctions of the tracheal epithelium in mice exposed to SO_2, but not into the intercellular spaces in the tracheas of mice sham-exposed to air.[13] Similar findings have been documented in the nasal epithelia of mice following SO_2 exposure. Using this model, mice were exposed to SO_2 for 3 hr at 500 ppm, and an HIV (VSV-G) vector was delivered onto the nasal epithelia drop by drop or to the tracheal epithelia by the double-tracheostomy technique.[23] Efficient reporter gene transfer was observed in respiratory epithelium lining the nasal septum of rats, whereas no gene transfer was detected in the nasal airway epithelia of vehicle-treated control rats. Similar findings were observed in mice, although the magnitude of enhanced gene transfer was less than that detected in rats. Gene transfer to murine trachea was more efficient following SO_2 exposure when vector was administered on the same day of exposure (~7% of cells transduced) compared to the day after SO_2 inhalation (~2% transduction of cells), consistent with preferential transduction of nondividing cells.[23] These data demonstrate that HIV vectors can efficiently transduce airway epithelia in vivo when access to basolateral receptors and/or the basolateral membrane is increased by injury techniques.

Transient permeabilization of tight junctions is another method by which to increase vector delivery the basolateral membrane and basal cells. Nonprimate lentiviral vectors have been coadministered with calcium chelators to airways to increase vector access to basolateral receptors, presumably by modulating paracellular permeability.[15,16,33] Wang et al. have reported development of FIV vectors for use in CF gene therapy.[16,33] These investigators applied FIV-CFTR vectors in combination with hypotonic solution and EGTA to the apical membrane of polarized, well-differentiated CF airway epithelial cells.[16,33] Restoration of chloride secretory function was achieved following infection with FIV-*CFTR* in primary CF airway epithelial cells that was similar to levels of correction achieved with an Ad*CFTR* vector. The correction of chloride secretory function mediated by FIV-*CFTR* persisted for up to six months in culture, whereas the Ad*CFTR*-mediated Cl⁻ correction had resolved by 21 days after transduction. Subsequently, these investigators demonstrated efficient transduction of ciliated and nonciliated cells in rabbit airways *in vivo* comprising ~5% of airway cells infected with vector at day 5, which decreased to ~2.5 % of cells at six weeks.[16,33] Thus, FIV-*CFTR* vectors are promising vectors for gene therapy of cystic fibrosis. However, transgene expression is attenuated over time.

Olsen and colleagues have developed a mammalian lentiviral vector based on equine infectious anemia virus.[15] Compared to HIV-1, EIAV has a much simpler genome. Horses infected with the wild-type EIAV virus typically survive the infection (~95%), and the EIAV promoter is not functional in human cells.[15] Olsen demonstrated efficient transduction of well-differentiated primary human airway epithelial cells after apical application of EIAV (VSV-G) *lacZ* vector in the presence of ethylenediaminetetraacetic acid (EDTA) or EGTA to increase access to basolateral receptors by permeabilizing the tight junction. Persistence of transgene expression *in vitro* lasted for up to 24 days post transduction, the longest period tested. In preliminary studies, EIAV vectors with internal promoters have been shown to express reporter genes in murine tracheal airway epithelia following SO_2 injury to increase delivery to basal cells and the basolateral membrane.[34] The efficiency of transduction was dose-related with minimal transduction at vector titers of 10^8 infectious units (IU)/ml, while vectors with ~10^{10} IU/ml yielded transduction efficiencies that were significantly greater than those observed at lower EIAV lentiviral titers.

Targeting receptors on the apical membrane is an alternative strategy to increase airway gene transfer. A number of investigators have begun to test a variety of naturally occurring, enveloped respiratory viruses for their ability to transduce polarized, well-differentiated airway cells across the apical membrane. The goal is to identify new envelope proteins that might be developed as pseudotypes for retroviral and lentiviral vectors that would target the apical membranes of polarized CF airway epithelia. Preliminary studies with respiratory syncytial virus, filaviruses, and corona viruses appear promising as potential lentiviral pseudotypes.[24,25,35]

CONCLUSIONS

Retroviral and lentiviral vectors fail to transduce airway epithelia when delivered to the apical surface of polarized airway epithelial cells. Methods that increase access to basal cells and the basolateral membrane of airway epithelial cells enhance retroviral- and lentiviral-mediated gene transfer. Relatively long-term transgene expression has been detected after lentiviral transduction *in vivo*, but is attenuated over time with current promoters. If retroviral approaches to gene therapy of CF are to become successful, better apical membrane-binding pseudotypes or safer, more consistent injury techniques in combination with better *in vivo* promoters will be required.

ACKNOWLEDGMENTS

The author thanks Ms. Marguerite Applin and Ms. Miriam Kelly for their assistance in the preparation of this manuscript. This work was supported by Grant HL58342 from the National Heart, Lung, and Blood Institute of the National Institutes of Health.

REFERENCES

1. COFFIN, J.M. 1996. Retroviridae: the viruses and their replication. *In* Fields Virology. Vol. 2. B.N. Fields, D.M. Knippe & P.M. Howley, Eds.: 1767–1847. Lippincott-Raven. Philadelphia, PA.
2. TRONO, D. 2000. Lentiviral vectors: turning a deadly foe into a therapeutic agent. Gene Ther. **7:** 20–23.
3. MILLER, A.D. & G.J. ROSMAN. 1989. Improved retroviral vectors for gene transfer and expression. Biotechniques **7:** 980–990.
4. NALDINI, L. 1998. Lentiviruses as gene transfer agents for delivery to nondividing cells. Curr. Opin. Biotechnol. **9:** 457–463.
5. NALDINI, L., U. BLOMER, P. GALLAY, *et al.* 1996. *In vivo* gene delivery and stable transduction of nondividing cells by a lentiviral vector. Science **272:** 263–267.
6. ZUFFEREY, R., D. NAGY, R.J. MANDEL, *et al.* 1997. Multiply attenuated lentiviral vector achieves efficient gene delivery *in vivo*. Nature Biotechnol. **15:** 871–875.
7. DELVIKS, K.A., W.-S. HU & V.K. PATHAK. 1997. Ψ-Vectors: murine leukemia virus-based self-inactivating and self-activating retroviral vectors. J. Virol. **71:** 6218–6224.
8. ZUFFEREY, R., T. DULL, R.J. MANDEL, *et al.* 1998. Self-inactivating lentivirus vector for safe and efficient *in vivo* gene delivery. J. Virol. **72:** 9873–9880.
9. PEAR, W.D., G. NOLAN, M.L. SCOTT, *et al.* 1993. Production of high-titer helper-free retroviruses by transient transfection. Proc. Natl. Acad. Sci. USA **90:** 8392–8396.
10. SONEOKA, Y., P.M. CANNON, E.F. RAMSDALE, *et al.* 1995. A transient three-plasmid system for the production of high titer retroviral vectors. Nucleic Acids Res. **23:** 628–633.
11. MCCRAY, JR., P.B., G. WANG, J.N. KLINE, *et al.* 1997. Alveolar macrophages inhibit retrovirus-mediated gene transfer to airway epithelia. Hum. Gene Ther. **8:** 1087–1093.
12. BATRA, R.J., J.C. OLSEN, D.K. HOGANSON, *et al.* 1997. Retroviral gene transfer is inhibited by chondroitin sulfate proteoglycans/glycosaminoglycans in malignant pleural effusions. J. Biol. Chem. **272:** 11736–11743.
13. JOHNSON, L.G., J.P. MEWSHAW, H. NI, *et al.* 1998. Effect of host modification and age on airway epithelial gene transfer mediated by a murine leukemia virus-derived vector. J. Virol. **72:** 8861–8872.
14. LEIGH, M.W., J.E. KYLANDER, J.R. YANKASKAS, *et al.* 1995. Cell proliferation in bronchial epithelium and submucosal glands of cystic fibrosis patients. Am. J. Resp. Cell Mol. Biol. **12:** 605–612.
15. OLSEN, J.C. 1998. Gene transfer vectors derived from equine infectious anemia virus. Gene Ther. **5:** 1481–1487.
16. WANG, G., V.A. SLEPUSHKIN, J. ZABNER, *et al.* 1999. Feline immunodeficiency virus vectors persistently transduce nondividing airway epithelia and correct the cystic fibrosis defect. J. Clin. Invest. **104:** R55–R62.
17. MILLER, D.G., M.A. ADAM & A.D. MILLER. 1990. Gene transfer by retrovirus vectors occurs only in cells that are actively replicating at the time of infection. Mol. Cell Biol. **10:** 4329–4242.
18. BURNS, J.C., T. FRIEDMANN, W. DRIEVER, *et al.* 1993. Vesicular stomatitis virus G glycoprotein pseudotyped retroviral vectors: concentration to very high titer and efficient gene transfer into mammalian and nonmammalian cells. Proc. Natl. Acad. Sci. USA **90:** 8033–8037.

19. WANG, G., B.L. DAVIDSON, P. MELCHERT, et al. 1998. Influence of cell polarity on retrovirus-mediated gene transfer to differentiated human airway epithelia. J. Virol. **72:** 9818–9826.
20. ZSENGELLER, Z.K., C. HALBERT, A.D. MILLER, et al. 1999. Keratinocyte growth factor stimulates transduction of the respiratory epithelium by retroviral vectors. Hum. Gene Ther. **10:** 341–353.
21. WANG, G., V.A. SLEPUSHKIN, M. BODNER, et al. 1999. Keratinocyte growth factor induced epithelial proliferation facilitates retroviral-mediated gene transfer to distal lung epithelia in vivo. J. Gene Med. **1:** 22–30.
22. FULLER, S., C.H. VON BONSDORFF & K. SIMONS. 1984. Vesicular stomatitis virus infects and matures only through the basolateral surface of the polarized epithelial cell line, MDCK. Cell **38:** 65–77.
23. JOHNSON, L.G., J.C. OLSEN, L. NALDINI, et al. 2000. Pseudotyped human lentiviral vector-mediated gene transfer to human airway epithelia in vivo. Gene Ther. **7:** 568–574.
24. RAI, S.K., J.C. DEMARTINI & A.D. MILLER. 2000. Retrovirus vectors bearing jaagsiekte sheep retrovirus env transduce human cells by using a new receptor localized to chromosome 3p21.3. J. Virol. **74:** 4698–4704.
25. KOBINGER, G.P., D. WEINER & J.M. WILSON. 2000. Pseudotyping HIV vectors with envelope proteins of divergent viruses allows for retargeting viral particle-mediated transduction [abstract]. Mol. Ther. **1:** S78–S79.
26. BAYLE, J.Y., L.G. JOHNSON, J. ST. GEORGE, et al. 1993. High efficiency gene transfer to primary monkey airway epithelial cells with retrovirus vectors using the GALV receptor. Hum. Gene Ther. **4:** 161–170.
27. YANG, Y., E.F. VANIN, M.A. WHITT, et al. 1995. Inducible, high-level production of infectious murine leukemia retroviral vector particles pseudotyped with vesicular stomatitis virus G envelope protein. Hum. Gene Ther. **6:** 1203–1213.
28. ORY, D.S., B.A. NEUGEBOREN & R.C. MULLIGAN. 1996. A stable human-derived packaging cell line for production of high titer retrovirus/vesicular stomatitis virus G pseudotypes. Proc. Natl. Acad. Sci. USA **93:** 11400–11406.
29. KAFRI, T., H. VAN PRAAG, L. OUYANG, et al. 1999. A packaging cell line for lentivirus vectors. J. Virol. **73:** 576–584.
30. PITT, B.R., M.A. SCHWARTZ, J.M. JILEWSKI, et al. 1995. Retrovirus-mediated gene transfer in lungs of living fetal sheep. Gene Ther. **2:** 344–350.
31. GOLDMAN, M.J., P.-S. LEE, J.-S. YANG, et al. 1997. Lentiviral vectors for gene therapy of cystic fibrosis. Hum. Gene Ther. **8:** 2261–2268.
32. HULBERT, W.C., S.F. MAN, M.K. ROSYCHUK, et al. 1989. The response phase—the first six hours after acute airway injury by SO_2 inhalation: an in vivo and in vitro study. Scanning Microsc. **3:** 369–378.
33. WANG, G., J. ZABNER, C. DEERING, et al. 2000. Increasing epithelial junction permeability enhances gene transfer to airway epithelia in vivo. Am. J. Resp. Cell Mol. Biol. **22:** 129–138.
34. OLSEN, J.C., M. PATEL, J.B. ROHLL, et al. 2000. An inducible first generation stable packaging cell line for equine lentiviral vectors [abstract]. Mol. Ther. **1:** 315.
35. SINN, P.L., G. WANG, J. NOSAKOWSKI, et al. 2000. Pseudotyping feline immunodeficiency virus (FIV)-based vectors to target the apical surface of differentiated human airway epithelia [abstract]. Ped. Pulmonol. Suppl. **20:** 233.

Regulated Gene Expression in Gene Therapy

PHILIP W. ZOLTICK[a,b] AND JAMES M. WILSON[a,b,c]

[a]Institute for Human Gene Therapy, [b]Department of Molecular and Cellular Engineering, University of Pennsylvania, Philadelphia, Pennsylvania 19104, USA

[c]The Wistar Institute, Philadelphia, Pennsylvania 19104, USA

ABSTRACT: The original model of gene therapy, that of efficient delivery, durable transfer, and stable expression of transgenes to correct a gene defect underlying an inherited disease, is limited in light of improved understanding of the processes involved. Techniques that enable regulated expression of transgenes may enhance safety and allow us to regulate the timing and level of expression with a goal of precisely targeting a therapeutic level between the extremes of suboptimal and supraoptimal thresholds. Using regulated systems to control protein expression has practical and possibly essential roles for the success of safe and effective gene therapy in a number of clinical situations. Pharmacologically regulated gene expression is an evolving tool, and no individual system may be effective in all clinical applications.

KEYWORDS: gene therapy; transgene; regulated gene expression; genetic diseases; ligand-based gene expression

INTRODUCTION

Gene therapy was initially envisioned as a form of molecular medicine to cure genetic diseases,[1–3] a consequence of improved understanding in the molecular and cellular basis of human disease. Conceptually, gene therapy is the transfer of a normal cDNA allele (transgene) to those affected cells in a patient with an inherited disease for which a single gene defect is believed to underlie the disease. The introduced transgene was to be restricted to somatic cells in the affected tissues and function in trans to correct or ameliorate the effect of the intrinsic defective gene.

For the success of gene therapy, initial practical considerations were paramount: efficient delivery, durable transfer, and stable expression of transgenes. These considerations remain crucial, but in the context of the improved understanding of the biology of genes, genetic diseases, and gene delivery, this model of gene therapy is limited in scope and potential. Most genetic diseases are caused by mutations affecting the protein-coding regions of genes, such as missense and frameshift mutations within exons, or mutations involving introns that disturb premessenger RNA processing.[4] However, many of these genes are expressed conditionally. Less frequent genetic diseases are associated with dysregulated expression at the level of transcription.[5–7] Mutations that increase or decrease efficiency of messenger RNA (mRNA) translation provide another mechanism in which the level of a gene product can con-

Address for correspondence: James M. Wilson, M.D., Ph.D., 204 Wistar Institute, 3601 Spruce Street, Philadelphia, PA 19104-4268. Voice: 215-898-3000; fax: 215-898-6588.
wilsonjm@mail.med.upenn.edu

tribute to disease.[8] The time to decode a transgene and the level of the encoded protein may be critical to convert a diseased phenotype to normal, an objective of gene therapy.

Current applications of gene therapy are no longer restricted to monogenetic diseases.[9] Gene therapy is being developed for cancer, acquired diseases, and as a vaccination or immunomodulating therapy. In a number of situations, strategies that permit the accurate control of transgene transcription are essential for the success of future clinical development of gene therapy. This review article will focus on regulating expression in gene therapy.

RATIONALE

Most gene therapy protocols have involved transfer of therapeutic genes without regulation because expression was designed to be transient, such as in cancer therapy, or there was a broad therapeutic index for the level of protein expression, such as in hemophilias, α_1-antitrypsin deficiency, and adenosine deaminase deficiency.[10] In these instances, efficient gene transfer, expression, and/or stability were limiting in preclinical models and/or clinical applications. Regulated expression may play a more important role as the above obstacles are overcome, transgenes encode proteins with narrower safety margins, and/or the desired effect is to regulate the timing and level of transgene expression for extended periods. In addition, regulated expression can add a level of safety and, in some circumstances, is required to control the expression levels of some proteins that have narrow therapeutic indices, such as cytokines and hormones. To improve the therapeutic index in cancer, for instance, regulating a "suicide gene" can provide an additional level of safety over that of gene targeting and promoter selectivity.

Two relevant categories of application for gene therapy in which regulated expression is crucial are (1) those diseases in which a narrow therapeutic window of protein expression is necessary to maintain cellular and host homeostasis and (2) those diseases in which a pharmacologic level of protein expression is required transiently in response to a dynamic of a disease. Regulated expression in this first category is to mimic a normal homeostatic program. The objective here is to control expression in response to a cellular or tissue disturbance to restore homeostasis. Examples of such diseases are erythropoietin-sensitive anemias. Transgene expression would be switched on or off contingent on a physiologic requirement. The second class of diseases would include autoimmune diseases and graft-versus-host disease, in which regulated expression of cytokines with antiinflammatory effects may modulate the severity of the disease. Regulated expression of cytokines and proteins that enhance immune or proinflammatory responses could be used as adjuncts to cancer therapy, immunodeficiency states, and chronic diseases such as chronic active hepatitis. In either application, transgene expression would be contingent on a clinical parameter.

Implicit in the importance of regulated expression is the concept of threshold. Transgene expression results in distribution into intracellular compartments. If the protein is secreted, it will also undergo a distribution phase in extracellular components followed by an elimination phase in which pharmacokinetic principles can be applied. Even if the protein is maintained within a cell, it will undergo accumulation and elimination phases. The rate of transgene expression will influence the level of the encoded protein. The objective of regulated expression is, optimally, to control not only the timing but the level of the transgene product; too little will be subtherapeutic, too much will be potentially toxic. A goal of regulated expression is the ability to precisely target a therapeutic level between these extremes of suboptimal and supraoptimal threshold. Even for a constitutively expressed protein, regulated expression may be able to fine-tune the protein level unique to an individual and permit adjusting the level appropriate to a changing clinical state.

An expression system endowed with an intrinsic physiologically responsive component in some circumstances would be an ideal. Such a system would be self-regulating. For instance, in erythropoietin expression, the mechanism would contain an oxygen sensor that would relay a signal to a responsive promoter leading to erythropoietin transcription. For a disease like diabetes, the regulated response rate at the level of transcription would be inadequate. To maintain the minute-to-minute glucose homeostasis, insulin would have to be regulated at the level of secretion. Therefore, such a system would need to mimic the physiology of a β-cell. Self-contained regulated systems are in their infancy, limited by our understanding of the complex components of their biology and the means to deliver those components. Even these physiologically responsive systems do not displace the need to have regulated systems that can be under the control and/or guidance of a clinician. A clinically guided, regulated system represents, in essence, a new pharmaceutical tool.

The prerequisites for an exogenous, controlled expression system have been based on several assumptions: (1) to turn on a transferred therapeutic gene, there needs to be an easy, safe, and reliable way to transmit the "on" signal to the target tissue containing the therapeutic gene; (2) the signal should be an "on" signal rather than a removal of an intrinsic repressive or "off" signal, thus decreasing the need for administering the signal continuously except when you want the therapeutic gene on; (3) the signal should be easy to deliver with a rapid "on" dynamic.

In the context of the above limitations, most regulated systems have been based on a pharmacologic model, that is, a ligand-dependent, transcription-regulated system. The method of transmitting an external signal is the use of a drug that serves as the ligand. The relay to the transgene will be dependent on the pharmacology of the drug. Alternative methods to communicate a signal include heat or light or radiation. For instance, a temperature-based system could use heat-shock protein promoters to regulate expression of a transgene. A light-mediated transduction signal could be used on the skin or retina, or in a more complex form, a prodrug that is light sensitive could be activated by light and then effect an "on" signal.

Based on current thinking, the state of the technology, safety, and criteria listed below, most work has centered on developing drug-inducible systems. Any regulated system, then, should have the following features: (1) ligand-induced expression, preferably with a dose–response kinetic; (2) specificity of the ligand to the regulated system (this is an important feature that may fail for other transducing signals such as heat); (3) a ligand that can be conveniently administered with a good safety and kinetic profile. The ligand-sensitive or inducible component should have the following features: (1) insignificant (subthreshold) basal levels; (2) reproducible "on–off" kinetics; (3) nonperturbing to the normal physiology of the target tissue or the host.

To satisfy this latter criterion, untoward host responses, such as immunogenicity of the system, will need to be evaluated. And such a response could be considered an adverse event.

Ligand-based, transcription-regulated systems fundamentally have been formulated on protein domain modularity principles established from the study of natural transcription factors. Design strategies for these systems derive from the following observations: (1) DNA-binding and transcriptional activation domains of transcription factors function independently and retain activity in a heterologous protein context[11]; (2) covalent or noncovalent interaction of these domains can reconstitute sequence-specific transcription activation; and (3) organic compounds can interact with appropriate domains to induce altered steric conformations (allostery) or induce protein–protein interactions.[12,13]

LIGAND-DEPENDENT INDUCIBLE EXPRESSION SYSTEMS

Regulated transcription systems in which expression of specific genes is directed by RNA polymerase II promoters have been attempted using the metallothionein and heat-shock protein gene promoters[14,15] and the mouse mammary tumor virus long-terminal repeat.[16] However, each of these systems has either required an inducing molecule (e.g., heavy-metal ion or glucocorticoid steroid) that had pleiotropic or toxic effects, an inducing event (e.g., stress/heat) that was difficult to modulate *in vivo*, and/or the basal activity of the inducible promoter in the noninduced state was elevated.

It has been difficult to design an endogenous system dependent on the mammalian RNA polymerase II that could be regulated by a specific exogenous signal and applicable to safe *in vivo* use. To resolve this dilemma, it was hypothesized that regulatory elements or inducers derived from species distant in evolution from higher eukaryotes would not interfere with the cellular physiology of mammals and therefore could provide the basis for a monospecific means to reversibly control the activity of a gene. The most effective gene switch systems for vertebrates have been modeled on and incorporated transcriptional control features from prokaryotes, fungi, or insects.

Operon-Based Regulated Systems

Features based on the *Escherichia coli lactose (lac)* operon[17] and the transposon 10–derived *tetracycline (tet)* operon[18–20] have been exploited to regulate gene activity in eukaryotic cells. The induction seen with the *lac* operon tends to be slow and partial (thermodynamic limitations) and may require concentrations of the inducer, isopropyl-D-thiogalactopyranoside (IPTG) that approach cytotoxic levels (pharmacologic limitations). The *tet* system does not have these limitations and has shown versatility in gene therapy models. Based on structure and function information, the initial *tet* system used the DNA-binding domain of the tet repressor fused to the eukaryotic transcriptional activation domain derived from the herpes simplex virus *VP16* gene (tTA) or the transactivation domain of NF-κB p65.[21] The tTA is under constitutive expression. The tTA-dependent promoter consists of multiple copies of the tet operator sequences upstream of a minimal promoter derived from the human

CMV immediate early promoter. The *tet* system demonstrated high-affinity pf tetra-cycline or doxycyline for the tTA and known pharmacology of *tet* and *tet* derivatives in which there is good tissue distribution and cell penetrance. Rapid induction is de-pendent on withdrawal of the effector molecule in the original *tet* system. This is nei-ther kinetically favored nor optimal in a gene therapy application. A *tet* repressor mutant was discovered that exhibits a reverse phenotype when fused to *VP16*. This altered chimeric protein, rtTA, binds to the *tet* operator sequences in the presence of doxycycline or anhydrotetracycline. This complementary property of the modified transactivator molecule reverses the system so that the drug activates gene expres-sion. Further modifications in the rtTA have improved ligand affinity, stability, and stringency of gene regulation.[22] How these changes translate to *in vivo* applications will require further study.

Basal level activity in the absence of inducer using the rtTA-based system has been observed. The Tn10 *tet* repressor, a class B *tet* repressor used in the tTA or rtTA molecules, contains the DNA-binding domain, a core ligand-binding domain, and a dimerization domain. Class E and G *tet* repressors derived from other gram-negative bacteria contain domains that permit dimerization specific to their class. This en-ables the construction of chimeric *tet* repressors with a class G dimerization domain fused with a eukaryotic transcriptional repressor domain that binds to the *tet* opera-tor in the absence of drug.[23,24] When that gene was coexpressed in cells containing the class B dimerization domain, the rtTA, the system showed improved regulated gene expression. In the absence of drug, gene expression was completely repressed. With addition of drug, there is complete gene induction. Such modifications add more complexity and the potential to induce transgene shutdown, a consequence of epigenetic effects, including methylation of the inducible promoter, histone deacety-lation, and chromatin compaction.[25]

Another complication is the presence of structural and functional interferon α-stimulated response elements in the *tet* operator sequences.[26] Their presence may re-sult in interferon-mediated promoter activation with loss of pharmacologically regu-lated gene expression. Removal of these response elements should abrogate the potential of cytokine promoter induction and improve the stringency of the *tet* system.

The *tet* system has been used in gene therapy models with variable success. How-ever, a number of improvements previously described have yet to be applied *in vivo.* The disadvantages in the "classical" rtTA system include the high dose of drug re-quired to induce gene expression, which may be problematic, and the deposition and/or slow clearance of drug from bone and liver.

Insect and Mammalian Nuclear Hormone Receptor-Based Systems

Development of steroid-based gene switch systems was partly motivated on the basis of the pharmacokinetic properties of steroids, small, highly lipophilic mole-cules with excellent tissue permeation, cell penetration, and rapid metabolism.[27] Two approaches have been developed to exploit this potential and avoid interfering with mammalian steroid biology. The first approach was based on ecdysone, an in-sect molting steroid hormone. A truncated *Drosophila melangaster* ecdysone recep-tor (EcR) containing the DNA and ligand-binding domains was fused to the transactivator domain of *VP16*.[28] Ecdysone-induced binding to the DNA response el-ement requires the heterodimerization of the EcR with the ultraspiral gene product, the insect homologue of the mammalian retinoid X receptor (RXR). The DNA binding domain of the EcR was mutated to bind a unique hybrid DNA response element that was recognized by the modified EcR-RXR heterodimer. The inducible system requires the constitutive expression of both the modified EcR-VP16 chimera and the human RXRα molecules and a transgene under the regulation of the ecdysone-responsive promoter. This system has been demonstrated in tissue culture cells and *in vivo*. Activation of the system depends on the overexpression of RXRα, which may alter the normal physiology in the mammalian cells. A chimeric nuclear receptor derived from *Bombyx mori* does not require exogenous expression of RXR because of the higher affinity for the endogenous RXR present in mammalian cells compared to that of the EcR.[29,30] Sequestration of the endogenous RXR by the constitutive expression of this modified EcR, however, may still disrupt mammalian physiology. Further complicating this system is the presence of phytoectosteroids, natural insecticides, and the potential development of chemically synthesized insecticides based on ecdysone. The presence of natural and artificial ectosteroids if present in the food chain would limit the specificity of a gene switch based on the EcR.

Because of the lack of specificity of inducer molecules, an estrogen nuclear receptor-based gene switch system for *in vivo* mammalian use has limited value in gene therapy. The exceedingly high affinity of progestin antagonists (e.g., mifepristone) for the mutated progesterone nuclear receptor contributed to the design of a progesterone receptor ligand-binding domain (Pr-LBD)-based system.[31] Similar to the previously described systems, the components are (1) the regulated activator composed of the yeast GAL4 DNA-binding domain fused to the truncated human Pr-LBD and a transactivator domain, *VP16,* or the activation domain of NF-κB p65 and (2) the inducible or responsive promoter composed of multiple copies of the GAL4 upstream activation sequence (UAS) fused to a minimal TATA box.[32,33] Specificity of the system results from the uniqueness of the UAS and the low dose of mifepristone (subthreshold for an anti-glucocorticoid or anti-progestin effect) required to activate the inducible promoter.[34] Stringency is dependent on the lack of interaction of the chimeric regulator protein with that of the UAS, which may depend on the intracellular concentration of the regulator protein. The system has shown promise in animal models requiring levels of mifepristone that theoretically would elude the development of adverse events in humans.

Chemically Induced Protein Heterodimerization

Protein–protein interactions mediate a number of biological phenomena, such as signal transduction, protein chaperoning, and transcriptional activation or repression. The ability to regulate protein oligomerization is the kernel of an idea for a gene switch system.[12,35] Rapamycin, a macrolide antibiotic produced by a *Streptomyces* sp., was observed to mediate the heterodimerization of the immunophilin, FK506-binding protein FKBP and the lipid kinase homologue FRAP (FKBP12-rapamycin-associated protein). A transcriptional regulator was devised using two separate chimeric protein molecules.[36] A novel DNA-binding domain was synthesized by fusing a zinc finger from Zif268 (identical to the corresponding region in the human *egr-1* gene) to that of the human *oct-1.*[37] This chimeric DNA-binding domain, termed ZHFD1, was fused to three copies of the human FKBP12 (FK506 binding protein with molecular mass 12 kDa). The other protein was composed of the

FKBP12 rapamycin-binding domain (FRB) of FRAP that was in continuity with the activation domain of the human NF-κB p65. The rapamycin-responsive inducible promoter contained multiple copies of the novel DNA-binding element upstream of a minimal promoter. These proteins are biologically inept until they form a complex mediated by the presence of rapamycin. This ternary drug–protein complex functions as a transcriptional activator recognizing a unique DNA sequence.

Gene therapy applications of the rapamycin-regulated system have been demonstrated.[38,39] A theoretical advantage is that the proteins composing the regulator are human derived and, except for junction sites and a directed mutation in the FRB domain, are likely to minimize the potential for host immune recognition. The system is based on rapamycin to interact with relatively natural protein domains. Therefore, for rapamycin to induce expression of the transgene, drug levels are required that will be immunosuppressive or have other adverse effects.[40–45] This may or may not be a significant problem depending on the clinical indications if a single, infrequent dose of rapamycin is required. Rapamycin derivatives with decreased immunosuppressive and other host-perturbing effects, but retaining the heterodimerization property, may alleviate this disadvantage.[46] To enhance the specificity and safety of a rapamycin analogue will require modifications in the binding domains of the associated protein components. Such changes will generate new epitopes and diminish a potential advantage.

LIMITATIONS

In the description of each system, there are differences and limitations. These differences may affect the kinetics, such as the response rate and duration of inducible gene expression following the transmission of the "on" signal and the decay rate in the return to basal levels. In addition, the available systems are a study in change. No system is without its flaws, and modifications are continuing. Though immunogenicity is considered a handicap, all the systems contain potential neoantigens. The rapamycin system may have the least immunogenic potential. However, some of the immunogenicity may be blunted in all the systems by the type of delivery system, the target tissue, and the use of tissue-specific promoters to drive the constitutive component(s) of the systems. *Ex vivo* bioengineering with subsequent transplantation may also alleviate some disadvantages and improve safety.

A potential problem with the systems is that basal or uninduced expressed levels of the transgenes may not be zero. This may be the result of many factors, some of which may in turn be the result of an intrinsic weakness of the system such as a low-level "on" state for the responsive component of the system or a consequence of the vector system used. For instance, the minimal CMV (human cytomegalovirus immediate early) promoter used in the *tet* system could be improved, though this has not been scientifically demonstrated. A more serious problem of the inducible promoter in that system has already been addressed.

Heteroconcatamerization, characteristic of recombinant adeno-associated vectors, may interfere with controlled expression systems when two vectors are needed because of the limited packaging size of the vector.[47–50] Theoretically, a segment of DNA containing the constitutive promoter with enhancer elements may be brought into continuity and influence the function of the inducible promoter. This problem may be alleviated by administering vectors sequentially. For the system to work, however, all the components from both vectors need to be in the same cell within the spatial limitations of overlapping nuclear domains if using a syncytium, or otherwise, within the same nucleus. In some circumstances, this may be difficult for somatic gene therapy to achieve. Targeting skeletal muscle using multiple vectors improves the success of this strategy. An alternative is *ex vivo* manipulation and testing of the systems before transplantation.

The immune system is complex and idiosyncratic. An assumption in the characterization of the regulated systems is the relative immune potential of the transactivator components. Using "humanized" components has been proposed as a means to decrease antigenicity. However, the components of the transactivators are in a heterologous context, flanked by novel epitopes and sometimes containing deliberate mutations. Are those modifications sufficient in some individuals to break tolerance to endogenous genes?[51–65]

CONCLUSION

The utility of ligand-based, regulated gene expression for studying the basic biology of genes in cell culture, in transgenic mice, and in somatic gene-transfer models is no longer theoretical. Applications for controlled expression are also pertinent in bioinformatics, functional genomics proteomics, and pharmacogenomics. Using regulated systems to control protein expression has practical and possibly essential roles for the success of safe and effective gene therapy in a number of clinical situations. Pharmacologically regulated gene expression is an evolving tool. No individual system may be effective in all clinical applications. As new systems develop and other systems evolve and improve, the safety and efficacy of the gene switches may require study in other models that more closely approximate humans. The systems controlling targeted gene expression may also be influenced by the vehicle used in gene transfer; vector configuration, such as the presence of insulator sequences or the transgene that is being regulated; and the tissue transduced. These variables and others require further study. There is much evidence to indicate that regulated expression is appropriate and may be necessary in gene therapy applications.

REFERENCES

1. ANDERSON, W.F. 1984. Prospects for human gene therapy. Science **226:** 401–409.
2. ANDERSON, W.F. 1994. Gene therapy for genetic diseases. Hum. Gene Ther. **5:** 281–282.
3. ECK, S.L. & J.M. WILSON. 1995. Gene-based therapy. *In* The Pharmacological Basis of Therapeutics. J.G. Hardman *et al.*, Eds.: 77–101. McGraw-Hill. New York.
4. LEWIN, B. 1997. Genes VI. Oxford University Press. Oxford, U.K.
5. SEMENZA, G.L. 1994. Transcriptional regulation of gene expression: mechanisms and pathophysiology. Hum. Mutat. **3:** 180–199.
6. KLEINJAN, D.J. & V. VAN HEYNINGEN. 1998. Position effect in human genetic disease. Hum. Mol. Genet. **7:** 1611–1618.
7. ROUX-ROUQUIE, M., *et al.* 1999. Human genes involved in chromatin remodeling in transcription initiation and associated diseases: an overview using the GENATLAS database. Mol. Genet. Metab. **67:** 261–277.

8. CAZZOLA, M. & R.C. SKODA. 2000. Translational pathophysiology: a novel molecular mechanism of human disease. Blood **95:** 3280–3288.
9. TEMPLETON, N.S. & D.D. LASIC. 2000. Gene Therapy Therapeutic Mechanisms and Strategies. Marcel Deker. New York.
10. 2000. Human gene marker/therapy clinical protocols (complete updated listings). Hum. Gene Ther. **11:** 2543–2617.
11. PTASHNE, M. & A.A. GANN. 1990. Activators and targets. Nature **346:** 329–331.
12. SPENCER, D.M., *et al.* 1993. Controlling signal transduction with synthetic ligands. Science **262:** 1019–1024.
13. AUSTIN, D.J., *et al.* 1994. Proximity versus allostery: the role of regulated protein dimerization in biology. Chem. Biol. **1:** 131–136.
14. MAYO, K.E., *et al.* 1982. The mouse metallothionein-I gene is transcriptionally regulated by cadmium following transfection into human or mouse cells. Cell **29:** 99–108.
15. BIENZ, M. & H.R. PELHAM. 1986. Heat shock regulatory elements function as an inducible enhancer in the Xenopus *hsp70* gene and when linked to a heterologous promoter. Cell **45:** 753–760.
16. MAJORS, J.E. & H.E. VARMUS. 1983. Nucleotide sequencing of an apparent proviral copy of env mRNA defines determinants of expression of the mouse mammary tumor virus env gene. J. Virol. **47:** 495–504.
17. LABOW, M.A., *et al.* 1990. Conversion of the lac repressor into an allosterically regulated transcriptional activator for mammalian cells. Mol. Cell. Biol. **10:** 3343–3356.
18. GOSSEN, M., *et al.* 1993. Control of gene activity in higher eukaryotic cells by prokaryotic regulatory elements. Trends Biochem. Sci. **18:** 471–475.
19. GOSSEN, M., *et al.* 1994. Inducible gene expression systems for higher eukaryotic cells. Curr. Opin. Biotechnol. **5:** 516–520.
20. GOSSEN, M., *et al.* 1995. Transcriptional activation by tetracyclines in mammalian cells. Science **268:** 1766–1769.
21. URLINGER, S., *et al.* 2000. The p65 domain from NF-κB is an efficient human activator in the tetracycline-regulatable gene expression system. Gene **247:** 103–110.
22. URLINGER, S., *et al.* 2000. Exploring the sequence space for tetracycline-dependent transcriptional activators: novel mutations yield expanded range and sensitivity. Proc. Natl. Acad. Sci. USA **97:** 7963–7968.
23. ROSSI, F.M., *et al.* 1998. Tetracycline-regulatable factors with distinct dimerization domains allow reversible growth inhibition by p16. Nature Genet. **20:** 389–393.
24. BLAU, H.M. & F.M. ROSSI. 1999. Tet B or not tet B: advances in tetracycline-inducible gene expression. Proc. Natl. Acad. Sci. USA **96:** 797–799.
25. WOLFFE, A.P., *et al.* 2000. Co-repressor complexes and remodelling chromatin for repression. Biochem. Soc. Trans. **28:** 379–386.
26. RANG, A. & H. WILL. 2000. The tetracycline-responsive promoter contains functional interferon-inducible response elements. Nucl. Acids Res. **28:** 1120–1125.
27. WILSON, J.D., *et al.* 1998. Williams Textbook of Endocrinology. W.B. Saunders. Philadelphia.
28. NO, D., *et al.* 1996. Ecdysone-inducible gene expression in mammalian cells and transgenic mice. Proc. Natl. Acad. Sci. USA **93:** 3346–3351.
29. SUHR, S.T., *et al.* 1998. High level transactivation by a modified Bombyx ecdysone receptor in mammalian cells without exogenous retinoid X receptor. Proc. Natl. Acad. Sci. USA **95:** 7999–8004.
30. HOPPE, U.C., *et al.* 2000. Adenovirus-mediated inducible gene expression in vivo by a hybrid ecdysone receptor. Mol. Ther. **1:** 159–164.
31. VEGETO, E., *et al.* 1992. The mechanism of RU486 antagonism is dependent on the conformation of the carboxy-terminal tail of the human progesterone receptor. Cell **69:** 703–713.
32. WANG, Y., *et al.* 1994. A regulatory system for use in gene transfer. Proc. Natl. Acad. Sci. USA **91:** 8180–8184.
33. TSAI, S.Y., *et al.* 1998. A novel RU486 inducible system for the activation and repression of genes. Adv. Drug Deliv. Rev. **30:** 23–31.

34. BURCIN, M.M., *et al.* 1999. Adenovirus-mediated regulable target gene expression in vivo. Proc. Natl. Acad. Sci. USA **96:** 355–360.
35. HO, S.N., *et al.* 1996. Dimeric ligands define a role for transcriptional activation domains in reinitiation. Nature **382:** 822–826.
36. MAGARI, S.R., *et al.* 1997. Pharmacologic control of a humanized gene therapy system implanted into nude mice. J. Clin. Invest. **100:** 2865–2872.
37. POMERANTZ, J.L., *et al.* 1995. Structure-based design of transcription factors. Science **267:** 93–96.
38. RIVERA, V.M., *et al.* 1999. Long-term regulated expression of growth hormone in mice after intramuscular gene transfer. Proc. Natl. Acad. Sci. USA **96:** 8657–8662.
39. YE, X., *et al.* 1999. Regulated delivery of therapeutic proteins after in vivo somatic cell gene transfer. Science **283:** 88–91.
40. SEHGAL, S.N. 1995. Rapamune (Sirolimus, rapamycin): an overview and mechanism of action. Ther. Drug Monit. **17:** 660–665.
41. PROUD, C.G. 1996. p70 S6 kinase: an enigma with variations. Trends Biochem. Sci. **21:** 181–185.
42. BURNETT, P.E., *et al.* 1998. Neurabin is a synaptic protein linking p70 S6 kinase and the neuronal cytoskeleton. Proc. Natl. Acad. Sci. USA **95:** 8351–8356.
43. SNYDER, S.H., *et al.* 1998. Neural actions of immunophilin ligands. Trends Pharmacol. Sci. **19:** 21–26.
44. ONDRIAS, K., *et al.* 1998. FKBP12 modulates gating of the ryanodine receptor/calcium release channel. Ann. N.Y. Acad. Sci. **853:** 149–156.
45. IVERY, M.T. 2000. Immunophilins: switched on protein binding domains? Med. Res. Rev. **20:** 452–484.
46. LIBERLES, S.D., *et al.* 1997. Inducible gene expression and protein translocation using nontoxic ligands identified by a mammalian three-hybrid screen. Proc. Natl. Acad. Sci. USA **94:** 7825–7830.
47. DUAN, D., *et al.* 1998. Circular intermediates of recombinant adeno-associated virus have defined structural characteristics responsible for long-term episomal persistence in muscle tissue. J. Virol. **72:** 8568–8577.
48. DUAN, D., *et al.* 1999. Structural analysis of adeno-associated virus transduction circular intermediates. Virology **261:** 8–14.
49. YANG, J., *et al.* 1999. Concatamerization of adeno-associated virus circular genomes occurs through intermolecular recombination. J. Virol. **73:** 9468–9477.
50. YAN, Z., *et al.* 2000. From the cover: *trans*-splicing vectors expand the utility of adeno- associated virus for gene therapy. Proc. Natl. Acad. Sci. USA **97:** 6716–6721.
51. JANEWAY, C.A. 1992. The immune system evolved to discriminate infectious nonself from noninfectious self. Immunol. Today **13:** 11–16.
52. MATZINGER, P. 1994. Tolerance, danger, and the extended family. Annu. Rev. Immunol. **12:** 991–1045.
53. MATZINGER, P. 1994. Immunology. Memories are made of this? Nature **369:** 605–606.
54. MEDZHITOV, R. & C.A. JANEWAY. 1998. An ancient system of host defense. Curr. Opin. Immunol. **10:** 12–15.
55. MEDZHITOV, R. & C.A. JANEWAY. 1998. Innate immune recognition and control of adaptive immune responses. Semin. Immunol. **10:** 351–353.
56. DITTEL, B.N., *et al.* 1999. Presentation of the self antigen myelin basic protein by dendritic cells leads to experimental autoimmune encephalomyelitis. J. Immunol. **163:** 32–39.
57. CARROLL, M.C. & C.A. JANEWAY. 1999. Innate immunity. Curr. Opin. Immunol. **11:** 11–12.
58. MEDZHITOV, R. & C. JANEWAY. 2000. Innate immunity. N. Engl. J. Med. **343:** 338–344.
59. MEDZHITOV, R. & C.A. JANEWAY. 2000. How does the immune system distinguish self from nonself? Semin. Immunol. **12:** 185–188; discussion 257–344.
60. MEDZHITOV, R. & C. JANEWAY. 2000. Innate immune recognition: mechanisms and pathways. Immunol. Rev. **173:** 89–97.

61. ANDERSON, C.C. & P. MATZINGER. 2000. Danger: the view from the bottom of the cliff. Semin. Immunol. **12:** 231–238; discussion 257–344.

62. ZINKERNAGEL, R.M. 2000. Assessing the mechanisms that give rise to autoimmunity. Science **290:** 11.

63. ZINKERNAGEL, R.M. 2000. Localization dose and time of antigens determine immune reactivity. Semin. Immunol. **12:** 163–171; discussion 257–344.

64. ANDERSON, C.C. & P. MATZINGER. 2001. Immunity or tolerance: opposite outcomes of microchimerism from skin grafts. Nature Med. **7:** 80–87.

65. HEATH, W.R. & F.R. CARBONE. 2001. Cross-presentation, dendritic cells, tolerance and immunity. Annu. Rev. Immunol. **19:** 47–64.

AAV-Mediated Gene Transfer for Hemophilia

KATHERINE A. HIGH

Department of Pediatrics, University of Pennsylvania School of Medicine, The Children's Hospital of Philadelphia, Philadelphia, Pennsylvania 19104, USA

ABSTRACT: Hemophilia is a particularly attractive model for developing a gene transfer approach for the treatment of disease. The protein is very well characterized, the genes are cloned and available, and there are large and small animal models of the disease. Moreover, in contrast to many diseases, there is no requirement for a specific target tissue for gene delivery, and the gene product itself does not require precise regulation of expression. Earlier efforts to establish a gene transfer approach to the treatment of hemophilia had failed to achieve the twin goals of *l*ong-term expression at levels that were adequate to result in phenotypic improvement of the disease. We have exploited advances in vector development that occurred in the mid-1990s to establish an experimental basis for an AAV (adeno-associated viral vector)-mediated gene transfer approach to the treatment of hemophilia B. Based on the observation that introduction of an AAV vector into skeletal muscle could result in sustained expression of β-galactosidase, we engineered an AAV vector expressing human factor IX and demonstrated in immunodeficient mice that intramuscular injection of the vector resulted in long-term expression of the secreted transgene product factor IX. Subsequently, we generated an AAV vector expressing canine factor IX; intramuscular injection into dogs with severe hemophilia B resulted in a dose-dependent increase in circulating levels of factor IX. The animal treated at the highest dose showed prolonged expression (>3 years and still under observation) at a level (70 ng/ml, 1.4% of normal circulating levels of factor IX) likely to result in phenotypic improvement in humans. Detailed studies in tissue culture using human myotubes have shown that muscle cells are capable of executing the posttranslational modifications required for activity of factor IX, and that the specific activity of myotube-synthesized factor IX is similar to that of hepatocyte-synthesized material, although some details of posttranslational processing differ. Based on these and other safety and efficacy studies, a clinical trial of AAV-mediated, muscle-directed gene transfer for hemophilia B has been initiated. The study has a dose-escalation design, with three subjects to be enrolled in three dose cohorts beginning with a dose of 2 x 10^{11} vg/kg. Results in the initial dose cohort showed no evidence of toxicity associated with vector administration or transgene expression. Analysis of muscle biopsies done on injected tissue showed clear evidence of gene transfer by PCR and Southern blot and of gene expression by immunocytochemistry. The general characteristics of muscle transduction appear similar in humans and in other animal models. The goal of dose escalation is to find a dose that is nontoxic but that results in circulating levels of factor IX >1% in all patients.

KEYWORDS: AAV; gene transfer; hemophilia B; factor IX

Address for correspondence: Katherine A. High, M.D., The Children's Hospital of Philadelphia, 3516 Civic Center Boulevard, Philadelphia, PA 19104. Voice: 215-590-4521; fax: 215-590-3660.

high@email.chop.edu

Gene transfer is a treatment approach in which the active agent is a nucleic acid sequence rather than a protein or a small molecule. Our laboratory has been working to develop an experimental basis for a gene transfer technique for the treatment of hemophilia. In this review I will summarize a number of lines of investigation, and demonstrate how these have been woven together to form the basis for an ongoing clinical trial of gene transfer for hemophilia. Hemophilia is a bleeding diathesis caused by mutations either in the gene for factor VIII (hemophilia A) or for factor IX (hemophilia B). Both of these genes are encoded on the long arm of the X chromosome, so that males are affected with the disease while women are carriers. The prevalence of the hemophilias is the same throughout the world, approximately one in 5,000 births. Hemophilia A is approximately five times more common than hemophilia B; the relative incidence of disease corresponds roughly with the relative sizes of the factor VIII and factor IX genes, 186 kb and 35 kb, respectively.

Clinically, the disease is characterized by frequent spontaneous bleeding episodes, most commonly into joints and soft tissues; the predilection for bleeds into joints is still not well understood. Bleeding into other critical closed spaces, such as the intracranial space or the retroperitoneal space, can be rapidly fatal. Indeed, before the era of AIDS, intracranial hemorrhage was the most common cause of death in persons with severe hemophilia. Hemophilia is divided into severe, moderate, and mild forms of the disease; severe disease is defined as circulating factor levels of <1%, moderate as levels of 1–5%, and mild as levels >5%. The largest category of disease in both hemophilia A and hemophilia B is severe.

Current treatment for hemophilia involves infusion of either recombinant or plasma-derived clotting factor concentrates, which can be given either in response to bleeds or prophylactically. Although the introduction of these concentrates into clinical practice in the 1970s resulted in a dramatic improvement in life expectancy for persons with severe disease, the current treatment strategy suffers from a number of disadvantages, which have fueled an interest in a gene-based approach to treating the disease. Some of the disadvantages of the current approach to treatment include the following: (1) the short half-life of the infused protein, which results in the necessity for fairly frequent infusions if one wishes to maintain a circulating level of factor, and (2) the risk of transmission of viral blood-borne diseases. Because the plasma-derived concentrates are prepared from large pools of human plasma, hepatitis and later HIV contaminated the earlier plasma-derived products. This resulted in infection of large numbers of hemophilic persons with hepatitis, HIV, or both. Current viral inactivation techniques have largely solved the problems related to hepatitis and HIV, but do not as effectively rid preparations of nonenveloped viruses, for example, and ongoing concerns remain about transmission of such diseases. (3) The products are very expensive; a person with severe disease may spend $50,000–$100,000 per year on concentrate alone. A corollary of this is that these products are not widely available except in North America, Europe, and Japan, and it is estimated that approximately two-thirds of the world's hemophilia population does not have access to clotting factor concentrates. (4) Intravenous infusion of a medication is an inconvenient way to treat any disease, particularly one that affects individuals from the time of birth. Finally, because of the factors cited above, including the expense and inconvenience of the product, most people with hemophilia are treated only in response to bleeds, rather than prophylactically, and during the inevitable delay between the time a bleed begins and the time a patient can infuse himself with factor, there is ongoing tissue damage that over a lifetime results in cumulative damage to the joints and disability on that basis. The advantage of a gene-based approach to treating hemophilia is that it would allow continuous maintenance of some level of clotting factor in the circulation, so that bleeds could be prevented rather than treated after they have occurred. The gene-based approach in which clotting factors are synthesized endogenously would avoid all the risks of plasma-derived material, would clearly be more convenient, and, it is hoped, would ultimately be less expensive and therefore more widely available.

Overall, clinical gene transfer has had mixed results in its first decade. Most approaches have proven safe, but evidence of efficacy for gene transfer is much rarer. One notable exception to this was the report last year of successful treatment of infants with X-linked severe combined immunodeficiency disease (SCID) through transduction of hematopoietic stem cells with a retroviral vector encoding the γc subunit of a cytokine receptor.[1] A key factor in this success is the marked *in vivo* proliferative advantage enjoyed by the transduced cells, a feature that does not characterize most diseases for which gene transfer has been attempted. Most authorities agree that judicious choice of the disease target will be a critical factor in early successes in gene therapy. Hemophilia has a number of attractive features as an experimental model in which to address problems of gene transfer. First, tissue-specific expression of the donated gene is not required. Although clotting factors are normally synthesized in hepatocytes, work by a number of investigators has clearly established that biologically active clotting factors can be synthesized in a wide variety of tissues, including muscle cells, endothelial cells, and fibroblasts.[2–5] Thus, as long as the gene product can gain access to the circulation, the site of synthesis is relatively unimportant. This affords latitude in the choice of target cells, always an advantage in developing a gene transfer strategy. Second, in contrast to a number of other inherited diseases, hemophilia does not require precise regulation of expression of the donated gene. Thus, in contrast to diseases like diabetes, where too much insulin is as harmful as too little, the clinical course of hemophilia can be greatly improved by a modest increase in the circulating levels of clotting factor, for example, into the range of 2–3%, while raising the level to 100% still leaves the patient with a value within normal limits. Thus the therapeutic window is wide. Third, there are well-characterized large and small animal models of hemophilia. There are genetically engineered mice with hemophilia A[6] and hemophilia B,[7–9] and naturally occurring dog models of both diseases as well.[10,11] For both species, murine and canine, the factor VIII[12] and factor IX genes[13,14] are cloned and available. The existence of these animal models, particularly of the large-animal model, allows safety and efficacy testing in a disease model that faithfully mirrors the human disease, insuring that only the most promising strategies reach clinical trials. Finally, again in contrast to other inherited diseases such as cystic fibrosis, the determination of therapeutic efficacy is straightforward and unequivocal in the setting of hemophilia. Many years of experience demonstrate that circulating levels of clotting factor correlate well with the clinical symptomology of the disease, and determination of circulating levels can be carried out through a simple clotting assay on a readily obtainable blood sample.

Gene therapy strategies can be characterized in terms of three basic parameters: the vector or gene delivery vehicle; the transgene or donated gene; and the target cells into which the vector is delivered. The goals of gene transfer for inherited diseases like hemophilia are twofold: (1) to achieve sustained expression and (2) to achieve protein expression at levels high enough to have a therapeutic effect. In the case of hemophilia, early work with retroviral and adenoviral vectors had been disappointing, since neither vector was able to achieve both goals.[15,16] An important observation in the mid-1990s was that a third class of vectors, adeno-associated viral (AAV) vectors, could achieve long-term expression of a donated gene following introduction of the vector into skeletal muscle. In 1996, two groups described long-term expression of a gene product following intramuscular injection with a recombinant AAV vector.[17,18] AAV serotype 2, the wild-type virus from which recombinant AAV is derived, is a member of the parvovirus family and has a single-stranded DNA genome of ~4.7 kb. AAV-2 is nonpathogenic; most individuals are infected with the wild-type virus during childhood, but there is no associated illness. It is also naturally replication-defective. The vector that has been derived from AAV-2 is devoid of all viral coding sequence, and in contrast to retroviral vectors, which require a dividing target cell, has been shown to efficiently transduce nondividing target cells such as skeletal muscle and liver.

To test the efficacy of an AAV approach, we generated a recombinant AAV vector expressing human factor IX (F.IX) under the control of the cytomegalovirus immediate early enhancer–promoter. We introduced the recombinant AAV-F.IX into the hindlimbs of Rag-1 mice, a strain of knockout mice that carry a defect in the recombinase activating gene-1, and lack functional B and T cells. (They thus do not generate an immune response to the circulating human factor IX gene product.) Following introduction of a dose of approximately 8×10^{12} vector genomes/kg into the hindlimbs of Rag-1 mice, we documented a gradual rise in circulating levels of human factor IX into the range of 250–350 ng/ml. These levels would correspond to factor IX levels in the range of 5–7% in human plasma.[19] Circulating levels were sustained for a period of approximately 1 year following injection, after which they declined slowly, dropping by approximately 30% over the next six months. However, all of these mice lived a normal life span, with no evident complications, and continued to express therapeutic levels of human factor IX until the time of death. Note that circulating levels of 5–7% would be sufficient to convert a person with severe hemophilia into one with mild disease. We examined muscle biopsies from the injected hindlimbs and stained these using an antibody to human factor IX. These showed several interesting features. First, the fibers were positive in a "checkerboard" pattern, that is, brightly positive fibers were found directly adjacent to clearly negative fibers. The explanation for this pattern was not apparent, but is now better understood, about which more later.[20] Another important finding was that, as one proceeds away from the center of the injection site, one no longer finds positive intracellular staining but still sees bright extracellular staining for factor IX, which is not seen in nonnjected control muscle sections. Although one would expect to see some extracellular staining for a secreted transgene product such as factor IX, the bright staining in the extracellular matrix surrounding muscle fibers had not been anticipated. The explanation for this was derived from another series of experiments. In 1996, Darrel Stafford and coworkers at the University of North Carolina–Chapel Hill had reported that collagen IV functions as a high-affinity binding site (K_d in the nM range) for factor IX in the subendothelium.[21] We hypothesized that collagen IV may also function as a binding site for factor IX in the extracellular matrix; indeed, collagen IV is known to be an abundant protein in the extracellular matrix of muscle. When injected murine muscle was stained with an antibody to collagen IV and with a second antibody to human factor IX, the dual localization experiment demonstrated that collagen IV and factor IX co-localized in the extracellular matrix of injected muscle. Thus, collagen IV may serve as a binding site for factor IX secreted from muscle cells. Although it does not block secretion entirely, it may retard secretion, as a portion of the muscle-synthesized factor IX is retained at these high-affinity binding sites and the remainder spills out into the circulation.

In the next series of experiments, we wished to determine whether these observations would also be confirmed in a large animal model of hemophilia. As noted above, the existence of large animal models permits more detailed efficacy studies in the setting of hemophilia before proceeding to clinical trials. In our particular case, there were at least at least three issues that we felt could be addressed more realistically in hemophilic dogs than in the mouse model. The first of these was simply the issue of scale-up of vector production. In recent years, rAAV vector production has improved by approximately 1 log per year, but at the time we initiated these studies, it was a challenge to produce enough vector to treat a series of hemophilic dogs, which can weigh as much as 20 kg each. Thus, these experiments allowed us to explore whether this was feasible. Secondly, it allowed us to assess whether factor IX could transit efficiently from the site of synthesis in the muscle into the circulation in an animal larger than a mouse. Note that a dog is approximately 400–800-fold larger than a mouse, whereas a human is only 3–10-fold larger than a dog, depending on the size of the dog and the person. Thus, success in the dog model would be much more predictive of success in humans than success in a mouse model. Finally, we wished to assess the immune response to the transgene product in a genetically deficient disease model, and this is more appropriately carried out using an outbred strain of hemophilic dog and a canine factor IX transgene than using inbred strains of immunodeficient mice and a human factor IX transgene.

With these challenges in mind, we began a collaboration with Dr. Ken Brinkhous and Dr. Tim Nichols at UNC-Chapel Hill. Dr. Brinkhous has maintained a colony of dogs with hemophilia B in Chapel Hill since the 1960s. These animals have a missense mutation in the factor IX gene that changes a glycine at 379 to a glutamic acid.[10] They have no circulating factor IX protein, but do have normal factor IX transcript levels in the liver. These animals have severe disease with <1% circulating factor IX, and clinically their disease mirrors human pathophysiology, with frequent soft tissue bleeds. To carry out these experiments, we constructed a canine factor IX vector, which was again driven by the CMV enhancer/promoter.[22] This vector was prepared using a triple transfection technique in which the therapeutic gene of interest (F.IX), an AAV rep-cap plasmid, and an adenoviral helper plasmid were all introduced into 293 cells, which were subsequently lysed to permit recovery of recombinant AAV through cesium chloride density centrifugation.[23] The experiments conducted in the hemophilic dogs were similar to those described in the mice, except that in the dogs a dose-escalation study design was used. Dogs ranged in size from 6 to 20 kg. They underwent intramuscular injection of vector at anywhere from 8 to 60 sites on day 1 of the protocol. Dogs were not covered with plasma for the injections, and most underwent injections uneventfully. After vector injection we followed a series of parameters including the whole blood clotting time, the factor IX antigen, and the activated partial prothrombin time (aPTT). Beginning with the lowest dose of 1.3×10^{11} vector genomes/kg, we have seen sustained correction of the whole blood clotting time. The whole blood clotting time is typically >60 minutes in hemophilic dogs and is 5–10 minutes in normal dogs. Following injection of even the lowest dose, the whole blood clotting time corrected into the range of 20 minutes and has remained shortened for a period of >31/2 years following the initial injection, with observation still ongoing. The whole blood clotting time is sensitive to even very low levels of factor IX; it was determined that higher doses, in the range of approximately 3×10^{12} vector genomes/kg, were required to correct the aPTT. Again, in these animals the aPTT is typically 50–80 seconds, while it is 10–20 seconds in normal dogs. Levels $<3 \times 10^{12}$ vector genomes/kg typically yielded aPTTs in the range of 30–40 seconds. In terms of factor IX levels, there was a dose-dependent increase in circulating levels of factors IX in the injected dogs. Injection of vector at a dose of 8.5×10^{12} vector genomes/kg resulted in circulating levels of factor IX of approximately 70 ng/ml, corresponding to about 1.4% in human with hemophilia. Note that levels >1% in humans are generally associated with an improved course of disease. It should also be noted that one of these animals, the one receiving the highest dose, did develop a transient inhibitory antibody to factor IX. This was documented both on Western blot, where it first becomes apparent two weeks after injection, peaks at about six weeks after injection, and then slowly recedes, and also through the use of a clinical assay, the Bethesda assay, which measures the inhibitory activity in a clotting assay. The titer of the inhibitory antibody peaked at approximately 7 Bethesda units and then receded in a time course consistent with the data generated on the Western blot. Inhibitory antibodies are the commonest complication of protein-based therapy for hemophilia; their presence precludes treatment with normal replacement therapy. Transient inhibitory antibodies were first extensively described and studied in the setting of the recombinant clotting factor trials,[24,25] but the factors that determine transient versus sustained inhibitory antibody production in the setting of protein-based therapy are not yet well understood. The occurrence of a transient inhibitory antibody in hemophilic dogs using this gene-based approach served as a cautionary note and indicated one of the safety concerns that would have to be carefully assessed in a human clinical trial.

A series of other clinical laboratory studies in hemophilic dogs revealed no evidence of toxicity associated with vector injection or transgene expression. Serial muscle biopsies at the injection sites have disclosed no evidence of damage or inflammatory infiltrate, and serial serum chemistries and CBCs have also shown no evidence of toxicity.

Another question that needed to be resolved before initiation of clinical trials was the biochemical characterization of factor IX synthesized in skeletal muscle cells. Factor IX is a highly posttranslationally modified protein. Under normal circumstances, before secretion from the hepatocyte into the circulation, the following posttranslational modifications take place: removal of the signal sequence and the propeptide; conversion of 12 glutamic acid residues at the NH_2-terminus to γ-carboxy glutamic acid residues; glycosylation of multiple residues; tyrosine sulfation at residue 155; serine phosphorylation at residue 158; and partial β-hydroxylation of the aspartic acid at 64. Whether all of these can take place accurately and efficiently in skeletal muscle was not clear, although it was clear that biologically active material was produced, since clotting studies in hemophilic animals were partially corrected.

In order to explore this question, we developed a cell culture system that utilized human myotubes.[5] These were obtained from muscle biopsies, after which myoblasts were grown in culture and differentiated into mature myotubes. The mature myotubes were then transduced with an AAV vector expressing human factor IX. Conditioned medium was collected, and recombinant factor IX synthesized in myotubes was purified using an ion-exchange column and an immunoaffinity column that made use of a monoclonal antibody directed against the heavy chain of human factor IX. This was done specifically to avoid selective recovery of the fraction of factor IX that is properly posttranslationally modified (since the heavy chain contains few posttranslational modifications). The myotube-synthesized factor IX was characterized using both plasma-derived factor IX and human factor IX purified from transduced HepG2 cells as controls. On SDS polyacrylamide gel, the myotube-synthesized factor IX migrates with a mobility identical to that seen with plasma-derived human factor IX or with HepG2 cell–derived factor IX. NH_2-terminal sequence analysis on the material recovered from myotube-conditioned medium reveals the normal sequence for mature factor IX, indicating that the signal sequence and propeptide have been accurately and efficiently removed before secretion. In addition, sequence analysis discloses that the glutamic acid residues at the NH_2-terminus are fully γ-carboxylated; γ–carboxy glutamic acid residues register as a blank on automated Edman degradation sequencing, whereas unmodified glutamic acid residues are detected as glutamic acid peaks. The absence of any detectable signal at the appropriate residues indicates that the glutamic acid residues are appropriately modified. On oligosaccharide analysis, myotube-synthesized factor IX shows extensive heterogeneity in N-linked carbohydrate residues and in this sense is similar to human hepatocyte-synthesized factor IX. The specific activity of the myotube-synthesized factor IX is similar to hepatocyte-synthesized material, with specific activities of 182 units/mg and 200 units/mg, respectively, at an MOI of 20,000 in tissue culture. Tyrosine sulfation and serine phosphorylation are much reduced in the myotube-synthesized material compared to human hepatocyte–synthesized material. It is of note that the specific activity of myotube-synthesized factor IX declines as the MOI is raised, indicating that one or more posttranslational modifications required for activity can be saturated in the myotube culture system. Thus, as doses are escalated in animals treated with vector, it is advisable to spread injectate over multiple sites, rather than to increase the amount of injectate at a single site, as this is likely to result in production of material that is not fully biologically active.

Although not discussed in this review, it should be noted that data generated by our group and by others[16,26,27] have demonstrated that similar levels of factor IX can be obtained following introduction of vector into the liver via the portal vein. Thus, when designing the initial hemophilia clinical trial with an AAV vector, it was necessary to determine which target tissue would be used at the outset. Several factors entered into this decision. Introduction of vector into skeletal muscle involves a procedure that is safe, familiar, and relatively noninvasive; whereas introduction of vector into liver requires an invasive procedure in which a catheter is introduced into the hepatic artery via an incision in the groin. Although this procedure can be carried out safely, its more invasive nature in a population of patients with a bleeding diathesis makes the intramuscular approach more attractive. Secondly, hepatitis has a high prevalence among persons with hemophilia. Although hepatitis would not be a contraindication to intramuscular administration of vector, very little data exist about the influence of hepatitis on transduction of hepatocytes; in fact, all of the preclinical data have been generated in animals with normal livers. Thus this represented an uncertainty for the liver-directed approach and again favored muscle as the initial target tissue. Third, detailed studies had been carried out defining the risk of germline transmission following introduction of AAV vector into skeletal muscle, and this appeared to be undetectable.[28] On the other hand, such studies had not yet been carried out for a liver-directed approach in which vector was introduced directly into the circulation. In favor of the liver, it is the normal site of synthesis of blood coagulation factors, and thus it is highly likely that all of the necessary posttranslational modifications would be executed accurately and efficiently, and preclinical studies had established that there was a clear dose advantage in favor of introduction of vector into the liver, probably because secretion from the hepatocyte into the circulation is a very efficient process. When all of these factors were taken together, however, it appeared that the safest course was to begin with introduction of vector into muscle. It is important to emphasize, though, that liver is clearly also an important target tissue, and one that merits further analysis in a clinical trial.

The overall design of the Phase I/II trial for AAV-mediated muscle-directed gene transfer is an open-label dose escalation design, with three subjects in each of three dose cohorts. Subjects undergo intramuscular injection of vector under coverage with factor IX protein concentrate, and at periodic intervals thereafter blood samples are drawn for analysis of serum chemistries and hematologic studies. Coagulation studies are also carried out, and muscle enzymes are analyzed. Built into the trial at periodic intervals are muscle biopsies that allow investigators to assess gene transfer and expression via the intramuscular route. The goals of this Phase I study were several: the first was to determine the safety of the procedure. It should be noted that at the time this trial was initiated, there was no experience with parenteral administration of AAV vectors; thus, the most important goal was to assess whether this procedure could be carried out safely in humans. The second goal was to determine the effect of preexisting immunity to AAV on gene transfer and expression. As noted earlier, perhaps 80% of individuals are infected with the wild-type virus from which the vector is derived during childhood. Whether antibodies to AAV serotype 2 would prevent gene transfer and expression following introduction of the vector into skeletal muscle was unknown. A third goal was to determine the level and duration of expression of vector in human skeletal muscle. An important goal of any new treatment for hemophilia is to determine the prevalence of clinically significant inhibitory antibodies. Finally it is important to determine the risk of germline transmission of vector sequences, which can be assessed by analyzing subject semen following injection. The major safety issues outlined in the consent form are first, the risk of inhibitory antibody formation, which had been highlighted in preclinical studies by the occurrence of a transient inhibitory antibody in one hemophilic dog; the risk of insertional mutagenesis, which refers to the theoretical possibility that the vector could integrate into a critical sequence, for example, a tumor suppressor gene, disrupt the function of that gene, and leave the cell with an undefined but increased risk of malignant transformation; and finally the risk that vector sequences would make their way into germ cells and thus cause a risk to potential offspring. The inclusion criteria for the trial are as follows: males with severe hemophilia B, factor IX level <1%; age >18 years; ability to give informed consent; >20 previous exposure days to treatment with factor IX protein; no history or presence of an inhibitor to factor IX protein; and willingness to practice birth control until three consecutive semen samples have been documented to be negative for AAV vector DNA. Exclusion criteria include the presence of active acute infections (but not chronic infections with

HIV or hepatitis); endstage renal or liver disease; a platelet count of <50,000; presence of inflammatory muscle disease; or patients who are unwilling to stop a regimen of factor IX prophylaxis, which would preclude determination of clinically relevant endpoints.

To date, six subjects have been enrolled in the trial; data are reported here on the first three subjects.[29] All have severe hemophilia B with baseline factor IX levels of <1%. Of the first three, one is CRM-positive and two others are CRM-negative. All subjects have distinct factor IX mutations, as is typical for this disease where no one mutation predominates. Of the first three subjects, one is HIV-positive, and two are hepatitis C–positive. Safety studies in the first three subjects have shown that vector is shed in urine and saliva for the first 24 hours following injection, and the serum is positive for the first 48 hours, but there is no evidence of positive body fluids after that time, and no semen samples have been positive to date. Studies to evaluate the risk of inhibitor formation have also been uniformly negative, including Western blot and Bethesda assays on all subjects. The safety studies have revealed no problems with the procedure to date. Muscle biopsies carried out in the first three subjects have shown evidence for gene transfer by either PCR or Southern blot on DNA harvested from muscle biopsies. In addition they have shown evidence of gene expression by immunohistochemical stains of biopsied muscle. Finally, one of the first three subjects showed factor IX levels >1% following injection, and two of the three have experienced at least a 50% reduction in the amount of exogenous factor IX infused over the first year following injection. In conclusion, at this early stage it would appear that intramuscular injection of AAV appears to be a safe and well-tolerated procedure, with no evidence of systemic or local toxicity. Muscle biopsies on the first three injected subjects demonstrate evidence for gene transfer and expressions of factor IX, and also indicate that the general properties of human skeletal muscle transduction by AAV-2 are similar to those that had been delineated in preclinical studies in animal models. Based on factor levels and on exogenous factor IX consumed, there would appear to be some early indications of efficacy from these studies, but confirmation of this will require additional study at higher vector doses. The goal of dose escalation is to identify a dose of vector that is nontoxic but results in circulating levels of F.IX >1% in all recipients.

It is likely that a successful gene transfer approach to the treatment of hemophilia can be developed, using this or some other strategy. We believe that the staged approach outlined here, with studies beginning in mice and progressing through the hemophilic dog model, can provide a strong experimental basis for the development and testing of gene transfer in humans.

REFERENCES

1. CAVAZZANA-CALVO, M., S. HACEIN-BEY, G. DE SAINT BASILE, *et al.* 2000. Gene therapy of human severe combined immunodeficiency (SCID)-X1 disease. Science **288:** 669–672.
2. PALMER, T.D., A.R. THOMPSON & A.D. MILLER. 1989. Production of human factor IX in animals by genetically modified skin fibroblasts: potential therapy for hemophilia B. Blood **73:** 438–445.
3. YAO, S.-N., J.M. WILSON, E.G. NABEL, *et al.* 1991. Expression of human factor IX in rat capillary endothelial cells: toward somatic gene therapy for hemophilia B. Proc. Natl. Acad. Sci. USA **88:** 8101–8105.

4. YAO, S.N. & K. KURACHI. 1992. Expression of human factor IX in mice after injection of genetically modified myoblasts. Proc. Natl. Acad. Sci. USA **89:** 3357–3361.
5. ARRUDA, V.R., J.N. HAGSTROM, R.W. HERZOG, et al. 2001. Post-translational modifications of recombinant myotube-synthesized human factor IX. Blood **97:** 130–138.
6. BI, L., A.M. LAWLER, S.E. ANTONARAKIS, et al. 1995. Targeted disruption of the mouse factor VIII gene: a model for hemophilia A. Nature Genet. **10:** 119–121.
7. WANG, L., M. ZOPPE, T.M. HACKENG, et al. 1997. A factor IX-deficient mouse model for hemophilia B gene therapy. Proc. Natl. Acad. Sci. USA **94:** 11563–11566.
8. LIN, H.F., N. MAEDA, O. SMITHIES, et al. 1997. A coagulation factor IX-deficient mouse model for human hemophilia B. Blood **90(10):** 3962–3966.
9. KUNDU, R.K., F. SANGIORGI, L.Y. WU, et al. 1998. Targeted inactivation of the coagulation factor IX gene causes hemophilia B in mice. Blood **92:** 168–174.
10. EVANS, J.P., K.M. BRINKHOUS, G.D. BRAYER, et al. 1989. Canine hemophilia B resulting from a point mutation with unusual consequences. Proc. Natl. Acad. Sci. USA **86:** 10095–10099.
11. MAUSER, A.E., J. WHITLARK, K.M. WHITNEY, et al. 1996. A deletion mutation causes hemophilia B in Lhasa Apso dogs. Blood **88:** 3451–3455.
12. CAMERON, C., C. NOTLEY, S. HOYLE, et al. 1998. The canine factor VIII cDNA and 5′ flanking sequence. Thromb. Haemost. **79:** 317–322.
13. WU, S.M., D.W. STAFFORD & J.L. WARE. 1990. Deduced amino acid sequence of mouse blood-coagulation factor IX. Gene **86:** 275–278.
14. EVANS, J.P., H.H. WATZKE, J.L. WARE, et al. 1989a. Molecular cloning of a cDNA encoding canine factor IX. Blood **74(1):** 207–212.
15. KAY, M.A., S. ROTHENBERG, C.N. LANDEN, et al. 1993. In vivo gene therapy of hemophilia B: sustained partial correction in factor IX-deficient dogs. Science **262:** 117–119.
16. KAY, M.A., L. MEUSE, A.M. GOWN, et al. 1997. Transient immunomodulation with anti-CD40 ligand antibody and CTLA4Ig enhances persistence and secondary adenovirus-mediated gene transfer into mouse liver. Proc. Natl. Acad. Sci. USA **94:** 4686–4691.
17. XIAO, X., J. LI & R.J. SAMULSKI. 1996. Efficient long-term gene transfer into muscle tissue of immunocompetent mice by adeno-associated virus vector. J. Virol. **70:** 8098–8108.
18. KESSLER, P.D., G.M. PODSAKOFF, X. CHEN, et al. 1996. Gene delivery to skeletal muscle results in sustained expression and systemic delivery of a therapeutic protein. Proc. Natl. Acad. Sci. USA **93:** 14082–14087.
19. HERZOG, R.W., J.N. HAGSTROM, Z.-H. KUNG, et al. 1997. Stable gene transfer and expression of human blood coagulation factor IX after intramuscular injection of recombinant adeno-associated virus. Proc. Natl. Acad. Sci. USA **94:** 5804–5809.
20. PRUCHNIC, R., B. CAO, Z.Q. PETERSON, et al. 2000. The use of adeno-associated virus to circumvent the maturation-dependent viral transduction of muscle fibers. Hum. Gene Ther. **11:** 521–536.
21. CHEUNG, W.-F., J.V.D. BORN, K. KÜHN, et al. 1996. Identification of the endothelial binding site for factor IX. Proc. Natl. Acad. Sci. USA **93:** 11068–11073.
22. HERZOG, R.W., E.Y. YANG, L.B. COUTO, et al. 1999. Long-term correction of canine hemophilia B by gene transfer of blood coagulation factor IX mediated by adeno-associated viral vector. Nature Med. **5:** 56–63.
23. MATSUSHITA, T., S. ELLIGER, C. ELLIGER, et al. 1998. Adeno-associated virus vectors can be efficiently produced without helper virus. Gene Ther. **5:** 938–945.
24. BRAY, G.L., E.D. GOMPERTS, S. COURTER, et al. 1994. A multicenter study of recombinant factor VIII (recombinate): safety, efficacy, and inhibitor risk in previously untreated patients with hemophilia A. Blood **83:** 2428–2435.
25. LUSHER, J.M., S. ARKIN, C.F. ABILDGAARD, et al. 1993. Recombinant factor VIII for the treatment of previously untreated patients with hemophilia A. N. Engl. J. Med. **328:** 453–459.
26. KAY, M.A. & K.A. HIGH. 1999. Gene therapy for the hemophilias. Proc. Natl. Acad. Sci. USA **96:** 9973–9975.
27. NAKAI, H., R. HERZOG, J.N. HAGSTROM, et al. 1998. AAV-mediated gene transfer of human blood coagulation factor IX into mouse liver. Blood **91:** 4600–4607.

Bone Marrow as a Source of Endothelial Cells for Natural and Iatrogenic Vascular Repair

JEFFREY M. ISNER, CHRISTOPH KALKA, ATSUHIKO KAWAMOTO, AND TAKAYUKI ASAHARA

Department of Medicine (Cardiology and Vascular Medicine), St. Elizabeth's Medical Center, Tufts University School of Medicine, Boston, Massachusetts 02135, USA

ABSTRACT: Postnatal neovascularization has previously been considered synonymous with angiogenesis, but the finding that circulating endothelial progenitor cells (EPCs) may home to sites of neovascularization and there differentiate into endothelial cells (ECs) is consistent with "vasculogenesis," through which the primordial vascular network is established in the embryo. Our findings suggest that growth and development of new blood vessels in the adult are not restricted to angiogenesis but encompass vasculogenesis as well, although the proportional contributions remain to be clarified. Likewise, augmented or retarded neovascularization probably involves enhancement or impariment of the vasculogenesis process.

KEYWORDS: endothelial cells; endothelial progenitor cells; angiogenesis; vasculogenesis; premature atherosclerosis; vascular endothelial growth factor; hematopoietic stem cells

Preliminary clinical findings in patients with critical limb ischemia established that the response to gene transfer of vascular endothelial growth factor (VEGF) was most robust and expeditious in young patients with premature atherosclerosis involving the lower extremities, so-called Buerger's disease.[1] This clinical observation was supported by experiments performed in live animal models, specifically young (4–5 months) versus old (6–8 years) rabbits and young (8 weeks) versus old (2 years) mice. In both cases, native neovascularization of the ischemic hindlimb was markedly retarded in old versus young animals. Retardation of neovascularization in old animals appeared in part to result from reduced expression of VEGF in tissue sections harvested from the ischemic limb.[2] Similarly, retarded neovascularization and reduced VEGF expression was observed in diabetic (NOD)[3] and hypercholesterolemic (ApoE$^{-/-}$)[4] mice. Cell-specific immunostaining localized VEGF protein expression to skeletal myocytes and infiltrating T cells in the ischemic limbs of C57 mice; in contrast, VEGF-expressing T-cell infiltrates were found to be severely re-

Address for correspondence: Takayuki Asahara, Vascular Medicine and Cardiovascular Research, St. Elizabeth's Medical Center, 736 Cambridge Street, Boston, MA 02135-2997. Voice: 617-789-3156.
asa777@aol.com

duced in ischemic limbs of mice in which angiogenesis was impaired. Transendo-thelial migration of human T cells has been previously shown to be compromised in elderly versus young subjects, although the basis for this defect in transmigration re-mains enigmatic.[5] The critical contribution of T cells to VEGF expression and col-lateral vessel growth has been reinforced by the finding of accelerated limb necrosis in athymic nude mice with operatively induced hindlimb ischemia.[4]

Reduction in endogenous VEGF expression, however, was not the only factor contributing to impaired neovascularization in these animals; older, diabetic, and hy-percholesterolemic animals—like human patients—also exhibit age-related endot-helial dysfunction, manifest as reduced vasodilation and decreased production of NO in response to endothelium-dependent agonists.[2] Endothelial dysfunction did not preclude a favorable response to cytokine replacement therapy: indeed, the ab-solute magnitude by which blood pressure ratio, angiographic score, and capillary density were increased in response to supplemental administration of recombinant VEGF protein was similar for young and old animals. In older animals, however, these indices failed to reach the ultimate levels recorded in younger animals, appar-ently reflecting the inherent limitations imposed by a less-responsive endothelial cell (EC) substrate.

This clinical experience and these animal studies have two implications. First, the findings suggest that the fundamental mechanism by which therapeutic neovascular-ization augments collateral development is to provide cytokine supplements to indi-viduals who—because of advanced age, diabetes, hypercholesterolemia, and/or other as-yet-undefined circumstances—are unable to appropriately upregulate cytokine expression in response to tissue ischemia. In this regard, ligand supplementation may be analogous to erythropoietin administration in patients with refractory anemia.

Second, cytokine administration clearly composes only one aspect of the thera-peutic intervention. Regardless of how much ligand is administered, the resident population of ECs that is competent to respond to an available level of angiogenic growth factors may also constitute a potentially limiting factor in strategies designed to promote neovascularization of ischemic tissues. A reasonable goal may therefore consist of developing a complementary strategy that would provide substrate togeth-er with ligand, a "supply side" version of therapeutic neovascularization.

POSTNATAL VASCULOGENESIS

The option of performing full-scale EC transplantation to optimize this therapeu-tic strategy is daunting if even feasible. Accordingly, we investigated an alternative strategy designed to exploit the conceptual notion that ECs and hematopoietic stem cells (HSCs) were ultimately derived from a common precursor, the putative heman-gioblast. HSCs had been shown previously to be present in circulating blood, in quantities sufficient to permit their harvesting and readministration for autologous—in lieu of bone marrow—transplantation. We therefore inferred that related descen-dents, endothelial progenitor cells (EPCs), might be present along with HSCs in the peripheral circulation. Flk-1 and a second antigen (CD-34) shared by angioblasts and HSCs were used to isolate putative angioblasts from the leukocyte fraction of peripheral blood.[6] *In vitro*, these cells differentiated into ECs. In animal models of ischemia, heterologous, homologous, and autologous EPCs were shown to incorporate into sites of active neovascularization.

More recently, we have utilized a bone marrow (BM) transplant (T) model to demonstrate incorporation of BM-derived EPCs into foci of neovascularization. Wild-type mice were lethally irradiated with 9.0 Gy and were transplanted with BM harvested from transgenic mice of the same genetic background in which constitutive *lacZ* expression is regulated by an EC-specific promoter, Flk-1 or Tie-2. Flk-1 (VEGFR-2) has been shown to be essential for EPC (angioblast) differentiation and blood vessel development during embryogenesis and postnatal neovascularization. The Tie-2 receptor has been shown to be expressed in endothelial lineage cells participating in angiogenesis, and in this regard is essential for blood vessel development and maturation. Consequently, β-galactosidase is constitutively overexpressed in the BM of the transplant recipient Flk-1 or *tie2/lacZ* mice but not in any other somatic cells. Application of a solution of X-gal to the BM renders it blue, and any blue cells that are detected at remote tissue sites can thus be inferred to have been derived from BM and delivered to those sites via the peripheral circulation. After a period of 4 weeks post-transplant, by which time the BM of the recipient mice is reconstituted, a variety of surgical experiments may be performed, all of which are intended to provoke neovascularization. For example, preliminary experiments performed in a mouse model of corneal injury disclosed BM-derived cells incorporated into neovascular foci at the corneal limbus. A similar approach may be used to investigate the contribution of circulating, BM-derived EPCs to neovascularization of ischemic hindlimbs, injured corneas, and tumor vasculature.

Previous investigators have shown that wound trauma causes mobilization of hematopoietic cells, including pluripotent stem or progenitor cells in spleen, BM, and peripheral blood. Consistent with EPC/HSC common ancestry, recent data from our laboratory has shown that mobilization of BM-derived EPCs constitutes a natural response to tissue ischemia.[7] In these experiments, we used the murine BMT model to establish direct evidence of enhanced BM-derived EPC incorporation into foci of corneal neovascularization following the development of hindlimb ischemia. Light microscopic examination of corneas excised 6 days after micropocket injury and concurrent surgery to establish hindlimb ischemia demonstrated a statistically significant increase in cells expressing β-galactosidase in the corneas of mice with versus those without an ischemic limb.[7] This finding indicates that circulating EPCs are mobilized endogenously in response to tissue ischemia, following which they may be incorporated into neovascular foci to promote tissue repair.

Given its regulatory role in both angiogenesis and vasculogenesis during fetal development, we subsequently investigated the hypothesis that VEGF may modulate EPC kinetics for postnatal neovascularization. Indeed, we observed that intraperitoneal injections of $VEGF_{165}$ recombinant protein administered to normal mice led to an increase in circulating EPCs.[8] VEGF-induced mobilization of bone marrow-derived EPCs resulted in increased differentiated EPCs *in vitro* and augmented corneal neovascularization *in vivo*. Similar increases in circulating EPCs were observed in human subjects undergoing VEGF gene transfer for limb[9] or myocardial[10] ischemia. Thus, constitutive overexpression of VEGF in mice and patients modulates EPC kinetics, suggesting that BM mobilization of circulating EPCs constitutes an alternative mechanism by which VEGF may promote neovascularization.

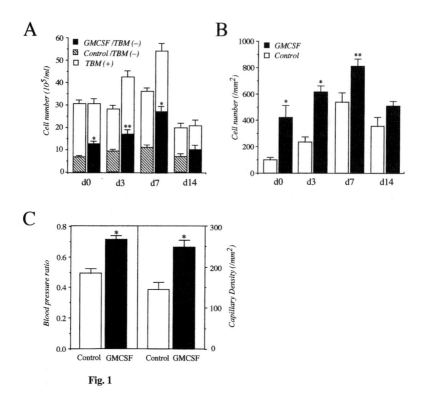

Fig. 1

FIGURE 1. Effect of GM-CSF-induced EPC mobilization on neovascularization in rabbit ischemic hindlimb model. Untreated (control) rabbit ischemic hindlimb demonstrated enhanced EPC kinetics as well. **(A,B)** Both circulating number of EPCs in peripheral blood and EPC differentiation (by culture assay) are increased at postoperative days 3 and 7 compared to day 0. Following pretreatment with GM-CSF, circulating EPC-enriched population (TBM⁻) is increased in number compared to control (ischemic, untreated) animals beginning at day 0 (before surgery) through day 7 **(A)**, as is EPC differentiation in culture **(B)** ($n = 5$ each time point). Two weeks after onset of rabbit ischemia, physiological assessment using blood pressure ratio of ischemic to healthy limb indicates significant improvement in GM-CSF versus control group **(C)**. Histologic examination with alkaline phosphatase staining demonstrates significant capillary density in GM-CSF group that exceeds control group **(C)** ($n = 9$ each group). (* = $p < 0.01$, ** = $p < 0.05$).

THERAPEUTIC VASCULOGENESIS

Having demonstrated the potential for endogenous mobilization of BM-derived EPCs, we considered that iatrogenic expansion and mobilization of this putative EC precursor population might represent an effective means to augment the resident population of ECs that is competent to respond to administered angiogenic cytokines. Such a program might thereby address the issue of endothelial dysfunction or depletion that may compromise strategies of therapeutic neovascularization in older, diabetic, and/or hypercholesterolemic animals and patients. This goal could be potentially accomplished indirectly, using cytokine mobilization, or directly by administration of supplemental EPCs.

As an example of an indirect strategy, we used GM-CSF, which stimulates hematopoietic progenitor cells and myeloid lineage cells, as well as nonhematopoietic cells including BM stromal cells and ECs.[7] To effect GM-CSF-induced EPC mobilization while avoiding a direct effect on ECs, rhGM-CSF was administered daily for 7 days *prior to* surgery to create hindlimb ischemia. GM-CSF pretreatment produced a statistically significant increase in the circulating population of EPCs and enhanced EPC differentiation versus controls. Moreover, capillary density analysis documented extensive neovascularization induced by GM-CSF pretreatment, and measurements of ischemic/normal hindlimb blood pressure ratio disclosed evidence of a corresponding increase in hindlimb blood flow. These results thus indicate that GM-CSF exerts a potent stimulatory effect on EPC kinetics and that such cytokine-induced EPC mobilization can enhance neovascularization of severely ischemic tissues as well as *de novo* vascularization of previously avascular sites (FIG. 1).

Direct repopulation of EPCs was investigated in murine and rodent models of hindlimb and myocardial ischemia, respectively. One day following operative excision of one femoral artery, athymic nude mice ($n = 17$), in which angiogenesis is characteristically impaired,[4] received an intracardiac injection of 5×10^5 culture-expanded human EPCs (hEPCs). Two control groups were identically injected with either human microvascular ECs (HMVECs) ($n = 12$) or medium from the culture plates employed for hEPC *ex vivo* expansion ($n = 14$). Serial examination of hindlimb perfusion by laser Doppler perfusion imaging (LDPI)[11] performed at days 3, 7, 14, 21, and 28 disclosed profound differences in the limb perfusion within 28 days after induction of limb ischemia. Three days post-operatively, limb perfusion was severely reduced in all three groups. Over the subsequent 28 days, however, substantial blood flow recovery in mice receiving hEPCs returned perfusion of the ischemic hindlimb to levels that were similar to those recorded in the contralateral nonischemic hindlimb. In contrast, limb perfusion remained markedly depressed in mice receiving either HMVECs or culture medium. By day 28, the ratio of ischemic/normal blood flow in hEPC-transplanted mice had improved to 0.69 ± 0.08 vs. 0.27 ± 0.08 and 0.34 ± 0.05 in mice receiving HMVECs and culture medium, respectively ($p < 0.003$). Such improvement in hindlimb perfusion in this animal model has been previously shown to reflect neovascularization, based on morphometric analyses of capillary density and EC proliferative activity.[11] Time-course studies demonstrated that peak hEPC incorporation into sites of neovascularization was achieved within 3 to 7 days post administration of hEPCs. Histologic evaluation of skeletal muscle sections retrieved from the ischemic hindlimbs of mice sacrificed at days 7, 14, and 28 showed that capillary density, an index of neovascularization, was markedly increased in hEPC-transplanted mice.

Enhanced neovascularization in mice transplanted with hEPCs led to important biological consequences. Among mice in which induction of hindlimb ischemia was followed by administration of HMVECs, limb salvage was limited to 1 (8.3%) of 12 animals, while the remainder developed extensive forefoot necrosis ($n = 5$, 41.7%), leading in 6 (50%) to spontaneous amputation. Likewise, a preserved limb was observed in only 1 (7.1%) of 14 mice treated with culture medium, while foot necrosis and/or autoamputation developed in 7 (50%) and 6 (42.9%) mice, respectively.

In contrast, hEPC transplantation was associated with successful limb salvage in 10 (58.8%) of 17 animals. Foot necrosis was limited to 5 (29.4%) mice, and only 2 (11.8%) experienced spontaneous limb amputation. The difference in outcome between the hEPC-treated mice and both control groups was statistically significant (for hEPC vs. HMVEC, $p = 0.006$; for hEPC versus control medium, $p = 0.003$). The outcomes in mice receiving HMVECs vs. culture medium were similar ($p = 0.9$).

Similar outcomes have now been demonstrated in rats with myocardial ischemia.[12] In this case, peripheral blood mononuclear cells obtained from healthy human adults were cultured in EPC medium and harvested 7 days later. Myocardial ischemia was induced by ligation of the left anterior descending coronary artery in male Hsd: RH-rnu (athymic nude) rats. In two rats, 10^6 EPCs labeled with Di I were injected intravenously 3 hours after induction of myocardial ischemia. Seven days later, fluorescence-conjugated BS-1 lectin was administered intravenously (i.v.), and the rats were immediately sacrificed. Fluorescence microscopy revealed that transplanted EPCs accumulated to the ischemic area and incorporated into foci of myocardial neovascularization.

To determine the impact on left ventricular function, five rats (EPC group) were injected i.v. with 10^6 EPCs 3 hours after induction of ischemia; five other rats (control group) received culture medium. Echocardiography, performed just before and 28 days after induction of ischemia, disclosed ventricular dimensions that were significantly smaller and fractional shortening (FS) that was significantly greater in the EPC versus control group by day 28 (diastole = 0.87 ± 0.03 vs. 0.93 ± 0.01 cm, $p < 0.05$; systole = 0.68 ± 0.03 vs. 0.79 ± 0.02 cm, $p < 0.01$; FS = 21.3 ± 0.6 vs. $15.3 \pm 2.2\%$, $p < 0.001$). Regional wall motion was better preserved in EPC versus control group (25.3 ± 0.8 vs. 30.6 ± 1.0, $p < 0.01$). Following sacrifice on day 28, necropsy exam disclosed that capillary density was significantly greater in the EPC group than in controls (290.1 ± 21.5 vs. 191.1 ± 17.8, $p < 0.001$). Moreover, extent of LV scarring was significantly less in rats receiving EPCs than in controls (8.9 ± 0.9 vs. $17.8 \pm 1.4\%$ of LV, $p < 0.01$). Immunohistochemistry revealed capillaries that were positive for human CD31 and UEA-1 lectin. Thus, ex vivo–expanded EPCs transplanted into ischemic myocardium incorporate into foci of myocardial neovascularization and have a favorable impact on preservation of LV function (FIGS. 2 and 3).

GENE-MODIFIED EPC THERAPY

The observation that circulating EPCs home to foci of neovascularization suggests potential utility as autologous vectors for gene therapy. For treatment of regional ischemia, neovascularization could be amplified by transfection of EPCs to achieve highly localized constitutive expression of angiogenic cytokines and/or provisional matrix proteins. For anti-neoplastic therapies, EPCs could be transfected with or coupled to anti-tumor drugs or angiogenesis inhibitors. Gene modification of EPCs has several advantages over conventional gene therapy. Ex vivo gene transfection of EPCs may avoid administration of vectors and vehicles into the recipient organism. Transcriptional or enzymatic gene modification may constitute effective means to maintain, enhance, or inhibit the capacity of EPCs to proliferate or differentiate. Preliminary findings utilizing a strategy of VEGF-gene transfer suggest that

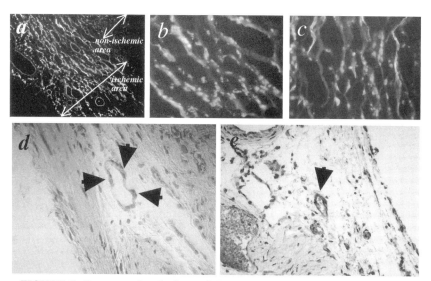

FIGURE 2. Representative findings of fluorescence microscopy 7 days after EPC transplantation (*a*: ×100; *b* and *c*: ×400) and immunohistochemistry using antibodies against human-specific ECs (*d*: ulex europaeus lectin type 1 [UEA-1] staining [×400]; *e*: human CD31 staining [×400]) in ischemic myocardium of nude rats treated with *ex vivo* expanded human EPCs. *d –e*: transplanted human EPCs differentiated to mature ECs (*arrows*) at sites of neovascularization.

gene-modified EPC therapy includes an additional advantage of reducing the numbers of EPCs required to achieve a given level of neovascularization.[13]

PHENOTYPIC MARKERS

Differential expression of phenotypic markers that permit isolation of EPCs, not only from HSCs but also from ECs, will facilitate strategies of therapeutic vasculogenesis. Antibodies to human CD34 identify a heterogeneous population of cells that includes both HSCs and EPCs. In our early experiments, putative EPCs were first permeabilized with 1% PFA and Triton X 1%, following which EPC selection was achieved using antibodies that recognized the intracellular domain of VEGFR-2 (Flk-1). More recently, we have used a monoclonal antibody directed against the extracellular domain of VEGFR-2 (Sigma, St. Louis, MO). Whereas VEGFR-2 is generally considered to distinguish EPCs from HSCs, there exists no epitope whose expression is restricted exclusively to either fully differentiated ECs or EPCs. There are at least three lines of evidence, however, which suggest that EPCs constitute the preponderance of such circulating BM-derived endothelial lineage cells. First, previous work has shown that freshly isolated CD34+ cells display a paucity of EC-specific markers, in contrast to plated cells cultured for 7 days.[6] Second, recent work from our own laboratory has shown that in contrast to EPCs, heterologously transplanted, differentiated ECs rarely incorporate into foci of neovascularization. Third,

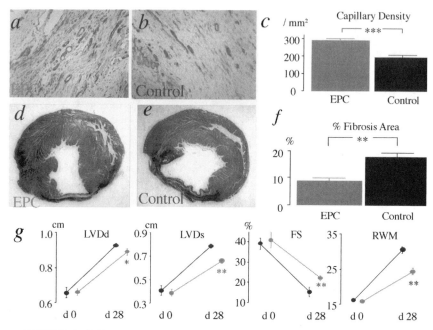

FIGURE 3. (*a,b*) Immunohistochemical findings using an antibody against isolectin B4 28 days after myocardial ischemia (×200). (*c*) capillary density in rats receiving *ex vivo* expanded EPCs versus controls 28 days after ischemia. Transplantation of *ex vivo* expanded EPCs enhanced myocardial neovascularization (***$p < 0.001$). (*d,e*) elastic tissue/ trichrome-stained tissues from rats receiving *ex vivo* expanded EPCs versus controls. (*f*) ratio of fibrosis area/ LV area in rats treated with EPCs versus controls (**$p < 0.01$). (*g*) serial changes in echocardiographic parameters from baseline (day 0) to day 28. ABBREVIATIONS: LVDd, left ventricular diastolic dimension; LVDs, left ventricular systolic dimension; FS, fractional shortening; RWM, regional wall motion score. *$p < 0.05$ vs. control; **$p < 0.01$ vs. control.

previous work suggests that the number of differentiated ECs circulating in peripheral blood identified using P1H12 antibody[14] ranges between 2 and 3 per milliliter, whereas the population of circulating EPCs in normal individuals based on work from our own laboratory is in the range of 0.5 to 1×10^3 per milliliter of blood.

IMPLICATIONS

These experimental findings call into question certain fundamental concepts regarding blood vessel growth and development in adult organisms. Postnatal neovascularization has previously been considered synonymous with proliferation and migration of preexisting, fully differentiated ECs resident within parent vessels, that is, angiogenesis.[15] The finding that circulating EPCs may home to sites of neovascularization and differentiate into ECs *in situ* is consistent with "vasculogenesis,"[16] a critical paradigm for establishment of the primordial vascular network in the embryo. Although the proportional contributions of angiogenesis and vasculogenesis to postnatal neovascularization remain to be clarified, our findings together with the recent reports from other investigators[17,18] suggest that growth and development of new blood vessels in the adult are not restricted to angiogenesis but encompass both embryonic mechanisms. As a corollary, augmented or retarded neovascularization—whether endogenous or iatrogenic—likely includes enhancement or impairment of vasculogenesis.

ACKNOWLEDGMENTS

Supported in part by National Institues of Health Grants HL57516, HL60911, and HL53354 (JMI); a Grant-in-Aid from the American Heart Association (TA); the Peter Lewis Foundation, Cleveland, OH; and a Grant-in-Aid from the Japanese Ministry of Education (AK).

REFERENCES

1. ISNER, J.M., I. BAUMGARTNER, G. RAUH, *et al.* 1998. Treatment of thromboangiitis obliterans (Buerger's disease) by intramuscular gene transfer of vascular endothelial growth factor: preliminary clinical results. J. Vasc. Surg. **28:** 964–975.
2. RIVARD, A., J-E. FABRE, M. SILVER, *et al.* 1999. Age-dependent impairment of angiogenesis. Circulation **99:** 111–120.
3. RIVARD, A., M. SILVER, D. CHEN, *et al.* 1999. Rescue of diabetes related impairment of angiogenesis by intramuscular gene therapy with adeno-VEGF. Am. J. Pathol. **154:** 355–364.
4. COUFFINHAL, T., M. SILVER, M. KEARNEY, *et al.* 1999. Impaired collateral vessel development associated with reduced expression of vascular endothelial growth factor in ApoE$^{-/-}$ mice. Circulation **99:** 3188–3198.
5. STOHLAWETZ, P., T. KOLUSSI, S. JAHANDIDEH-KAZEMPOUR, *et al.* 1996. The effect of age on the transendothelial migration of human T lymphocytes. Scand. J. Immunol. **44:** 530–534.
6. ASAHARA, T., T. MUROHARA, A. SULLIVAN, *et al.* 1997. Isolation of putative progenitor endothelial cells for angiogenesis. Science **275:** 965–967.
7. TAKAHASHI, T., C. KALKA, H. MASUDA, *et al.* 1999. Ischemia- and cytokine-induced mobilization of bone marrow–derived endothelial progenitor cells for neovascularization. Nature Med. **5:** 434–438.
8. ASAHARA, T., T. TAKAHASHI, H. MASUDA, *et al.* 1999. VEGF contributes to postnatal neovascularization by mobilizing bone marrow-derived endothelial progenitor cells. EMBO J. **18:** 3964–3972.
9. KALKA, C., H. MASUDA, T. TAKAHASHI, *et al.* 2000. Vascular endothelial growth factor-165 gene transfer augments circulating endothelial progenitor cells in human subjects. Circ. Res. **86:** 1198–1202.
10. KALKA, C., H. TEHRANI, B. LAUDENBERG, *et al.* 2000. Mobilization of endothelial progenitor cells following gene therapy with VEGF$_{165}$ in patients with inoperable coronary disease. Ann. Thorac. Surg. **70:** 829–834.
11. COUFFINHAL, T., M. SILVER, L.P. ZHENG, *et al.* 1998. A mouse model of angiogenesis. Am. J. Pathol. **152:** 1667–1679.
12. KAWAMOTO, A., H-C. GWON, H. IWAGURO, *et al.* 2000. Therapeutic potential of *ex vivo* expanded endothelial progenitor cells for myocardial ischemia. Circulation **103:** 634–637.
13. ASAHARA, T., H. IWAGURO, C. KALKA, *et al.* 1000. Gene therapy of endothelial progenitor cell for vascular development in severe ischemic disease. (Abstr.) Circulation **100:** 1–481.

14. SOLOVEY, A., Y. LIN, P. BROWN, *et al.* 1997. Circulating activated endothelial cells in sickle cell anemia. N. Engl. J. Med. **337:** 1582–1590.
15. FOLKMAN, J. 1971. Tumor angiogenesis: therapeutic implications. N. Engl. J. Med. **285:** 1182–1186.
16. RISAU, W., H. SARIOLA, H-G. ZERWES, *et al.* 1988. Vasculogenesis and angiogenesis in embryonic stem cell-derived embryoid bodies. Development **102:** 471–478.
17. SHI, Q., S. RAFII, M.H-D. WU, *et al.* 1998. Evidence for circulating bone marrow-derived endothelial cells. Blood **92:** 362–367.
18. HATZOPOULOS, A.K., J. FOLKMAN, E. VASILE, *et al.* 1998. Isolation and characterization of endothelial progenitor cells from mouse embyros. Development **125:** 1457–1468.

DRUG-RESISTANT TUBERCULOSIS
FROM MOLECULES TO MACRO-ECONOMICS

Introduction

PETER DAVIES

Consultant Respiratory Physician, Cardiothoracic Centre, Liverpool L14 3PE, U.K.

For two days in March 2001, approximately 200 people—medical doctors, scientists, legal experts, anthropologists, nurses, and others—met to discuss the problem of drug-resistant, and specifically multidrug-resistant, tuberculosis. The topics covered were exhaustive. They varied from the purely medical and scientific to the legal and economic implications of the disease.

A summary of topics is provided in the roundup article at the end of the section on multidrug-resistant tuberculosis. As ever in the rapidly changing fields of science and medicine, events have moved on, even in the few months it has taken to compile the manuscripts from the meeting. In particular the concern about costs raised by Farmer's enthusiastic support of the "DOTS-plus" strategy have been partially answered by the willingness of pharmaceutical companies to reduce the costs of second-line drugs used in the treatment of drug-resistant tuberculosis.[1]

There still remains an immense task in convincing governments and other funding organizations of the importance of developing new strategies for the prevention and control of this disease, the most important of these being the development of new vaccines and drugs. In the meantime, the practicalities of management with what we have at our disposal remain a problem. The implications for society as a potentially fatal communicable disease increases its incidence have not been fully explored. In particular the issues of human rights and detainment of patients in the face of an incurable condition need wider debate.

We hope that these papers will be of value in moving the debate forward and eventually will play a part in controlling and even eradicating this deadly problem.

REFERENCE

1. COGHLAN, ANDY. 2001. Lives before profit. Drug companies slash the cost of treating resistant TB. New Sci. **171(2298):** 6.

The Burden of Drug-Resistant Tuberculosis and Mechanisms for Its Control

MARIO C. RAVIGLIONE, RAJESH GUPTA, CHRISTOPHER M. DYE, AND MARCOS A. ESPINAL

Communicable Diseases, Stop TB, World Health Organization, Geneva 27, Switzerland

ABSTRACT: Drug resistance in tuberculosis is largely a man-made phenomenon caused by erroneous prescribing practices on the part of physicians and non-compliance on the part of patients. The global epidemiology of drug-resistant TB, the impact of standardized short-course chemotherapy (SSC), and the potential future evolution of MDR TB are discussed in this chapter.

KEYWORDS: tuberculosis; drug-resistant tuberculosis; TB control programs; standardized short-course chemotherapy; global epidemiology

INTRODUCTION

Drug-resistant tuberculosis (TB) and, particularly, multidrug-resistant (MDR) TB (defined as disease due to strains of *M. tuberculosis* resistant to at least isoniazid and rifampicin, the two most powerful anti-TB drugs) have recently received heightened attention in the media. This has not only helped foster advancement within the field of MDR TB, but it has also brought TB to the forefront of discussions in public health. Drug resistance in TB is primarily created by two man-made mechanisms. The first is erroneous prescribing practices combined with the inability to implement systems to foster patient adherence to treatment, as is often seen with private practitioners not fully aware of TB control procedures.[1] For instance, one study in India revealed 80 different treatment regimens were being recommended for difficult-to-trace patients in a single slum in Bombay.[2] The second is patient-related, whereby patients do not follow the prescribed regimen or are affected by other diseases (such as co-infection with HIV) that interfere with the mechanisms of anti-TB drugs.[3] These factors place selective pressure on the bacilli in a patient, thereby increasing the growth (in terms of rate and quantity) of resistant bacilli.[4] However, these two factors simply reflect the overriding principle that drug resistance tends to arise when national TB programs (NTPs) do not adhere to international recommendations for TB control.[5] This paper reviews three major topics that help comprise the discourse surrounding MDR TB: the global epidemiology of drug-resistant TB, the impact of standardized short-course chemotherapy (SCC) on drug-resistant TB, and the potential future evolution of MDR TB.

Address for correspondence: Mario Raviglione, World Health Organization, Communicable Diseases—StopTB, 20 Avenue Appia, CH 1211 Geneva 27, Switzerland.
raviglionem@who.int

GLOBAL EPIDEMIOLOGY OF DRUG-RESISTANT TB

Since 1994, the World Health Organization (WHO) and the International Union Against TB and Lung Disease (IUATLD) have conducted a global project on drug resistance surveillance. The project builds upon internationally recommended methods for drug resistance surveillance and drug susceptibility testing to four first-line anti-TB drugs: isoniazid, rifampicin, ethambutol, and streptomycin.[6,7] The project distinguishes between drug resistance among new cases (presence of resistant strains of *M. tuberculosis* in a newly diagnosed patient who has never received TB drugs or has received them for less than one month of treatment) and drug resistance among previously treated cases (presence of resistant strains of *M. tuberculosis* in a patient who has previously received treatment for at least one month).[8]

Data from the two surveys conducted in 1994–1997 and 1997–2000 confirm the existence of drug resistance among new cases in all countries surveyed. Data also show that MDR TB is present in 58 of 67 sites surveyed.[9,10] In the most recent survey (1997–2000), the median prevalence of drug resistance among new cases was 10.7% (range 1.7–36.9%), and the median prevalence of MDR TB among new cases was 1.0% (range 0–14.1%). The median prevalence of resistance to each drug was as follows: isoniazid, 6.2%; rifampicin, 1.2%; ethambutol, 0.6%; streptomycin, 5.2%. Surveys in countries such as Botswana, Cuba, Chile, Slovenia, Uruguay, and Venezuela showed low prevalence of drug resistance among new cases. This was expected, because these countries are also known for the high quality of their TB control programs. However, surveys in other countries (such as those having recently undergone political and economic transition or those with a previous history of poor TB control practices) demonstrated higher levels of drug resistance among new cases. These countries include those of the former Soviet Union (Russia, Estonia, and Latvia), Bolivia, Thailand, Sierra Leone, and some settings in China and India. The WHO/IUATLD Global Project has revealed the existence of several "hot spots" for MDR TB (defined conventionally as those where the prevalence of MDR TB among new cases was 3% or above) including Dominican Republic, Estonia, Iran, Ivory Coast, Latvia, Mozambique, and selected areas in China, India, and the Russian Federation (FIG. 1). Of particular note is the high prevalence of MDR TB among new cases in the two provinces of China (11% and 4.5%) not implementing DOTS, the WHO-recommended strategy for TB control, as opposed to the lower prevalence in the three provinces (1.4–2.9%) implementing DOTS.

Trends analysis from those countries that had more than one survey done over the years clearly outlines the importance of sound TB control practices in preventing the emergence of drug resistance. For instance, Cuba and Chile have successfully implemented the DOTS strategy for more than 20 years.[11] As a result, Cuba had a prevalence of MDR TB among all TB cases varying from 0 to 1% between 1995 and 1998, and Chile maintained a prevalence of MDR TB of less than 1% from 1980 to 1998. However, Ivanovo Oblast in the Russian Federation reported a prevalence of MDR TB of 6% in 1995, which reached 9% in 1998. In the case of Estonia, an even more alarming situation has been described in which MDR TB among new cases gradually increased from 10% in 1994 to 14% in 1998. These high levels require direct management of MDR TB cases within a proper DOTS setting in order to contain transmission and reduce the high burden imposed by MDR TB.

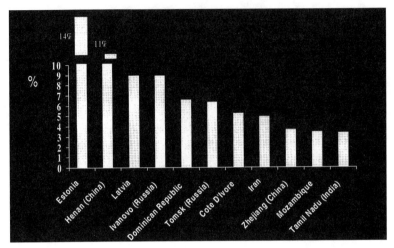

FIGURE 1. Prevalence of MDR TB among new cases in selected settings, 1994–1999.[7–10]

Given the recent trend of transnational migration and the potential spread of MDR TB across continents,[12] industrialized countries have begun to examine national policies of TB control in foreign-born populations.[13] The WHO/IUATLD project also attempted to determine whether foreign-born populations, generally immigrating from high-TB prevalence areas, have a higher or lower level of MDR TB than indigenous populations. Not surprisingly, all industrialized countries examined showed a higher prevalence of drug resistance among foreign-born new cases (FIG. 2). A similar trend was observed with MDR TB among foreign-born new cases. For example, Germany in 1998 reported 0.6% MDR TB prevalence among indigenous cases and 1.5% among foreign-born cases; Norway in 1997 reported 0 and 1.4%, respectively; and the United States in 1997 reported 1.1 and 1.9%, respectively. Finally, in Israel, a MDR TB prevalence of 2.5% among indigenous people and of 9% among recent immigrants was reported, the latter being largely due to recent waves of immigration from the former Soviet Union.[14]

Previously treated cases have a much higher likelihood of being infected with drug-resistant strains, mostly as a result of the patient's infecting strains having acquired resistance during improper treatment in the past.[15] In the most recent survey (1997–2000), the median prevalence of resistance among previously treated cases was 23.3% (range 0–93.8%), and that of MDR TB was 9.3% (range 0–48.2%).[10] Recognizing that some of these cases were infected with drug-resistant TB or MDR TB at the outset, however, the term "acquired resistance" was abandoned after the first survey and replaced with "resistance among previously treated cases." The use of "acquired resistance" should be limited to settings that possess the capability (technically and financially) to perform drug-susceptibility testing and DNA fingerprinting on all new TB cases to determine whether a resistant strain, once isolated in a case for retreatment, is the same that produced the disease in the previous episode and acquired drug resistance during treatment, or is a new strain that re-infected the patient after the first episode was diagnosed and treated.

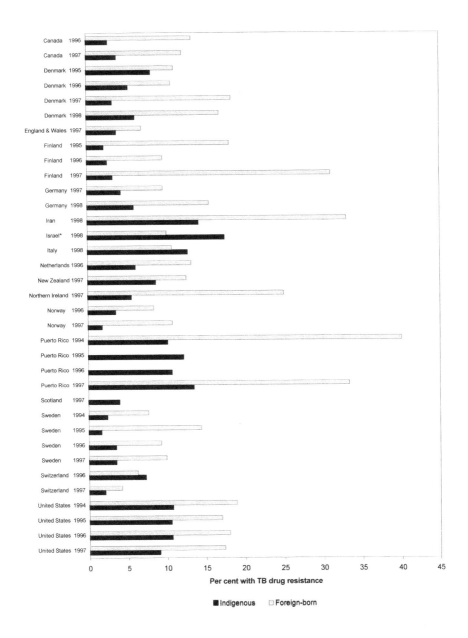

FIGURE 2. Drug resistance (inclusive of MDR TB) among indigenous (black bars) and foreign-born (gray bars) new TB patients in selected settings, 1994–1998.[8,10]

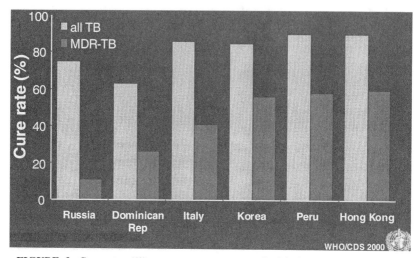

FIGURE 3. Cure rates (%) among new cases treated with short-course chemotherapy in six progammatic settings. The left columns (lighter) refer to all cases with TB except MDR TB. The columns on the right (darker) refer to MDR TB cases only. (From Espinal *et al.*[18] Used with permission.)

IMPACT OF SHORT-COURSE CHEMOTHERAPY ON THE TREATMENT OF DRUG-RESISTANT TB

Short-course chemotherapy (SCC), recommended as part of the DOTS strategy, can generate treatment success rates as high as 98% in new cases.[16] However, this high level of cure was observed in settings with minimal levels of primary drug resistance. Among cases resistant to a single drug, SCC may achieve cure rates as high as those in pan-susceptible cases. Evidence also suggests that for new cases of TB resistant to one or more anti-TB drugs, including isoniazid, ethambutol, or streptomycin, rates of failure are comparable to those of new drug-susceptible cases. However, new cases of TB resistant to rifampicin experience significantly higher failure rates than drug-susceptible cases.[17,18] For patients with MDR TB, SCC is not appropriate for treatment (FIG. 3).[18] In settings where effective DOTS is implemented (Korea, Peru, Hong Kong), the cure rate achieved with SCC is no greater than 59% in new MDR TB cases compared to 85–89% among new drug-susceptible cases and 76–87% among new isoniazid-resistant (non-MDR) cases. For regions and countries with generally poorer TB control programs (Ivanovo Oblast of the Russian Federation and the Dominican Republic), cure rates in MDR TB cases range from 10 to 20%.[18] As expected, increasing levels of resistance correlate directly with decreasing rates of treatment success.[19] For MDR TB cases, failure rates to SCC have reached up to 40% in some settings.[18] Not only do these cases continue to remain infectious, but also such cases may undergo amplification of resistance to the drugs to which they were exposed in the regimen on which they failed.[20] This "amplification" phenomenon is simply the well-described mechanism of acquired drug resistance. In conclusion, these data indicate that alternative strategies for the

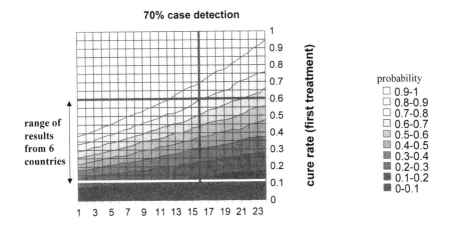

70% case detection

duration of infectiousness (months)

FIGURE 4. Model of the probability of containing MDR TB using the duration of infectiousness (*x*-axis) and the cure rate of new cases of MDR TB (*y*-axis). As a reference, a 70% case detection rate corresponds to 16 months of infectiousness (vertical, thick, black line). Cure rates for new cases of MDR TB using short-course chemotherapy (as presented in FIG. 3) ranges from 11 to 60% (horizontal, thick, black and white lines). The shaded regions correspond to varying levels of probability of containing MDR TB. To reach a high probability (denoted by white or very lightly shaded areas), high cure rates and/or short duration of infectiousness (i.e., early identification of cases or increased case detection) are required.[23]

management of MDR TB cases, including use of regimens containing second-line anti-TB drugs, should be considered in those settings where MDR TB is frequent and where there is a need to treat cases at a programmatic level.[21] WHO and its partners are currently piloting a strategy called "DOTS-Plus" that aims to develop global policy recommendations for the management of MDR TB with second-line anti-TB drugs.[22] This strategy must be based on the existence of an effective DOTS program.

POTENTIAL FUTURE EVOLUTION OF MDR TB

Critical questions for the future evolution of MDR TB include what indicators for control efforts will be needed and will levels of MDR TB rise globally or only in some settings? To address these issues, mathematical models were created based on current knowledge of the epidemiology of MDR TB.

Two important measures of the success of chemotherapy are the case detection rate (which is inversely related to the duration of infectiousness) and the proportion of cases cured at first treatment. The first model[23] quantifies the combinations of these two variables that are required, in principle, to eliminate MDR TB. FIGURE 4 shows, for example, that if only 50% of patients is cured at first treatment, these cases must be found and treated within seven months of becoming infectious to maintain a high chance of elimination, exceeding 90%. If the cure rate is 70%, then the

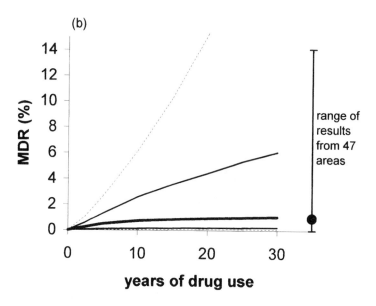

FIGURE 5. Results from a projected spread of MDR TB in relation to the spread of MDR TB calculated empirically. Prevalence of MDR TB among new cases (%) is depicted on the *y*-axis and number of years of rifampicin use is on the *x*-axis. The projected median spread of MDR TB over 30 years corresponds to the measured median range of results from the WHO/IUATLD global project (1994–1999) (large dot). The thin solid lines represent the 95% confidence intervals for the projections, while the dashed lines represent the complete range of outcomes of 10,000 Monte-Carlo simulations used to generate the projections.[25]

tolerable delay to first treatment is about 17 months, equivalent to removing 70% of TB cases from the prevalent, infectious pool each year. Less favorable combinations of case detection and cure not only lower the probability of eliminating MDR TB, but also greatly magnify the time scale for elimination. It becomes less certain that MDR TB can be contained and, even if it can, the process could take decades.

This first model was constructed under the assumption that multidrug-resistant infections are almost as transmissible as drug-susceptible infections. However, some recently published data suggest that MDR strains, in one part of Mexico at least, have markedly lower fitness than drug-susceptible strains, being found much less frequently than susceptible strains in RFLP clusters (odds ratio 0.16, 95% CI 0.04–0.6).[24] The second model[25] made use of these new data to predict the evolution of the MDR TB epidemic after 30 years of joint isoniazid and rifampicin use (FIG. 5). The best forecast is very near the median prevalence of MDR TB as measured empirically in 47 areas. Under these assumptions, MDR TB arises mainly as the by-product of poor treatment given to patients presenting with drug-susceptible disease. If the assumptions underpinning this analysis apply widely, then MDR TB is unlikely to become a significant obstacle to global TB control.

These models do not yet explain why a relatively large fraction of new cases (>10%) in some countries, notably the Baltic states and Russia, carries multidrug-resistant strains. They do, however, identify possible mechanisms. The first is that

MDR TB is mostly acquired by drug-susceptible cases as a result of persistently poor treatment. There is some transmission of MDR TB, but these drug-resistant forms cannot spread in self-sustained cycles. The second, a less likely hypothesis, is that MDR TB, once created, is highly transmissible. It could be transmissible because MDR genotypes tend to be more virulent; they generate more cavities, cause greater respiratory difficulties leading to more coughing, or produce higher bacterial loads. More likely, MDR TB cases tend to remain infectious for long periods in some settings because they are poorly managed; that is, the patients default from treatment, or inadequate regimens are prescribed. Considering this last possibility, we would expect to see rather variable results from studies of MDR TB fitness carried out in different parts of the world. These two kinds of explanation for the spread of MDR TB are not mutually exclusive; indeed, we would expect to see consistently good (or bad) practice in treatment throughout a national control program, applied to drug-susceptible and drug-resistant patients alike.

CONCLUSIONS

Drug-resistant TB and MDR TB are ubiquitous, and the prevalence is alarming in some settings, although in most countries prevalence is at a low level and does not pose a potential problem for TB control programs. In parts of eastern Europe, MDR TB has increased to a prevalence that threatens TB control as a whole. The prevalence of MDR TB appears to be correlated with the duration of implementation of effective TB control programs, and some evidence supports this notion.[9] The prevalence of drug-resistant TB in industrialized countries is generally higher among the foreign-born than the indigenous populations, reaffirming that TB control is a global issue. Second-line anti-TB drugs to manage MDR TB must be contemplated, provided proper systems exist to deliver these drugs. However, TB control programs that cannot achieve high cure rates and cannot keep patients on treatment for six months with SCC are unlikely to be able to keep patients adherent to treatment when using more toxic agents for 18–24 months. Such programs should not embark on the use of second-line drugs until they are capable of doing so. Otherwise, these settings face the additional problem of creating *M. tuberculosis* resistant to second-line anti-TB drugs. Given the uncertainties above, the critical questions for further analysis are when and how to introduce second-line anti-TB drugs? To decide when, we need to know more about MDR TB transmission under current management practices. If transmission is frequent even with the best possible use of first-line anti-TB drugs, then second-line anti-TB drugs will be needed soon. To decide how, we need to identify the efficacy of various treatment regimens using second-line anti-TB drugs against the range of resistance patterns.

Given these conditions, what should be the future course of action to address MDR TB in this new century? The first priority is to strengthen TB control programs to properly manage new, mostly drug-susceptible TB cases in order to minimize the creation of drug resistance. Second, access to second-line drugs should be increased to make them available where they are needed. The high prices of these drugs are essentially prohibitive to poor countries. The issue of cost is being addressed through a multiagency "Green Light Committee" hosted by WHO that screens proposals and provides access to concessional prices of second-line anti-TB drugs that are up to

99% lower than open market costs.[26] However, this increased access must be compounded by increased control on the use of drugs that can be achieved only through implementation of sound TB control practices, as recommended by WHO. Third, technical capacity to use these drugs under proper case management conditions needs to be developed. DOTS-Plus pilot projects are being established to foster proper management of MDR TB and to help develop sound policy on MDR TB case management in resource-limited settings. The key point is that management of drug-susceptible cases (which can take up to six months) serves as a foundation in TB control; otherwise, management of MDR TB cases via second-line anti-TB drugs (which can take up to two years) will not be successful. The issue of the "hot spots" is complicated, because these are usually settings where TB control is weak but MDR TB management should be contemplated. Such settings should be considered true public health emergencies, where the international community together with the government should act quickly and implement DOTS to be rapidly followed by DOTS-Plus. Fourth, where MDR TB cases are known or suspected to be numerous, reliable laboratories must be established to test for resistance to first-line anti-TB drugs in order to regularly monitor and assess the effectiveness of the activities undertaken to address MDR TB. Finally, continued advocacy is needed to maintain the momentum created by years of efforts to raise the TB issue in the global political agenda. MDR TB is a useful tool with which to do so, given characteristics that continue to maintain the attention of decision-makers. This tool must be properly used within the boundaries of scientific evidence, so that a balanced view of the constraints to TB control can be maintained.

ACKNOWLEDGMENT

The authors are grateful to Dr. Mohamed Aziz of WHO for providing useful comments on this manuscript.

REFERENCES

1. MAHMOUDI, A. & M.D. ISEMAN. 1993. Pitfalls in the care of patients with tuberculosis. JAMA 270: 65–68.
2. UPLEKAR, M.W. & D.S. SHEPARD. 1991. Treatment of tuberculosis by private practitioners in India. Tubercle 72: 284–290.
3. KOCHI, A., B. VARELDZIS & K. STYBLO. 1993. Multidrug-resistant tuberculosis and its control. Res. Microb. 144: 104–110.
4. PABLOS-MENDEZ, A. & K. LESSNAU. 2000. Clinical mismanagement and other factors producing antituberculosis drug resistance. In Multidrug-resistant Tuberculosis. I. Bastian & F. Portaels, Eds.: 59–76. Kluwer Academic Publishers. Dordrecht.
5. WORLD HEALTH ORGANIZATION. 1997. Treatment of Tuberculosis: Guidelines for National Programmes. WHO/TB/97.220. Geneva.
6. WORLD HEALTH ORGANIZATION, INTERNATIONAL UNION AGAINST TUBERCULOSIS AND LUNG DISEASE. 1997. Anti-tuberculosis drug resistance in the world: the WHO/IUATLD Global Project on Anti-tuberculosis Drug Resistance Surveillance. WHO/TB/97.229. Geneva.
7. WORLD HEALTH ORGANIZATION/INTERNATIONAL UNION AGAINST TUBERCULOSIS AND LUNG DISEASE. 1997. Guidelines for the Surveillance in Drug Resistant Tuberculosis. WHO/TB/96.216. Geneva.

8. WORLD HEALTH ORGANIZATION, INTERNATIONAL UNION AGAINST TUBERCULOSIS AND LUNG DISEASE. 2000. Anti-tuberculosis Drug Resistance in the World: The WHO/IUATLD Global Project on Anti-tuberculosis Drug Resistance Surveillance. Report No. 2. WHO/TB/2000.278. Geneva.

9. PABLOS-MÉNDEZ, A., M.C. RAVIGLIONE, A. LASZLO, *et al.* 1998. Global surveillance for antituberculosis drug resistance, 1994–1997. N. Engl. J. Med. **338:** 1641–1649.

10. ESPINAL, M.A., A. LASZLO, L. SIMONSEN, *et al.* 2001. Global trends in resistance to antituberculosis drugs. N. Engl. J. Med. **344:** 1294–1303.

11. WORLD HEALTH ORGANIZATION. 2001. Global Tuberculosis Control: WHO Report 2001. WHO/CDS/2001.287. Geneva.

12. BECERRA, M.C., P.E. FARMER & J.Y. KIM. 1999. The problem of drug-resistant tuberculosis. *In* The Global Impact of Drug-resistant Tuberculosis. pp. 1–38. Program in Infectious Disease and Social Change. Department of Social Medicine, Harvard Medical School. Boston.

13. TALBOT, E.A., M. MOORE, E. MCCRAY & N.J. BINKIN. 2000. Tuberculosis among foreign-born persons in the United States, 1993–1998. JAMA **284:** 2894–2900.

14. GILAD, J., A. BORER, K. RIESENBERG, *et al.* 2000. Epidemiology and ethnic distribution of multidrug-resistant tuberculosis in southern Israel, 1992–1997: the impact of immigration. Chest **117:** 738–743.

15. WORLD HEALTH ORGANIZATION. 1997. Guidelines for the Management of Drug-resistant Tuberculosis. WHO/TB/96.210 (rev.2). Geneva.

16. FOX, W. 1981. Whither short-course chemotherapy. Br. J. Dis. Chest **75:** 331–357.

17. MITCHISON, D.A. & A.J. NUNN. 1986. Influence of initial drug resistance on the response to short-course chemotherapy of pulmonary tuberculosis. Am. Rev. Resp. Dis. **133:** 423–430.

18. ESPINAL, M.A., S.J. KIM, P.G. SUAREZ, *et al.* 2000. Standard short-course chemotherapy for drug-resistant tuberculosis: treatment outcome in six countries. JAMA **283:** 2537–2545.

19. CONINX, R., C. MATHIEU, M. DEBACKER, *et al.* 1999. First-line tuberculosis therapy and drug-resistant *Mycobacterium tuberculois* in prisons. Lancet **353:** 969–973.

20. FARMER, P.E. 1999. Managerial successes, clinical failures. Int. J. Tuberc. Lung Dis. **3:** 365–367.

21. ESPINAL M.A., C. DYE, M.C. RAVIGLIONE & A. KOCHI. 1999. Rational DOTS-Plus for the control of MDR-TB. Int. J. Tuberc. Lung Dis. **3:** 561–563.

22. WORLD HEALTH ORGANIZATION. 2000. Guidelines for Establishing DOTS-Plus Pilot Projects for the Management of Multidrug-Resistant Tuberculosis (MDR-TB). R. Gupta & T. Arnadottir. WHO/CDS/TB/2000.279. Geneva.

23. DYE, C. & B.G. WILLIAMS. 2000. Criteria for the control of drug-resistant tuberculosis. Proc. Natl. Acad. Sci. USA **97:** 8180–8185.

24. GARCIA-GARCIA, M.L., A. PONCE-DELEON, M.E. JIMENEZ-CORONA, *et al.* 2000. Clinical consequences and transmissibility of drug-resistant tuberculosis in southern Mexico. Arch. Intern. Med. **160:** 630–636.

25. DYE, C. & M.A. ESPINAL. 2001. Will tuberculosis become resistant to all antibiotics? Proc. R. Soc. London B **268:** 45–52.

26. GUPTA, R., J.Y. KIM, M.A. ESPINAL, *et al.* 2001. Responding to market failures in tuberculosis control. Science **293:** 1049–1051.

India's Multidrug-Resistant Tuberculosis Crisis

ZARIR F. UDWADIA

Hinduja Hospital and Research Centre, Parsee General Hospital, Breach Candy Hospital and Research Centre, Bombay, India

ABSTRACT: India has the highest number of tuberculosis cases of any country in the world, and many of these cases are MDR TB. A combination of contributing factors has led to the current public health crisis: a failing National Tuberculosis Programme, denial and lack of compliance on the part of patients, lack of regulation of doctors in private practice, governmental policy failure and corruption, social and economic problems, and a growing HIV epidemic. This situation must be combatted on several fronts, including promoting social change; increasing government funding; seeking global aid; implementing DOTS, non-DOTS, and NGO programs; integrating TB and HIV programs; funding research; enacting regulatory legislation; and establishing continuing medical education programs among private practitioners.

KEYWORDS: epidemiology of MDR TB; HIV; DOTS; national tuberculosis program; India

INTRODUCTION

Tuberculosis is endemic in India. The facts speak for themselves: 300 million Indians are infected, 13 million with active disease, and 22% of the world's smear-positive cases reside here, making this the largest TB concentration in the world.[1] Indeed, India bears the burden of the most TB cases in the world, more than twice as many as second-ranked China (FIG. 1).

Pulmonary tuberculosis is without doubt India's biggest public health crisis; 9% of all Indian deaths are TB deaths. Overall, TB results in about 500,000 to 750,000 deaths annually, or one death per minute, a grim statistic that has remained unchanged over the last four decades. Deaths from TB far outweigh combined deaths from HIV, malaria, and all infectious diseases in India put together. At a conservative estimate, 64,000 hospital beds are used exclusively for TB patients, and the loss of economic output accruing from this single disease is a staggering $400 million per year. The focus of this article is on multidrug-resistant (MDR) TB in India, and I will attempt to raise and answer a number of questions on the extent and epidemiology of the problem, the factors that allowed MDR TB to get entrenched in India, what steps have been taken to overcome MDR TB to date, and whether these measures will work.[2]

Address for correspondence: Dr. Zarir Udwadia, Hinduja Hospital and Research Centre, Veer Savarkar Marg, Mahim, Mumbai 400 016, India.
zfu@vsnl.com or zfu@vsnl.net.in

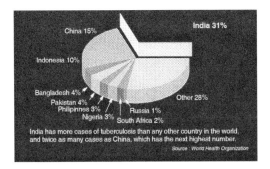

FIGURE 1. India has the most TB cases in the world.

EPIDEMIOLOGY OF MDR TB IN INDIA

The epidemiology of tuberculosis in India is bedeviled by a number of confounding factors. Notification is seldom if ever performed, few laboratories in the country reliably perform sensitivity testing, lab techniques are not standardized, and most existing Indian studies fail to reliably distinguish primary from secondary drug resistance. Indeed, India's TB data recording is woefully bad. In a study by Mario Raviglione, India was the only one of eight world regions with less than 2% of its population covered (in 1997) by the WHO control strategy.[3] It was also the region with the worst kept data on case holding, cure, and outcome rates. These circumstances must be kept in mind whenever the epidemiology of MDR TB is discussed.

India fared poorly in the two global studies on MDR TB conducted by the WHO/IUATLD Global Surveillance Project. In the first, conducted by Cohn *et al.*, Indian MDR TB rates in the four Indian studies included in this Medline search varied from 0.9% in Jaipur to 33.8% in Gujarat.[4] These rates were the second highest worldwide after Nepal. This study can be criticized, however, for including only 7939 isolates from four laboratories of widely varying standards. Besides, primary resistance was not reliably distinguished from secondary resistance in any of these samples. The second study, conducted by A. Pablos-Mendez, was a major global coordinated effort including data from 35 countries between 1994 and 1997. Here too, India emerged with the second highest MDR rates globally after Latvia.[5] The combined MDR TB rate from India was 13.3%. This study too can be criticized for including small numbers of isolates (2240) from only one region in the country (New Delhi). Again, as in Cohn's study, primary resistance could not be reliably distinguished from acquired resistance.

It is my opinion that both these global studies underestimate the extent of the MDR TB problem in India. A closer search reveals several other Indian MDR prevalence studies, with primary prevalence rates varying from 0.9% to 36.6% and acquired resistance rates varying from 6.3 to 56.6%.[6] The highest prevalence rates ever reported have been from our center at the Hinduja Hospital in Bombay.[7] Here, our Level 2 mycobacterial laboratory, which serves as a reference lab for the teeming metropolis of Bombay, currently reports around 60% of all isolates it receives as MDR.

MDR-TB IN INDIA: THE CO-CONSPIRATORS

MDR-TB took root in India as the result of a combination of the following factors: (1) a failing National Tuberculosis Programme (NTP), (2) patient-related factors, (3) doctor-related factors, (4) government apathy, (5) social factors, and (6) the spread of the HIV virus. These will be discussed in greater detail in the following sections.

A Failing National Tuberculosis Program

India's NTP, which originated in 1962, was conceived on sound scientific and social grounds. It was poorly implemented, however, and made no epidemiological impact over three decades. Indeed, it begat and bred multidrug resistance. Alarm bells were slow to ring, and it was only in 1992 that the Indian government finally conceded the NTP had failed. A joint panel of experts from WHO, SIDA, and the Indian government concluded it be abandoned in favor of the Revised National Tuberculosis Control Programme (RNTCP).[8] This was funded by a soft loan of $142 million and based on the five DOTS (directly observed treatment, short course) principles.[9]

Patient-Related Factors

TB is not an easy topic for an Indian patient to discuss. There is a large amount of secrecy, denial, and unfortunately even ostracism of Indian patients with tuberculosis. These attitudes are borne out of ignorance. Compliance remains poor, with no more than 30% of patients completing their treatments. "Doctor shopping" is a peculiar Indian trait with work by Uplekar showing that the average urban patient with tuberculosis visits 2.5 doctors and the average urban patient visits 4 before even starting treatment.[10] Indian patients switch doctors and systems of medicine with impunity, so there is little continuity of care.

Doctor-Related Factors

India has a huge and often unregulated private health sector including 1.25 million doctors. Seventy percent of hospitals are privately run, and 76% of doctors engage in private practice. In addition, Indian doctors are a heterogeneous mix with a good 50% being nonallopaths who practice a number of alternative forms of medicine, including homeopathic, ayurvedic, and unani systems. Besides these an unknown number of "doctors" practice without any qualifications at all (hakims, tantriks, vaids). Uplekar has commented on the poor prescribing practice of Indian doctors.[11] He asked 143 doctors practicing in the Dharavi slum area of Bombay what prescription they would give a sputum-positive patient weighing 50 kgs with no prior history of treatment. Of the 102 respondents, 80 different regimes were conjured up, the majority being inappropriate and expensive. Interestingly, the prescribing habits of allopaths were no better than those of nonallopaths. Unfortunately, doctors in India are of greatly varying standards. They perform unnecessary tests, have little formal training in community health, do not keep adequate records, do not notify public health authorities about cases of TB, and do not feel it is their duty to bother with contact tracing.

Government Factors

Many of India's health problems have arisen from policy failure and government callousness, corruption, and bureaucratic shortsightedness. TB is no exception. Lack of funding and failure to grasp the scale and severity of India's TB crisis are other ways in which the country has been let down by successive governments that have passively allowed the TB situation to escalate to its current epidemic proportions.

Social Factors

The harsh fact that tuberculosis is a social disease is brought into sharp focus in a country like India, which is plagued with seemingly insurmountable social and economic problems. The facts speak for themselves: a population in excess of 1 billion, with 46% below the poverty line. Adult literacy rates presently run at 51%, childhood malnutrition at 47%, and the infant mortality rates are among the highest in the world at 47%. While the RNTCP waxes eloquent about providing free short-course chemotherapy (SCC) to the entire country, one should not loose sight of the fact that 25% of the population do not even have access to safe drinking water.

The HIV Epidemic

India now has the highest absolute numbers of HIV cases of any country in the world (around 5 million). The HIV epidemic in this country is now established and mature: all ages, both sexes, and all social strata are affected. There has been a frightening speed of escalation, with HIV rates increasing from 1% to 51% among prostitutes in Bombay and from 8% to 36% among STD clinic patients in a period of 5 years. Ignorance about AIDS remains profound, with several polls showing only a minority of Indian women of reproductive age had even heard about AIDS. AIDS will cost India an estimated $11 billion by the end of 2001, impoverishing this country even more deeply. It will prove an extraordinary threat to development. A huge, dually infected population is emerging, some of them with MDR strains. This will pose an enormous additional strain on the overstretched national TB program in India.

DOTS AND ITS IMPACT IN INDIA

Most DOTS principles originated in Indian studies that emerged from research arising from the Tuberculosis Research Centre in Madras and the National Tuberculosis Institute in Bangalore.[12] These two centers contributed truly pioneering research in the 1950s and 60s that helped shape not only India's TB control programs but also those of many developed nations. It was in 1993 that DOTS began in India, starting with pilot studies covering 2.35 million people in five states. The numbers covered have steadily increased so that 250 million were covered by the end of 2000, and further coverage of 100 million people each year is planned until the entire population is eventually covered. This makes the Indian DOTS program the second largest in the world after China. Case detection rates are higher than those reported from China and Bangladesh, and success rates are comparable to those from Southeast Asia and Africa. Where DOTS is used in India, TB patients are twice as likely to be cured. Where DOTS is not used, patients are seven times more likely to die of TB.

A recent report by Khatri and Frieden reveals that detection rates in all Indian states have steadily increased over time with treatment outcomes also steadily improving from 72% in 1993 to 90% in 2000. Overall failure rates run at an impressive 3.5%, default rates at 9%, and death rates at 4%.[13]

Thus, the initial gains made by DOTS in India have undoubtedly been impressive, but I doubt whether DOTS success can be sustained to cover the entire country. In the words of Mukund Uplekar, a noted TB health researcher; "DOTS will be as good and as effective as the general health services in the country." Thomas Frieden, currently WHO director for S.E. Asia, is cautiously optimistic about DOTS but admits that "The key challenge is to balance the urgent need for rapid expansion with the paramount importance of ensuring quality of implementation." I remain unconvinced DOTS can ever eradicate TB in India and would like to point out the many practical stumbling blocks DOTS faces in this country.

Practical Problems DOTS Faces in India

A verifiable address is mandatory before an Indian patient can be registered at an Indian DOTS center. Where does this policy leave the homeless, the slum dweller, the pavement dwellers, and the migrants that form up to 50% of the population of big Indian cities like Bombay?

Women are more hesitant to attend DOTS centers in India, finding them too intrusive. Indeed, tuberculosis in India robs Indian women of the little respect and standing they have in society. Visiting a DOTS clinic is something Indian women are reluctant to do for fear of being stigmatized further. It is less conspicuous for them to visit a private doctor, and as a consequence many Indian DOTS clinics have a skewed male-to-female ratios of 3:1.

"Difficult" patients seem to be deliberately weeded out in an attempt to make results appear more impressive. Thus, the alcoholics, the drug addicts, and the marginalized, all of whom DOTS centers should be striving to incorporate, find themselves being excluded.

Patients complain that DOTS clinic hours are too rigid and inflexible. A daily-wage laborer often ends up going without pay, and his family therefore without food on the days he visits a DOTS clinic. Travelling large distances across harsh terrain in a country as vast as India is a real problem for DOTS clinics located in more remote parts of the country. This becomes particularly difficult for the old, the sick, the invalid, and the poor. The incentives, which are an important component of DOTS programs in the developed world, are an unaffordable luxury in India.

Private patients are outside the purview of DOTS. Private practitioners rarely refer their patients to DOTS centers, because this would mean loss of control. Because at least 50% of TB patients would choose first to visit a private practitioner over attending a government clinic, a large segment of the population is excluded.

The extra workload imposed by DOTS may overwhelm the system. The pre-DOTS system struggled to cope with the large numbers of patients it faced. Each patient registered at a DOTS clinic needs 40 episodes of supervision over the course of his or her 6-month SCC. This may prove an unmanageable additional load that understaffed and underfunded DOTS centers may eventually buckle under. Successful implementation of DOTS would need much more in terms of staff, infrastructure,

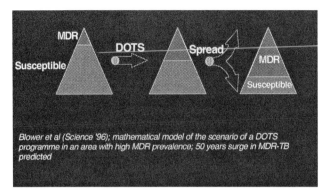

Blower et al (Science '96); mathematical model of the scenario of a DOTS programme in an area with high MDR prevalence; 50 years surge in MDR-TB predicted

FIGURE 2. MDR-TB may alter the pyramid in India.

and funds than can be presently afforded. This is currently estimated to run into an incremental recurrent cost of $100 million a year.

Finally, special mention must be made of the impact MDR-TB will have on DOTS and vice versa.

Effect of SCC/DOTS in India with Its High Existing MDR-TB Burden

- *Unacceptable failure rates.* Even the most carefully supervised DOTS and SCC program following WHO category 1 or category 2 guidelines will not be successful in patients who have MDR-TB. Several studies from Russian jails in Baku and Kemerovo have confirmed this, and Espinal's recent study in JAMA also demonstrated that SCC was unsuccessful in curing MDR-TB in six countries that had high pre-existing MDR rates.[14] India has higher MDR rates than any of the six countries in this study, and almost certainly SCC would result in an even more dismal outcome. As Horsburgh says in an accompanying editorial; "Achieving control of MDR-TB through establishment of DOTS alone in such countries was a false hope."[15]

- MDR cases would indeed persist, increase, and eventually represent a larger proportion of cases (FIG 2).

- By means of the amplifier effect, resistance would develop to additional drugs.[16]

- Nosocomial spread of MDR-TB could occur when MDR patients are confined in close proximity with other patients, family members, and medical personnel in crowded DOTS clinics.

Thus to conclude, the dilemma of MDR-TB in India is that a large and ever-expanding MDR-TB population exists that currently is accorded the status of untreatable, undesirable, and untouchable. The RNTCP has turned a blind eye to these patients while the WHO strategy, focusing on DOTS to the exclusion of all else, also ignores this large and hopeless group of patients. Individual treatment is extremely expensive and not considered cost-effective in a poor country. As a national strategy, this is shrugged off as acceptable public health realpolitic. This is a myopic approach, however, because there will be an even greater price to pay if procrastination continues and this pool of patients swells. It is also ultimately morally reprehensible, for as Paul Farmer points out, "our mission must be to treat the sick, not just the sick who can pay. Our mission must be to treat TB regardless of resistance patterns."[17]

SUGGESTIONS FOR THE FUTURE

"There is no point having sharp images when you have fuzzy ideas" said Jean Luc Goddard. The following are my suggestions for the future:

(1) *Social change.* It is stating the obvious, but the TB situation in India will never improve until the grinding poverty, the desperate overcrowding, and unhygienic sanitation improve. Malnutrition must be overcome, and demographic control over India's escalating population must be quickly achieved. Living standards must be raised, the people educated about tuberculosis, and the disease destigmatized. The per-capita Indian income (Rs. 11,000) falls 50 times short of the amount needed to successfully cure a patient with MDR disease (Rs. 450,000).

(2) *Government funding.* The 2001 Indian budget announced at the beginning of this year allotted 17% of total expenditure on defense, whereas only 0.67% was allocated for health. That India spends only 0.10% of its GDP on health is scandalous.

(3) *Global aid.* The containment of tuberculosis is impeded by a global attitude of silent fatalism. The gross inequities of wealth and health care must be addressed. Direct aid and debt relief are both needed from the developed world. Indeed, at present just 0.1% of all external aid to developing countries is devoted to TB control. If even 5% of the domestic TB budget of the world's richer countries were diverted to Asia and Africa, the epidemic could be reversed.

(4) *DOTS, non-DOTS, NGOs.* We need to build on the impressive initial gains of DOTS, but try to make DOTS more adaptive and user-friendly and less disruptive. DOTS should be integrated with the general health services of the country. In the quest to expand DOTS, we should not forget the paramount importance of ensuring quality of implementation. Instead of letting DOTS become a hollow dogma, it would be worthwhile considering non-DOTS options and comparing them in formal trials with DOTS to ascertain whether DOTS is really worth the extra costs, effort, and labor. The Bangladesh BRAC model is an inspiring idea that could easily be applied to India with the help of committed NGOs.[18]

(5) *Integrate TB and HIV programs.* Ultimately, it is what happens concerning TB in the HIV-positive group that will have the greatest impact on the future epidemiology of TB in India. We need to accept that current approaches to TB control are inadequate in the HIV era. Instead of pretending these two epidemics exist in isolation, we need to integrate their control programs. This includes more resources, enhanced surveillance, and a minimal package of care for HIV-positive patients (e.g., isoniazid and septran prophylaxis at the least).

(6) *Research.* We need to marry the molecular wizardry of the West with the huge patient load and unquenchable thirst for knowledge of the developing world. Research collaborations such as our recent Hinduja Hospital–Oxford University collaboration benefit both sides.[19]

(7) *Legislation.* Strict legislation should be enforced to ensure prescriptions are standardized according to guidelines, and only allopathic doctors prescribe TB

drugs. Second-line drugs should only be available on the prescription of a specialist. Only a few drugs and fixed drug combinations of proven quality and bioavailability should be allowed in the market.

(8) *Private medical practitioners.* There remains the vexing issue of private medical practitioners. These cannot be wished away. Instead, every effort should be made to educate and inform them and involve them in government-run TB programs.[19] In a democracy like India, there will always be patients who choose to go private and those who decide to go public. These two divergent streams of patients should be integrated inasmuch as possible.

REFERENCES

1. WORLD HEALTH ORGANIZATION. 1998. Report on the tuberculosis epidemic, 1998. WHO/TB/98. 237. WHO. Geneva.
2. UDWADIA, Z.F. 1998. India. *In* Clinical Tuberculosis, 2nd ed. P.D.O. Davies, Ed.: 591–605. Chapman and Hill. London.
3. RAVIGLIONE, M.C., C.M. DYE, S. SCHMIDT & A. KOCHI. 1997. An assessment of worldwide tuberculosis control. Lancet **350:** 624–628.
4. COHN, D., F. BUSTREO & M.C. RAVIGLIONE. 1997. Drug-resistant tuberculosis: review of the worldwide situation. Clin. Infect. Dis. **24:** s121–s130.
5. PABLOS MENDEZ, A., M.C. RAVIGLIONE, A. LASZLO, *et al.* 1998. Global surveillance for anti tubercuosis drug resistance 1994–1997. N. Engl. J. Med. **338:** 1641–1648.
6. GOTHI, G.D. 1996. Tuberculosis: an overview. P.K. Sen Tuberculosis Association of India oration, Bangalore.
7. UDWADIA, Z.F., A. HAKINIYAN, C. RODRIGUEZ, *et al.* 1996. A profile of drug-resistant tuberculosis in Bombay. Chest **110:** 228s.
8. GOVERNMENT OF INDIA, SIDA & WORLD HEALTH ORGANISATION. 1992. Review committee report. WHO. Geneva.
9. SARIN, R. & L.B.S. DEY. 1995. Indian National Tuberculosis Programme, revised strategy. Ind. J. Tuberc. **42:** 95–99.
10. UPLEKAR, M.W., S. RANGAN & T.B. TACKLING. 1996. The Search for Solutions. The Foundation for Research in Community Health. Bombay.
11. UPLEKAR, M.W. & D.S. SHEPARD. 1991. Treatment of tuberculosis by private general practitioners in India. Tubercle **72:** 284–290.
12. BAYER, R. & D. WILKINSON. 1995. Directly observed therapy for tuberculosis: history of an idea. Lancet **345:** 1545–1548.
13. KHATRI, G.R. & T.R. FRIEDEN. 2000. The status and prospects of tuberculosis control in India. Int. J. Tuberc. Lung Dis. **4(3):** 193–200.
14. ESPINAL, M.A., S.J. KIM, P.G. SUAREZ, *et al.* 2000. Standardised short course chemotherapy for drug resistant tuberculosis: treatment outcomes in 6 countries. JAMA **283(19):** 2537–2545.
15. HORSBURGH, C.R. 2000. The global problem of MDRTB: the genie is out of the bottle. JAMA **283(19):** 2575–2576.
16. BASTIAN, J., N. RIGONITI, A. VAN DEUN & F. PORTAELS. 2000. Directly observed treatment, short course strategy and multidrug resistant tuberculosis: are any modifications required? Bull. WHO **78:** 238–248.
17. FARMER, P. 1998. The dilemma of MDRTB in the global era. Int. J. Tuberc. Lung Dis. **2:** 869–876.
18. CHOUDHARY, A.M.R., S. CHOUDHARY, M.D. ISLAM, *et al.* 1997. Control of tuberculosis by community health workers in Bangladesh. Lancet **350:** 169–172.
19. LALVANI, A., P. NAGVENKAR, Z.F. UDWADIA, *et al.* 2001. Enumeration of T cells specific for RD1-encoded antigens: a novel approach to estimating the prevalence of latent *M. tuberculosis* infection. J. Infect. Dis. **183:** 469–477.
20. UPLEKAR, M. 1999. Involving the private medical sector in tuberculosis control: practical aspects. *In* Tuberculosis. An Interdisciplinary Perspective. J.D.P. Porter & J.M. Grange, Eds. Imperial College Press. London.

Drug-Resistant Tuberculosis in Africa

A. MWINGA

Department of Medicine, University of Zambia, Lusaka, Zambia

ABSTRACT: Africa has the highest incidence rate per capita of tuberculosis, although the rate varies among the African countries from 17.8% in Cameroon to 70% in Botswana, Zambia, and Zimbabwe. Nevertheless, the levels of drug resistance are relatively low, compared to countries like Russia and Estonia. Because treatment of MDR TB is beyond the reach of most African countries, prevention of the development of resistance should be a major priority. Establishment of programs to ensure prompt diagnosis of TB and adequate treatment with supervision should be undertaken by national governments with cooperating partners.

KEYWORDS: initial drug resistance; acquired drug resistance; Africa

Tuberculosis was declared a global emergency by the World Health Organization (WHO) in 1993, in recognition of the large increase in the number of notified cases worldwide. Though this increase was noted in many areas of the world, by far the largest increase occurred in the developing countries of Southeast Asia and sub-Saharan Africa, where 95% of the cases occurred. It has been estimated that in 1997 about 1.86 million people, or 32% of the world's population, were infected with *Mycobacterium tuberculosis*, whereas the number of new cases totaled 7.96 million, with 1.87 million reported deaths. Eighty percent of all the reported incident cases were said to have occurred in 22 countries, and eight of the ten countries with the highest incidence were found in Africa. This increased burden of disease from tuberculosis globally, in an era when effective drug treatment exists, has been ascribed to factors like poor control in areas such as Southeast Asia, eastern Europe and sub-Saharan Africa and co-infection with HIV in some African countries.[1]

Though Southeast Asia and the Western Pacific regions had the highest number of reported cases of TB, Africa had the highest incidence rate per capita with an average of 259/100,000. This region also has the highest rate of HIV infection in TB patients, with an average of 32%,[1] though this figure varies from 17.8% in Cameroon[2] to as high as 70% in Botswana, Zambia,[3] and Zimbabwe. The case fatality rate for tuberculosis in Africa is high, exceeding 50% in some African countries, compared to a global figure of 23%.[4] The high rate of HIV co-infection has contributed to this high case fatality rate.

In order to ensure that TB is brought under control, the WHO has recommended that a target be set of detection of 70% of infectious cases and a treatment success

Address for correspondence: Dr. Alwyn Mwinga, Department of Medicine, University of Zambia, P.O. Box 50110, Lusaka, Zambia.
amwinga@zamnet.zm

TABLE 1. Drug resistance in patients with no history of prior treatment expressed as a percentage of case

Country	Year	Sample	Overall	Resistance to 1 drug	2 drugs	3 drugs	4 drugs	Polyresistance/ Any	MDR
Benin	1994–97	333	8.4	6.0	2.1	0.3	0.0	2.4	0.3
Botswana	1994–97	407	3.7	3.4	0.2	0.0	0.0	0.2	0.2
Botswana	1998	638	6.3	5.3	0.8	0.2	0.0 0	0.9	0.5
Cameroon	1995		31.8						
Central African Republic	1999	464	16.4	10.8	3.7	1.7	0.2	5.6	1.1
Ethiopia	1995	167	15.6						
Ghana			54.5						
Guinea	1998	539	14.7	9.8	4.3	0.6	0.0	4.8	0.6
Ivory Coast	1994–97	320	13.4	5.3	6.3	1.6	0.3	8.1	5.3
Kenya	1994–99	445	6.3	5.4	0.9	0.0	0.0	0.9	0.0
Lesotho	1994–97	330	8.8	6.1	2.4	0.3	0.0	2.7	0.9
Mozambique	1999	1028	20.8	12.2	5.8	2.3	0.5	8.7	3.5
Sierra Leone	1994–97	463	28.1	16.6	1.1	1.1	0.2	11.4	1.1
Sierra Leone	1997	117	24.8	17.9	6.0	0.9	0.0	6.8	0.9
South Africa (Hlabisa)	1996		8.9						
South Africa (Mpumalanga)	1997	661	8.0	5.9	1.2	0.5	0.5	2.1	1.5
Swaziland	1994–97	224	11.7						
Uganda	1997	374	19.8	12.8	6.7	0.3	0.0	7.0	0.5
Zimbabwe	1994–96	676	3.3	1.3	1.2	0.1	0.6	1.9	1.9

NOTE: Adapted from the WHO/IUATLD Global Project on Anti-Tuberculosis Drug Resistance Surveillance and other available data.

rate of 85% and that this should be achieved by 2005.[5] One of the biggest barriers for the successful treatment of TB is poor adherence on the part of the patient. Therefore, in 1995 WHO urged the use of DOTS (directly observed treatment, short course) as a priority for effective TB control and as a means of reducing the development of drug resistance. The ability of the DOTS strategy to improve the treatment outcome was demonstrated in a survey conducted by WHO between 1994 and 1998, in which 85% of patients evaluated under DOTS successfully completed treatment compared to a treatment success of 37% in non-DOTS areas.[3] Drug resistance is, however, a threat to the potential success of TB control efforts.

The development of drug resistance has always been a concern with the use of chemotherapy, and in the case of tuberculosis this became evident soon after the introduction of streptomycin. The use of multidrug therapy as a means of preventing the emergence of drug resistance therefore became standard practice in the treatment of tuberculosis. An increase in the number of drug-resistant isolates was noted in New York City in 1991, primarily due to inadequate treatment. Within a couple of years, however, the number of drug-resistant cases had decreased by 21%, mainly due to improved case management with the use of directly observed treatment.[5]

The levels of drug resistance in a country are generally indicative of the quality of TB control and the use of short-course chemotherapy. Drug resistance may arise as a result of a lack of standardized treatment regimens, poor implementation of the regimens, shortages of drugs, and use of drugs of questionable quality. Other factors include failure to monitor the patients' treatment and nonadherence on the part of the patients. In particular, the level of multidrug resistance provides an indicator of the performance of the national TB program in the country.

The available data on the rates of drug resistance in Africa are not extensive, as many countries have not conducted nationwide surveillance of the level of drug resistance. The available reports generally cover a small area of the country, or the sample size is small and hence can not be considered to be representative of the country as a whole. In collaboration with the International Union Against Tuberculosis and Lung Disease (IUATLD), WHO has conducted a major surveillance of the global rates of drug resistance between 1994 and 1996,[6] and this exercise was repeated between 1997 and 1999.[7] During the surveillance, 16% of the countries were sampled. In the first round 8 countries from the AFRO region (sub-Saharan Africa) were included: these were Benin, Botswana, Ivory Coast, Kenya, Lesotho, Sierra Leone, Swaziland, and Zimbabwe. In the second surveillance, seven African countries were included (Botswana, Central African Republic, Guinea, Mozambique, Sierra Leone, South Africa, and Uganda). Thus, only Botswana and Sierra Leone were assessed in both surveys.

The recommended definition of drug resistance by WHO now applies either to drug resistance among new cases or to drug resistance among previously treated cases.[7] However, because a history of prior treatment for tuberculosis may be difficult to exclude completely, it is more appropriate to classify the resistance as either initial or acquired. The levels of primary drug resistance in Africa vary according to the country assessed. The presence of drug resistance is an indicator of the quality of the treatment delivery process, and resistance occurring in patients with no prior history of treatment reflects poor treatment in the past. The rate of drug resistance in patients with a previous history of treatment for tuberculosis is always much higher than in patients with no history of previous treatment for tuberculosis.

In general, the levels of drug resistance in Africa are low when compared to other parts of the world. This is despite the HIV-associated increase in TB cases and political strife and wars. This is probably a reflection of the presence of relatively well-functioning control programs; 61% of the countries in the WHO's African Region were covered by the DOTS strategy compared to the global average of 42.6%. The more recent introduction of rifampicin may also contribute to this lower incidence of drug resistance.

TABLE 2. Levels of drug resistance to each drug in selected African countries

| Country | Sample | Overall | Resistance | | | | Polyresistance/ | |
			1 drug	2 drugs	3 drugs	4 drugs	Any	MDR
Benin								
Botswana	114	14.91	7.0	2.6	0.9	4.4	7.9	6.1
Botswana	145	22.8	12.4	6.2	4.1	0.0	10.3	9.0
Cameroon								
CAR	33	36.4	12.1	6.1	5.2	3.0	24.2	18.2
Ethiopia								
Ghana								
Guinea	32	50.0	9.4	12.5	15.6	12.5	40.6	28.1
Ivory Coast								
Kenya	46	37.0	30.4	6.5	0.0	0.0	6.5	0.0
Lesotho	53	34.0	20.8	5.7	5.7	1.9	13.2	5.7
Mozambique	122	45.1	22.1	21.3	0.8	0.8	23.0	3.3
Sierra Leone	172	52.9	16.3	24.4	5.2	7.0	36.6	12.8
Sierra Leone	13	61.5	30.8	7.7	23.1	0.0	30.8	23.1
South Africa (Hlabisa)								
South Africa (Mpumalanga)	100	22.0	11.0	11.0	0.0	0.0	11.0	8.0
Swaziland	44	20.5	9.1	4.5	2.3	4.5	11.4	9.1
Uganda	45	51.1	28.9	20.0	2.2	0.0	22.2	4.4
Zimbabwe	36	13.9	5.6	5.6	2.8	0.0	8.3	8.3

NOTE: Adapted from the WHO/IUATLD Global Project on Anti-Tuberculosis Drug Resistance Surveillance and other available data.

In the first survey conducted by WHO and IUATLD, the overall level of resistance among new cases for the African countries was as follows: Zimbabwe, 3.3%; Botswana, 3.7%; Kenya, 6.3%; Benin, 8.4%; Lesotho, 8.8%; Swaziland, 11.7%; Ivory Coast, 13.4%; and Sierra Leone, 28.1%.[7] In this survey, the Dominican Republic had the highest level of resistance to any drug, with a rate of 40.6%. Overall drug resistance to any drug in the second survey, conducted between 1996 and 1999,[7] in the African countries was as follows: Botswana, 6.3%; South Africa's Mpumalanga Province, 8.0%; Guinea, 14.7%; Central African Republic, 16.4%; Uganda, 19.8%; Mozambique, 20.8%; and Sierra Leone, 24.8%. Between the two surveys, the level of resistance in Botswana increased from 3.7% to 6.3%, while for Sierra Leone the rate reduced from 28.1% to 24.8%. The rate of resistance in other countries not included in the WHO survey varies widely from country to country. The available figures are as follows: Malawi, 11.8%; Cameroon, 31.8%[2]; Ghana, 54.5%; Ethiopia, 15.6%[8]; Tanzania, 2.8%[9]; and Senegal, 37%.

TABLE 3. Levels of drug resistance among patients with a history of prior treatment

Country	Year	Sample size	INH		RMP		EMB		SM	
			mono	any	mono	any	mono	any	mono	any
Benin		333	3.3	5.4	0.0	0.3	0.0	0.6	2.7	4.8
Botswana		407	1.2	1.5	0.7	1.0	0.0	0.0	1.5	4.5
Botswana	1999	638	3.6	4.4	0.2	0.6	0.0	0.2	1.6	2.2
Cameroon										
CAR	1998	464	4.1	9.5	0.2	1.3	0.0	2.4	6.5	11.0
Ethiopia										
Ghana										
Guinea	1998	539	4.5	9.3	0.2	0.7	0.0	0.6	5.2	9.5
Ivory Coast		320	3.1	11.3	0.0	5.3	0.0	0.3	2.2	6.9
Kenya		445	5.4	6.3	0.0	0.0	0.0	0.0	0.0	0.9
Lesotho		330	5.2	7.9	0.0	0.9	0.0	0.0	0.9	0.3
Mozambique	1999	1028	7.9	16.5	1.8	5.3	0.0	0.5	2.5	10.5
Sierra Leone		463	2.6	13.0	0.2	1.3	0.6	2.4	13.0	24.0
Sierra Leone	1997	117	3.4	10.3	0.0	0.9	0.0	0.0	14.5	21.4
South Africa (Hlabisa)										
South Africa (Mpumalanga)	1997	661	3.5	5.6	0.2	1.7	0.0	0.5	2.3	3.8
Swaziland		334	3.9	9.0	0.0	0.9	0.3	0.9	2.4	7.2
Uganda	1997	374	6.2	12.5	2.0	5.8	3.0	8.0	5.6	11.2
Zimbabwe		676	6.7	20.0	1.1	3.6	0.2	1.1	11.1	24.1

The levels of resistance to isoniazid in new patients, or primary resistance, varied from 1.2% in Ivory Coast to 12.4% in Cameroon. Resistance to streptomycin ranges from 0% in Kenya to 20.5% in Cameroon. Levels of mono-resistance to rifampicin are low, being less than 1% in most countries where it has been reported (Botswana, Benin, Sierra Leone, Central African Republic, Guinea, and Cameroon) and only Mozambique (1.8%) and Ethiopia (1.8%) had higher rates. Only Sierra Leone (0.6%), Swaziland (0.3%), Cameroon (0.4%), and Uganda (2.4%) have reported any mono-resistance to Ethambutol. The low levels of mono-resistance to rifampicin reflect the recent introduction of rifampicin-containing regimens as well as the tendency to use rifampicin as a combined tablet with isoniazid.

Available data on drug resistance indicates that the rates of resistance are higher to one drug than to two or more drugs. The level of multidrug resistance (MDR) in Africa is relatively low compared to the highest level reported for Ivory Coast (5.3%),[10] Mozambique (3.5%), Zimbabwe (1.9%), South Africa's Mpumalanga Province (1.5%), Sierra Leone (1.1%),[7] and other countries reporting less than 1% of

MDR TB (Botswana, Benin, Lesotho, Swaziland, Guinea, Uganda, and Tanzania). In Kenya no multidrug resistance was reported in the WHO survey conducted between 1994 and 1997, though in the refugee population the level of MDR was 2.9%.[11] It should be noted, however, that the countries included in the WHO surveys are countries that have reasonably well-functioning programs. In countries lacking a well-functioning program, the levels of MDR TB may be much higher. In a survey conducted in Cameroon, where there is no functioning control program, multi-drug resistance was observed in 27.6% of the patients with a previous history of treatment.[12]

The level of drug resistance is substantially higher among patients with a history of prior treatment with antituberculosis drugs than in patients with no previous treatment for tuberculosis. This fact supports the impression that the development of drug resistance is primarily associated with irregular medication and poor control of tuberculosis. In Durban, South Africa, the strongest predictor of drug resistance was a history of prior treatment with antituberculosis therapy (ATT).[13] In Hlabisa, Kwa Zulu-Natal, South Africa, resistance to isoniazid was 6.4% in cases with no prior history of treatment compared to 13.6% in cases with a history of prior treatment.[14] In Uganda, resistance to isoniazid in cases with no history of prior treatment was 6.7% compared to 37.8% in those cases with prior treatment. Rates of MDR TB are similarly higher in cases with prior treatment (4.4%) compared to those with no prior treatment (0.5%).[15]

No significant association has been observed between the level of resistance to TB drugs and HIV serostatus in several studies[2,13,16,17] However, the presence of the increased rates of infection due to co-infection with HIV has placed a strain on the existing control measures for tuberculosis and the ensuing decrease in quality of control can lead to an increase in the overall levels of drug resistance and of MDR TB in particular. The health system has been overburdened by the high levels of HIV infection. In some countries up to 75% of the hospital admissions are due to HIV-related infections: Hospitals are overcrowded, bed-occupancy rates are very high, and isolation of infectious cases may not be possible. Hence, s situation exists in which a patient with active TB may be next to a patient with HIV-related complications, making the possibility of nosocomial infections high. Under these conditions, drug-resistant strains of TB can easily spread within the community.

Although the levels of drug resistance in Africa are relatively low compared to countries such as Russia and Estonia, it is vitally important that every effort be made to maintain a low incidence. Many African countries with high levels of tuberculosis are currently unable to fund tuberculosis control efforts adequately without external support from cooperating partners. Although treatment for tuberculosis is one of the most cost-effective strategies, in some countries the cost is more than the per capita expenditure available for the entire health budget. It therefore follows that treatment of MDR TB will be beyond the reach of most countries.[18] Thus, prevention of the development of resistance should be viewed as a major priority for these countries. Increasing the availability of drugs and putting a mechanism in place to ensure prompt diagnosis of cases and adequate treatment with supervision are important weapons in the battle against increasing multidrug resistance. National governments should therefore work closely with cooperating partners to ensure that tuberculosis remains high on the agenda for the health system through the provision of adequate resources—material, financial, and human—for the fight against tuberculosis.

REFERENCES

1. DYE, C., S. SCHEELE, P. DOLIN, *et al.* 1999. Global burden of tuberculosis estimated incidence: prevalence and mortality by country. JAMA **282:** 677–689.
2. BERCION, R. & C. KUABAN. 1997. Initial resistance to anti-tuberculosis drugs in Yaounde, Cameroon in 1995. Int. J. Tuberc. Lung Dis. **1:** 110–114.
3. ELLIOTT, A.M., B. HALWINDII, R.J. HAYES, *et al.* 1995. The impact of human immuno-deficiency virus on mortality of patients treated for tuberculosis in a cohort study in Zambia. Trans. R. Soc. Trop. Med. Hyg. **89:** 78–82.
4. WORLD HEALTH ORGANISATION. 2001. WHO Report 2001: Global Tuberculosis Control. WHO/CDS/2001.287. WHO. Geneva.
5. FREIDEN, T.R., P.I. FUJIWARA, R.M. WASHIKO & M.A. HAMBURG. 1995. Tuberculosis in New York City—turning the tide. N. Engl. J. Med. **333:** 229–233.
6. WORLD HEALTH ORGANISATION. 1997. Anti-tuberculosis Drug Resistance in the World. WHO. Geneva.
7. WORLD HEALTH ORGANISATION. 2000. Anti-tuberculosis Drug Resistance in the World. Report No 2: Prevalence and Trends. The WHO/IUATLD Global Project on Anti-tuberculosis Drug Resistance Surveillance 2000. WHO. Geneva.
8. DEMISSIE, M., M. GEBEYEHU & Y. BERHANE. 1997. Primary resistance to anti-tuberculosis drugs in Addis Ababa, Ethiopia. Int. J. Tuberc. Lung Dis. **1(1):** 64–67.
9. RANGE, N.S., G. MFINANGA, T.M. CHONDE & H. MASANJA. 2000. Anti-TB drug resistance patterns and the relationship with HIV prevalence among TB patients in Tanzania. Int. J. Tuberc. Lung Dis **3(9):** S120.
10. DOSSO, M., D. BONARD, P. MSELLATI, *et al.* 1999. Primary resistance to antituberculosis drugs: a national survey conducted in Cote d'Ivoire in 1995–1996. Int. J. Tuberc. Lung Dis. **3(9):** 805–809.
11. GITHUI, W.A., M.P. HAWKEN, E.S. JUMA, *et al.* 1999. Drug resistance survey in refugee and non-refugee populations in north-eastern Kenya. Int. J. Tuberc. Lung Dis. **3(9):** S118.
12. KUABAN, C., R. BERCION, G. JIFON, *et al.* 2000. Acquired drug resistance in Yaoude, Cameroon. Int. J. Tuberc. Lung Dis. **4(5):** 427–432.
13. ANASTASIS, D., G. PILLAI, V. RAMBIRITCH, *et al.* 1997. A retrospective study of human immunodeficiency virus infection and drug resistant tuberculosis in Durban, South Africa. Int. J. Tuberc. Lung Dis. **1(3):** 220–224.
14. DAVIES, G., M. PILLAY, A.W. STRUM & D. WILKINSON. 1999. Emergence of multi-drug resistant tuberculosis in a community-based daily observed treatment program in South Africa. Int. J. Tuberc. Lung Dis. **3(9):** 799–804.
15. BERTZEL, G., M. AZIZ, U. WENDL-RICHTER, *et al.* 1999. Anti-tuberculosis drug resistance surveillance in Uganda 1996–1997. Int. J. Tuberc. Lung Dis. **3(9):** 810–815.
16. CHURCHYARD, G.J., E.L. CORBETT, I. KLEINSCHMIDT, *et al.* 2000. Drug-resistant tuberculosis in South African gold miners: incidence and associated factors. Int. J. Tuberc. Lung Dis. **4(5):** 433–440.
17. BRAUN, M., J.O. KILBURN, R.W. SMITHWICK, *et al.* 1992. HIV infection and primary resistance to antituberculosis drugs in Abidjan, Cote d'Ivoire. AIDS **6:** 1327–1330.
18. SCHLUGER, N.W. 2000. The impact of drug resistance on the global tuberculosis epidemic. Int. J. Tuberc. Lung Dis. **4(2):** 271–275.

Problems in Prisons Worldwide, with a Particular Focus on Russia

VIVIEN STERN

International Centre for Prison Studies, Kings College, London

ABSTRACT: The link between prisons and disease has existed as long as prisons have been used for punishment. The prisons of the world still have high rates of infection with hepatitis, HIV, mental illness, and tuberculosis. TB is a major cause of death in prisons, mainly as a result of overcrowding, poor physical conditions, and lack of adequate treatment. The priorities of prisoners and of public health officials are often at odds with the priorities of prison administrators and prosecutors. Prison health care should be independent of prison administration and should be answerable only to the national public health program. Efforts should be made in those countries with the highest inprisonment rates to find other solutions to maintaining order in the interests of improving public health.

KEYWORDS: tuberculosis; epidemiology; prisons; Russia; Brazil; United States; prison health care services; human rights; imprisonment rates

Prisons and disease have been inextricably linked ever since prisons became the main repository of society's unwanted or deviant members. In 1666 an English Act of Parliament noted that when prisoners came to court for their trials they often infected those in court with them.[1] In 1750 some Old Bailey judges died of gaol fever.[2] The great prison reformer John Howard died in 1790 from typhus he contracted after visiting a sick prisoner in the Ukraine.[3] It was after attending to a prisoner with typhus at Kherson in the Ukraine that Howard became ill. He died January 20, 1790 at the age of 64 and was buried in Russia.

The world's prisons, jails, police cells, and detention centers are still unhealthy places where persons with HIV infection, hepatitis, mental illness, or TB are concentrated. A study carried out in Puerto Rico in 1999 showed that 94% of the prisoners were infected with hepatitis C.[4] A study of the prison system of the state of Sao Paulo in Brazil, carried out in 1995, showed 14.4% of prisoners to be HIV-positive.[5] A 1997 study carried out in England and Wales found that 90% of all prisoners had some symptoms of mental illness.[6]

Rates of TB infection in prisons are also very high. The data are fairly limited, but what information is available shows that the concentration of TB cases in prisons is remarkable. Studies show TB infection is 100 times more common in prison than

Address for correspondence: Baroness Vivien Stern, International Centre for Prison Studies, School of Law, Kings College, London, 8th floor, 75-79 York Rd., London, SE1 7AW United Kingdom. Voice: 44(0) 207 401 2559; fax: 44(0) 207 401 2577.

icps@kcl.ac.uk

TABLE 1. Tuberculosis infection rates in prisons and civilian populations

Country	Prison cases per 100,000 (year)	Civilian cases per 100,000 (year)
Brazil	5714 (1992–93)	55.9 (1992)
Georgia	5995 (1997–98)	155 (1997)
Malawi	5142 (1996)	209 (1996)
Rwanda	3363 (1996–98)	79.3 (1997)
Spain	2283 (1992–93)	24 (1993)

SOURCE: Based on Bone et al.[12]

outside prison, and up to a quarter of any country's TB cases may be found in prison.[7] The International Committee of the Red Cross (ICRC), while announcing its program in Georgia in 1998, noted that the rate of TB infection in prison was 60 times that in civilian society and that TB was a major cause of death in prisons there.[8] In Kazakstan in 1997, 1034 of the 1491 prisoner deaths that year were from TB,[9] but by 2000 the number of prisoner deaths from TB was down to 202 (personal communication to author May 2001), a figure estimated to be 20 times higher than among the general population.[10] In 1996, Medecins sans Frontieres began working in a special prison for TB-infected prisoners in Kemerovo in Russia, where prisoners were dying at a rate of two to three a day. By the end of 1998, deaths were running at two to three a month.[11]

TABLE 1 shows that such disproportionate rates are not limited to the former Soviet Union. High prison infection rates are also found in countries in Africa, Latin America, and Western Europe. The first outbreak at a British prison of 14 cases, all resistant to the drug isoniazid, was reported in May 2001.[13]

How is this gross disproportion explained? A combination of contributing factors can be suggested. The literature makes it clear that TB is a disease of substandard social conditions—poverty, malnutrition, and overcrowding. Because prisons are places where persons from these social conditions, with backgrounds of poverty, are concentrated under one roof, usually in very overcrowded conditions and with limited resources for food and care, TB will be an ever-present danger.

Who are the people in the prisons of the world? Everywhere, in both rich and poor countries, prison inmates are drawn from the poor and the marginalized.[14] Of Swedish prisoners, one-quarter are homeless, one-half are unemployed, and one-half abuse narcotics.[15] In some countries with corrupt justice systems, it is only the poor who end up in pretrial detention or with a prison sentence. Those who can afford it buy their way out of detention or secure the services of a competent lawyer.[16]

So they come to prison in poor health, with a high vulnerability to infection. Although prison could be a place where untreated conditions are discovered and dealt with so that prisoners leave healthier than they were when they came in, this happens only rarely. Usually prisons are unhealthy places. Most prisons in the world are overcrowded, some desperately so. Overcrowding in the prisons of the Russian Federation has been so bad that prisoners have had less than one square meter each, and there are not enough beds to go round. Beds are used many times over and sleeping is organized in three shifts.[17] In some prisons in Brazil, prisoners tie themselves to the window bars so that they can sleep standing up.[18]

TABLE 2. Rates of multidrug-resistant TB in prison populations

Country and year	Rate
Azerbaijan (1997)	23%
Georgia (1997–98)	13%
Russia (1998)	at least 20%

SOURCE: Based on Bone *et al.* 2000.

What about the buildings, the physical conditions? Many prison buildings are old and dilapidated, damp and unhygienic. Light and air are important for disease prevention, but prison cells do not usually have large picture windows with good access to air and light. Mostly they have small windows, high in the wall and covered with bars. In many prisons of American design, the cells have no direct access to natural light at all. The cells open out onto a corridor, and the windows are in the corridor.

If the treatment of TB in such an environment is not prompt and well-organized, multidrug-resistant (MDR) TB can result. Information on the levels of MDR TB in prisons worldwide is also limited, but some figures are available. WHO suggests that in some prisons the level is up to 24%.[19] TABLE 2 shows some estimates of the rates for MDR TB among imprisoned tuberculosis patients.

Clearly the countries of the former Soviet Union are particularly at risk of seeing high rates of MDR TB infection in their prison populations. The ICRC study in Georgia found that 69% of the patients examined in prison were resistant to at least one TB drug.[21] Comparable figures for MDR TB rates in civilian populations are not available, although WHO suggests that high rates are to be found in Estonia, Latvia, and the oblasts of Ivanovo and Tomsk in the Russian Federation.[22] The high cost of the treatment of MDR TB means that most of the infected prisoners in the developing world and in the former Soviet Union are unlikely to receive any treatment, though one pilot project in Tomsk in Russia involves 50 prisoners.[23]

To understand these rates, it is important to take into account the explanations given by WHO for the growth of drug resistance generally, that is, inconsistent or partial treatment, wrong prescribing or unreliable drug supply[24] and set them against the particular circumstances of imprisonment. First, there is the background described above—the many prisoners from a background of poverty, with poor health services and a drastic lack of resources. Furthermore, one needs to understand what sort of a place a prison is and who sets the priorities. There will be two sets of major and competing priorities—the priorities of the system and the priorities of the prisoners.

Consider, for example, an enormous system like that of the Russian Federation with nearly a million prisoners. The system is under enormous pressure and will find it very difficult to be concerned with the care or treatment of individuals. Every day in the pretrial prisons, prisoners arrive and have to be processed quickly. Some have to go to court for hearings. Some have already been tried and sentenced. These prisoners have to be shipped out to the place for sentenced prisoners so that there is room for the next group of arrestees. All the time people need to be moved on to make room for others. Then in prisons all over the world there is always the potential for trouble. Prison is not happy place. It is a place into which people bring the violence of the home or the street, and trouble can break out. The prison authorities will deal with the trouble by effecting transfers; that is, they will move the prisoners designated as troublemakers to somewhere else. The priorities are, therefore, keeping the system going by moving people through it and maintaining control.

The prisoners also have their priorities. A class structure exists inside the prison as it does outside, with some persons at the top and some at the bottom—the strong and the weak. For many prisoners, prison is a place of fear, and the best strategy is to get protection from someone stronger. The prisoners' priorities will be their own survival inside the prison and their families' welfare outside.[25]

The perception of the prison health care service about what needs to be done will come a poor third in the prison world's order of priorities. In spite of good intentions, many prisoners will not be screened at entry. There are too many of them, and the length of their stay is unpredictable. Treatment starts and stops, for many reasons. A great deal of movement occurs within the system. Corruption is common. It is easy to see why: A poorly paid health worker or one who has not had wages paid for months can be persuaded by a powerful prisoner to provide some medication, even though the health worker knows there may not be enough to complete the treatment. Prisoner priorities can also defeat the efforts of the best-organized health workers. Weak prisoners might give their medications to someone else in exchange for protection, or a prisoner concerned about a sick parent might save them up and give them to the family when they visit. Such processes can lead to the occurrence of drug-resistant TB. More than being the result of incompetence, bad management, stupidity, and irresponsibility, they are a rational reaction by all players to the situation in which they have been placed.

Therefore, it is the situation that needs to change. This situation, in which the sick are subject to many priorities other than those of the treatment they need, leads to an increase in disease; for some, it even leads to death. For all it is a threat to public health as well as a gross abuse of human rights. International human rights treaties and covenants require all participating countries to treat prisoners with respect for the inherent dignity of the human person. Furthermore, the International Covenant on Civil and Political Rights states (Article Six):

> Every human being has the inherent right to life. This right shall be protected by law. No one shall be arbitrarily deprived of his life.

In addition the international human rights instruments make it clear that prisoners must be given access to proper health care while they are imprisoned. Principle 9 of the UN Basic Principles for the Treatment of Prisoners provides the following:

> Prisoners shall have access to the health care services available in the country without discrimination on the grounds of their legal situation.

When prisoners are denied health care, or their health care needs are subordinated to other pressures, such as security or length of the prison sentence, a human rights abuse is taking place.

In prison systems throughout the world, the requirements of health are subordinated, relegated to a position of less importance than the requirements of the criminal justice system, and the rules of the prison authorities, the prosecutors, and police. For example, in all the pretrial prisons of the former Soviet Union, the cells have the same size of windows. The size is larger than in many other countries. There are bars, of course, but unfortunately hardly any light or air comes through these windows because they are covered on the outside with heavy shutters made of wood or steel. These shutters keep out most of the air and most of the light. Because so many prisoners are sick and TB is an ever-present danger, a wise policy would be to remove them from the windows. Sadly, the law prevents removal. The shutters are there to prevent pretrial prisoners involved in the same case from communicating with each other. The possibility that prisoners will catch a deadly disease as a result of poor ventilation is less important to the system than that a criminal investigation is deemed to require such a measure. Thus, the prosecutors enforce it.

Another example of legal and prison priorities competing with health priorities is in the prevention of HIV. The presence of HIV infection increases the risk of developing TB. It is estimated that in prisons HIV infection is 75 times more common than in the community at large.[26] Those prisons with the most extreme TB epidemics are also those with the fastest growing rates of HIV infection. In Russia at the end of March 1999, 12,332 cases of infection were reported. By the beginning of August 2000, that number had grown to 52,427. (Personal communication from the Moscow office of Médecins Sans Frontiers. [One year health promotion in the Russian prison system—an update.]) Not unexpectedly, HIV infection rates inside Russian prisons are also increasing rapidly: 3,500 HIV-positive prisoners were identified in Russia at the end of May 2000,[27] compared to 2,661 one year previously.[28]

Sexual activity takes place in prison and puts many prisoners at risk for HIV infection. Injecting drugs also takes place in prisons in spite of strong efforts by the authorities to prevent it. Harm-reduction strategies dictated by public health concerns would suggest that a policy of access to condoms, bleach, and clean needles would be a wise step; but for many prison systems that is a step too far in the direction of sanctioning such activities. It is therefore particularly noteworthy that the penitentiary system in the Ukraine makes condoms available,[29] and the Russian Federation has provided in recent legislation for condoms and bleach to be available in prisons under certain circumstances.[30]

There is wide agreement that, in order to provide adequate prison health care and to protect public health, prison health care has to be linked with the national health services. Two major reasons are put forward to support this position. The first has to do with the relationship between the prison and the outside world and the permeability of the prison walls. Many people enter and leave prisons every day—prison personnel, other workers, and prisoners' family members. Many prisoners leave prison after serving a short sentence or in the middle of a course of treatment. Unless treatment can be continued once the prisoner has been released, the risks of creating drug resistance are great. The closer the links between the care inside and outside the prison, the more effective for promoting public health.

The second reason for the public health link brings into question the independence of action of the prison health service workers. Health care should be independent of the prison authorities, and prison doctors should be employees of the health ministry or the health services. From such a position of independence, the doctors can press with greater authority for measures conducive to public health, such as the removal of shutters and the distribution of condoms, bleach, and clean needles. They can press for prisoners not to be transferred in the middle of treatment and for a policy prohibiting the withholding of medicines as disciplinary punishment. From such a position of independence, they are also better able to point out the public health consequences of prison overcrowding.

Prison overcrowding is, of course, a product of the decision to use imprisonment as a punishment and of the limited resources available for the implementation of that decision. The level of use of imprisonment varies greatly between different countries for reasons only marginally related to the crime rate. Deciding factors are more likely to be the political and cultural environment of the country. Imprisonment rates are measured per 100,000 of the general population. The highest rate of imprisonment in the world is the United States, with 702 prisoners per 100,000. Canada has 122 prisoners per 100,000. Russia used to have the highest rate of imprisonment in the world, but measures taken by the Russian government have achieved a reduction to 675 per 100,000. The figure in England and Wales is 124, and that is the second highest among the countries of the European Union. Five of the 15 countries of the former Soviet Union also have very high rates, that is, over 400 per 100,000, but two-thirds of the world's countries have rates of 150 per 100,000 or below.[31]

It is clear that these high imprisonment rates are not necessary for the preservation of law and order because most countries manage to maintain order with far lower rates. Furthermore, high rates of imprisonment have adverse public health implications. When imprisonment can lead to the contracting of a deadly disease like MDR TB and its spread into the community, it is incumbent upon those who care about public health to involve themselves in the debates about the penal systems of their societies.[32]

NOTES AND REFERENCES

1. HARDING, C., B. HINES, R. IRELAND & P. RAWLINGS. 1985. Imprisonment in England and Wales: A Concise History. Croom Helm. London. p. 95.
2. Ibid., 115.
3. http://www.acjnet.org/jhsa/
4. *Puerto Rico Daily News*, Tuesday, May 16, 2000.
5. BONE, A., *et al.* 2000. Tuberculosis Control in Prisons: A Manual for Programme Managers. World Health Organisation. Geneva. p. 22 (text version).
6. SINGLETON, *et al.* 1998. Psychiatric Morbidity among Prisoners: Summary Report. Office for National Statistics. London. p. 23.
7. See Tuberculosis in Prisons, World Health Organisation, March 2000, p. 1, and "Armenia: agreement signed for TB-control programme in prisons," *ICRC News*, 31 August 2000.
8. 1998. "Georgia: ICRC TB programme in prisons under way," *ICRC News*, 4 June 1998.
9. KAZAKSTAN PENAL REFORM INTERNATIONAL CENTRAL & EASTERN EUROPE AND CENTRAL ASIA PROGRAMME. 1999. Information Pack 1: Measures to Reduce Overcrowding in Prisons.
10. Tuberculosis in Prisons Roundtable. Press releases. 1 December 2000. United States Embassy Kazakstan.
11. MÉDECINS SANS FRONTIERES. 17 July 2000. Anti-TB program in Siberia, Russia.
12. Based on Bone, A., *et al.* 2000. Tuberculosis Control in Prisons: A Manual for Programme Managers. WHO. Geneva. p. 19 (prepublication text).
13. MEIKLE, JAMES. 2001. "Screening plan after TB outbreak at jail." *The Guardian*, London, 7 May 2001.
14. See Stern, Vivien. 1998. A Sin Against the Future. Penguin Books. London. pp. 105–136.
15. See Kriminalvarden, Swedish Prison and Probation Service. 1999. The Link to a Life Free of Crime, p. 7.
16. See Narayan, Deepa, with Patel, Schafft, Rademacher and Koch-Schulte. 2000. Voices of the Poor. Can Anyone Hear Us? Oxford, for a description of corruption in justice systems in poor countries.

17. STERN, VIVIEN. 1999. Introduction: An overview and some issues. *In* Sentenced to Die? The Problem of TB in Prisons in Eastern Europe and Central Asia. Vivien Stern, Ed.: 12. ICPS. London.
18. AMNESTY INTERNATIONAL. 1999. No-One Sleeps Here Safely: Human Rights Violations Against Detainees. Amnesty International, para. 3.1.
19. WORLD HEALTH ORGANISATION. 2000. Tuberculosis in Prisons. WHO. Geneva. p. 2.
20. "Georgia: ICRC TB programme in prisons under way," *ICRC News,* 4 June 1998.
21. See WHO Anti-Tuberculosis Drug Resistance in the World - Report No. 2. 2000.
22. "TB epidemic to cost Russian $1bn," *Moscow News*, 30 August 2000.
23. Tuberculosis Fact Sheet. 2000.
24. See Reyes, Hernan & Rudi Coninx. 1999. Pitfalls of tuberculosis programmes in prisons. *In* Sentenced to Die? The Problem of TB in Prisons in Eastern Europe and Central Asia. Vivien Stern, Ed.: 12. ICPS. London.
25. BONE, A., *et al.* 2000. Tuberculosis Control in Prisons: A Manual for Programme Managers. World Health Organisation, p. 21 (text version). WHO. Geneva.
26. Ibid., 20 (text version published by UNAIDS, Geneva).
27. Russian Criminal Correction System Overview, May 2000, Public Health Research Institute.
28. See Best Practice Case Study: Joint Project of the Ministry of the Interior and UNAIDS for the Reduction of HIV and AIDS in the Prison System of the Ukraine. UNAIDS (in press).
29. Newsletter-Penal Reform Project in Eastern Europe and Central Asia, No. 10. Autumn 2000. Penal Reform International and the International Centre for Prison Studies. London.
30. See Walmsley, Roy, World Prison Population List, 2000, Home Office, London, and World Prison Brief on www.prisonstudies.org.

The Impact of Worldwide Drug Resistance on the United Kingdom

JOHN WATSON

PHLS Communicable Disease Surveillance Centre, London NW9 5EQ, UK

ABSTRACT: **The incidence of tuberculosis in the United Kingdom, which declined beginning in the middle of the 19th century, began to increase in the late 1980s. The distribution of tuberculosis by geographic area, age, and ethnic group is discussed. Drug resistance is high among U.K. residents born abroad, but the proportion of drug-resistant cases is remaining stable.**

KEYWORDS: **multidrug-resistant tuberculosis; tuberculosis; Mycobnet; distribution of tuberculosis; worldwide drug resistance**

RECENT TUBERCULOSIS TRENDS IN THE UNITED KINGDOM

In the 19th century, tuberculosis was common throughout the United Kingdom and was one of the main causes of death. A decline in death from tuberculosis, however, was apparent beginning in the middle of the 19th century, and that decline continued once tuberculosis became a notifiable disease in 1912. The decline in tuberculosis continued throughout most of the 20th century, preceding the introduction of specific antituberculosis chemotherapy in the 1940s and the wide-scale use of BCG immunization from the 1950s. In recent decades, however, the rate of decline has slowed, and in the late 1980s tuberculosis incidence numbers began to increase. In England and Wales notifications had dropped to 5085 in 1987, but had risen to 6572 by the year 2000.

The distribution of tuberculosis varies substantially across the country. Whereas the overall rate for England and Wales in 1998 was 10.9 per 100,000 population, the rate in the southwestern region (predominately rural) was 4.4 per 100,000, and the rate in London was 32.0 per 100,000. In general, rates in urban areas are higher than other areas. The high rate of incidence and the increases in rates in London have led some to compare the situation to that seen in New York 10 years earlier. At that time, the tuberculosis rate rose to high levels in New York, and only very substantial interventions with tuberculosis services reversed this.[1]

In addition to the variation in distribution by geographic area, the occurrence of tuberculosis also varies substantially by age and ethnic group. Having been predominately a disease of the older age groups for many years, the majority of cases now occur in young adults. The proportion of cases occurring in the white indigenous population has declined over the last two decades to less than 40%. Cases in those

Address for correspondence: John Watson, PHLS Communicable Disease Surveillance Centre, 61 Collindale Avenue, London NW9 5EQ, U.K.
  jwatson@phls.org.uk

TABLE 1. Resistance to first-line drugs in initial isolates of *M. tuberculosis* complex in the U.K. 1998 and 1999

Initial isolates by type	1998	1999
Total number initial isolates reported	3827	4241
(*M. tuberculosis*)	(3782)	(4185)
(*M. africanum*)	(5)	(15)
(*M. bovis*)	(40)	(41)
Number resistant to at least one first-line drug	246 (6.4%)	267 (6.3%)
Number resistant to isoniazid alone	124 (3.2%)	167 (3.9%)
Number resistant to isoniazid with or without other drugs	229 (6.0%)	251 (5.1%)
Number multidrug-resistant (MDR)	49 (1.3%)	33 (0.8%)

persons of Indian subcontinent ethnic origin have remained approximately stable at 40%. The proportion of cases occurring in the black African population, however, has increased substantially since the late 1980s to reach 13% in 1998.[2] Whereas the rate of disease in the white indigenous population is between 4 and 5 per 100,000 population, the rate in the Indian subcontinent ethnic group is estimated at approximately 120, and in the black African population at about 200 per 100,00 population. Fifty-nine percent of all cases now occur in persons who were born abroad.[2]

TUBERCULOSIS DRUG RESISTANCE SURVEILLANCE METHODS

The U.K. mycobacterial resistance network ("Mycobnet") was formed in 1993. It is based on a collaboration among all the U.K. mycobacteriology reference laboratories with data collated by the PHLS Communicable Disease Surveillance Centre in London. It is based on initial isolates (i.e., isolates obtained at the time of diagnosis) from all culture-confirmed tuberculosis cases in the United Kingdom.

In 1998–1999 the results on over 8,000 isolates were submitted to Mycobnet (TABLE 1). Most of these were *Mycobacterium tuberculosis,* and a very small number were identified as *Mycobacterium africanum.* Approximately 40 isolates each year were identified as *Mycobacterium bovis.* Between 3 and 4% of isolates were reported as being resistant to isoniazid alone and approximately 1% as being multidrug resistant (MDR—resistant to isoniazid and rifampicin with or without resistance to other drugs). Monoresistance to rifampicin or ethambutol was very low.

Overall, 5.9% of isolates were resistant to isoniazid with or without resistance to other drugs, but the rate was a little higher in England (6.1%) than in Wales (5.2%), Scotland (4.3%), or Northern Ireland (3.0%). Similarly, in 1998–1999 rates of multidrug resistance were higher in England (1.1%) than in Wales (0.4%), Scotland (0.9%), or Northern Ireland (0).

Among the isolates reported for 1998 and 1999 combined, 7.6% were resistant to isoniazid in London compared with 5.0% in the remainder of the United Kingdom. The corresponding figures for multidrug resistance were 1.3% and 0.8%. As expected, both isoniazid resistance and multidrug resistance were more common in those

TABLE 2. Resistance to first-line drugs in initial isolates of *M. tuberculosis* complex, U.K. 1993–1999

Year	Isoniazid resistant[a]	MDR
1993	157 (4.6%)	19 (0.6%)
1994	181 (5.6%)	43 (1.3%)
1995	197 (6.1%)	49 (1.5%)
1996	221 (6.1%)	60 (1.7%)
1997	193 (5.4%)	45 (1.3%)
1998	229 (6.0%)	49 (1.3%)
1999	251 (5.9%)	33 (0.8%)

[a]With or without resistance to other drugs.

with a previous history of tuberculosis (11.3% and 7.4%, respectively) compared with those with no history of previous tuberculosis (5.9% and 0.5%, respectively.). Both isoniazid resistance and multidrug resistance were more common in children and rates of incidence decrease with increasing age. Drug resistance was less common in those born in the United Kingdom and nearly twice as common in those born abroad. Both isoniazid resistance and multidrug resistance were more common in those known to be HIV seropositive.

Between 1993 and 1999, levels of drug resistance in the United Kingdom have remained approximately stable (TABLE 2), although the number of isoniazid-resistant isolates and multidrug-resistant isolates has increased in line with the increasing total number of cases of tuberculosis in the United Kingdom.[3]

Using data from the Mycobnet system in 1993–1994, Hayward *et al.* have estimated the proportion of isoniazid and multidrug resistance likely to have been acquired in the U.K. on the basis of the patients' history of previous treatment and place of birth.[4] They estimated that, although over 50% of isolated isoniazid resistance was acquired abroad, at least 32% of such resistance was homegrown.

OUTBREAKS OF DRUG-RESISTANT TUBERCULOSIS IN THE UNITED KINGDOM

Two outbreaks of drug-resistant tuberculosis have been reported in the United Kingdom in association with hospitals. The first occurred in London in 1995 and involved eight cases in a unit for HIV-infected patients. A multidrug-resistant strain of tuberculosis was responsible for the outbreak, which originated from an index case from Portugal.

Both diagnostic delay and infection control problems contributed to the incident.[5] The second hospital outbreak also occurred in London in 1995–1996. The source case was an individual who was HIV-negative and came from Africa. Isolates from the case were initially susceptible but subsequently became multidrug resistant. Following a stay by the index case in hospital, multidrug-resistant tuberculosis occurred in seven HIV-infected hospital contacts. Problems with the supervision of therapy and infection control were identified as factors in the incident.[6]

An outbreak of isoniazid-resistant tuberculosis was identified in North London in 1995–2001. Although the earliest case with the same strain of *Mycobacterium tuberculosis* was ill in 1995, the main outbreak "source" case occurred in 1999. By March 2001, 43 linked cases had been identified in the outbreak. Transmission among young adults of various ethnic groups in North London was identified to be occurring in this outbreak.[7]

CONCLUSION

Tuberculosis case numbers are increasing in the United Kingdom. Cases occurring in persons originating outside the United Kingdom are a major contributor to the recent increases. Drug resistance is high among those born abroad. Although the proportion of drug-resistant cases in the U.K. is remaining stable, the number of drug-resistant cases is rising. Drug resistance in the U.K. originates not only in infection acquired abroad but is also homegrown. Outbreaks of drug-resistant tuberculosis have revealed some deficiencies in aspects of treatment prevention and control in the U.K. In order to reduce the problem of drug resistance in the U.K., efforts must be made to avoid diagnostic delay. Drug resistance should be suspected in the groups identified as being at increased risk of drug-resistant disease, and therapy should be supervised, at least in all infectious patients. Control of infection is a final important element, particularly in hospitals where other vulnerable patients are based.

REFERENCES

1. HAYWARD, A.C. & R.J. COKER. 2001. Could a tuberculosis epidemic occur in London as it did in New York? Emerg. Infect. Dis. **6:** 12–16.
2. ROSE, A.M.C., J.M. WATSON, C. GRAHAM, *et al.* 2001. Tuberculosis at the end of the 20th century in England and Wales: results of a national survey in 1998. Thorax **56:** 173–179.
3. IRISH, C., J. HERBERT, D. BENNETT, *et al.* 1999. Database study of antibiotic resistant tuberculosis in the UK 1994/6. Br. Med. J. **318:** 497–498.
4. HAYWARD, A.C., J. HERBERT & J.M. WATSON. 2000. Tuberculosis drug resistance in England and Wales. How much is home grown? Epidemiol. Infect. **125:** 463–464.
5. ANONYMOUS. 1995. Outbreak of hospital acquired multidrug resistant tuberculosis. Comm. Dis. Rep. Wkly. **5:** 161.
6. BREATHNACH, A.S., A. DE RUITER, G.M. HOLDSWORTH, *et al.* 1998. An outbreak of multi-drug resistant tuberculosis in a London teaching hospital. J. Hosp. Infect. **39:** 111–117.
7. ANONYMOUS. 2001. Comm. Dis. Rep. Wkly.

Specific Features of the Spread of Tuberculosis in Russia at the End of the 20th Century

MARGARITA V. SHILOVA

Department of Epidemiology and TB Control, Research Institute of Phthisiopulmonology (RIPh), Moscow Sechenov Medical Academy, Moscow 101478, Russia

ABSTRACT: This study shows the dynamics of the epidemiological process over the last decade and presents the causes of the deterioration in TB control. Explanations are given for the TB mortality rate increase, the trustworthiness of the data, and the factors influencing its formation. The present-day TB epidemiological situation in Russia is characterized by an increase in exogenous infection. Peaks of epidemiological deterioration were registered in 1993 and 1999. Marked deterioration of the epidemiological situation in 1999 resulted from an economic crisis in August 1998 and a consequent dramatic decrease in the living standards of the population. In the 1990s this trend has changed. TB infection spreads according to trends that are quite similar to those at the beginning of 20th century. The official TB morbidity rate does not reflect the true level of incidence because of undetected TB cases (approx. 10%).

KEYWORDS: tuberculosis; epidemiology; diagnostics; drug resistance; Russia

INTRODUCTION

The end of 20th century was characterized by a marked increase in the prevalence of TB infection, both worldwide and in Russia. The deterioration of the TB epidemiological situation in Russia started in the mid-1980s. The reason for this was a worsening of standards of living: Tuberculosis is a disease that is bound to social conditions. A general deterioration of the living conditions of the population, hostilities in several territories of Russia and the Confederation of Independent States (CIS), increased migration, an increase in the number of socially disfunctioning population groups, and the existence of a large reservoir of TB infection in the penitentiary system have all led to a marked increase in TB prevalence. Underfunding of the TB service and poor distribution of TB services among the population have also influenced the epidemiological process unfavorably.

The rate of morbidity depends on several factors, such as the number of new cases and the quality of diagnostics. This study demonstrates the reliability of the morbidity rate and its linkage to a variety of factors. There is a possibility of a growth of recorded TB incidence in the near future because of better active detection and registration of new cases and a general improvement of the service.

Address for correspondence: Professor M.V. Shilova, Department of Epidemiology and TB Control, Research Institute of Phthisiopulmonology (RIPh), Moscow Sechenov Medical Academy, 4 Dostoyevsky Street, Moscow 101478, Russia. Voice: 7 095 2811720 or 2843170; fax: 7 095 9711515.

Oxana.Gouli@kingshc.nhs.uk

RESEARCH METHODS AND MONITORING OF TB

We have undertaken analysis of the TB morbidity rate in the Russian population within the period from 1970 to 2000 on the basis of official medical statistics. Registration of new TB cases in Russia is performed by institutions of the specialized TB service to which patients are referred if TB is detected. Newly detected cases of TB ("new cases") include patients with characteristic radiographic signs of TB with or without sputum smear positivity for acid-fast bacilli (AFB). Patients with TB relapse are not included in the number of new cases. A final diagnosis of TB is either confirmed or rejected jointly by the members of the Central Medical Commission of Experts, which has representatives based in every major TB dispensary (regional, territorial, republican) in all areas of the Russian Federation (RF). There are a total of 80 of these dispensaries, where the most skilled phthisiatrists and x-ray specialists are available. As soon as the diagnosis is verified, the recording form N 089/y is completed for every patient with active TB diagnosed for the first time. On the basis of these recording forms, every administrative territory compiles a report on TB incidence using forms N 8 and N 33. These form the basis of the official state statistics and are submitted to the Ministry of Public Health of the RF in both electronic and paper formats. The staff of Russian TB Department of Epidemiology and TB Control perform their verifications and compile summary reports on every administrative territory of the country. Form N 33 reports mainly those patients with TB who are residents of the given territory and are covered by the TB service of the Ministry of Public Health. Form N 8 records all new cases of TB including residents of the given region, immigrants, refugees, forced resettlers, homeless and unemployed people (vagrants), persons under investigation and prisoners (Ministry of Justice system), and patients detected and followed up by other departments as well as those in whom TB was detected postmortem. Methods of compiling the reports on form N 33 have not changed greatly in the last 30 years. Before 1995 the data on immigrants, refugees, forced resettlers, vagrants, and persons under investigation and prisoners were not considered while calculating morbidity rates. The incidence calculation is performed per 100,000 average annual population in the corresponding groups. Annual growth or decrease of morbidity rates is calculated as a percentage for a certain time period. The mortality rate is calculated by State Statistics Committee and is based on death certificates filed for every person who dies (form N 106/y).

The treatment outcomes of new TB cases are assessed by two criteria: sputum conversion, both smear and culture, and cavity closure (by x-ray and mandatory tomography). Indicators are calculated in relation to the corresponding group of new cases detected in the previous year, that is, 1.5 years after the beginning of treatment. We have studied a few other indicators of TB case monitoring as well.

A total of 132,000 new cases of active TB were detected in the year 2000, which is 8,000 more than in 1997, yielding a rate of 90.7 per 100,000. The TB incidence among the population covered by the health care system (relatively permanent population) has grown within last year from 60.0 to 65.5 per 100,000. The TB incidence among men is 2.5 times higher than among women. The highest TB incidence is registered in people from 25 to 34 years of age—159.5 per 100,000—and in children from 3 to 6 years—26.2 per 100,000 children in the population. The incidence of TB in all children is 17.9 per 100,000 and remains at the level of 1999.

A total of 29,000 people died of TB in 2000, which is 300 more cases than in the previous year. The mortality rate has grown from 20.2 per 100,000 in 1999 to 20.4 in 2000.

In 2000 the proportion of the population actively screened for TB increased from 56.9% in 1999 to 57.1% in 2000. But the proportion of TB cases actively detected by fluorographic screening, microbiological examination, and tuberculin skin testing declined slightly, from 52.0% to 51.4%, probably as a result of a deterioration in the quality of the detection and registration methods.

Treatment outcomes of new cases are about the same compared to the previous year's indicators, although there are some slight differences: Sputum conversion declined from 72.9 to 72.2%, and cavity closure from 61.8 to 61.3% of cases.

Since 1999, data on MDR in new cases have been added to official state statistics. Multidrug resistance (MDR) means resistance to isoniazid and rifampicin, and does not depend on resistance to other TB drugs. MDR is detected in 2.9% of all new cases and in 7.1% of sputum smear–positive patients.

RESULTS AND DISCUSSION

TB prevalence in Russia at the end of 20th century is characterized by an increase in exogenous infection and superinfection in the epidemiologic process. In 2000 the TB mortality rate went back to 1966 levels (20.4 per 100,000), and the morbidity rate returned to 1967 levels (90.7 per 100,000).

The deterioration of the TB epidemiological situation in Russia started in the mid-1980s. This conclusion is based on the analysis and comparison of several traditional and nontraditional indicators.[1] The period from 1990 to 1992 showed growth in all basic indicators of TB prevalence in Russia. Though the TB epidemiological situation continued to worsen in 1993–1998, its rate of increase slowed down (FIG. 1). A new upward leap of the major indicators appears to have occurred in 1999, depending on which TB epidemiological indicator is assessed. The period from 1986 to 1991 was falsely favorable, because TB case detection was not very active at that period. Thus, the recorded incidence rate was artificially low.

The basic reasons for TB prevalence growth are as follows: a general deterioration of socioeconomic status; hostilities in several territories of Russia and the CIS; increasing migration; an increase in the number of socially disfunctioning groups of population and occupants of penitentiary institutions; underfunding of medical and preventive activities of TB institutions; and a poor distribution of TB services among the population.

What groups of the population have a major influence on the worsening of epidemiological process? To consider this problem, we have studied the mortality dynamics of the whole population and have identified two large groups: TB patients registered at TB health care institutions (a relatively permanent group of residents) and TB patients at other departments, including occupants of the penitentiary system of the Ministry of Justice and those with postmortem TB diagnoses who are not registered at any institutions.

The analysis of mortality dynamics shows that after quite a long period of significant growth of the death rate from TB, some slight decrease of this indicator was

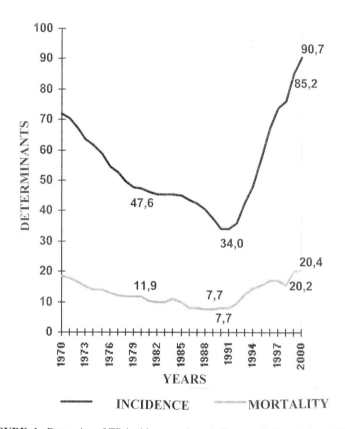

FIGURE 1. Dynamics of TB incidence and mortality rates in Russia (per 100,000).

first registered in 1997. This decrease happened because of a slight reduction of TB death rates among the population covered by the health care system. The year 1998 demonstrated a noticeable reduction of the level of TB mortality, which was caused by quite a remarkable decrease of TB mortality rates among the rest of population. This decrease is caused by mortality reduction among prisoners and persons under investigation who compose most of this population group. In 1999 there was a remarkable upward change in the level of TB mortality, especially among the population covered by the health care system. In 2000 the TB death rate remained at the same level.

Similar tendencies can be traced while studying the dynamics of TB morbidity. The overall TB incidence as well as the TB incidence among the population covered by the health care system continued to increase in 1997–1998, while the incidence among prisoners and the number of cases diagnosed postmortem decreased slightly. Insignificant growth of the overall TB incidence in 1998 (compared to the previous year) can be explained by the decrease in morbidity rate among the latter group of the population. In 1999 TB morbidity rates increased again.

Thus, before 1998 positive changes in both TB mortality and morbidity rates of the whole population were to a certain extent caused by the decrease in TB mortality and morbidity rates among persons under investigation and prisoners. These comprise 88.7% of new TB cases registered by other departments and 24.8% of all new TB cases. The significant growth of TB incidence and mortality in 1999 was caused by the growth of these indicators in both groups of the population.

What were the most unfavorable periods in the TB epidemiological process? Our conclusions about the most unfavorable periods were based on an assessment of the indicators of changing rates. The period of stabilization in 1988–1989 with a TB mortality rate of 7.7 per 100,000 population was followed by a period of gradual growth of this indicator. The maximum growth in TB mortality rate was registered in 1993 and reached 34.4% within one year. Then a gradual decrease in the growth rate occurred, with just a small increase in 1996. The first slight decrease of mortality rate was registered in 1997 (1.2%), which in 1998 became 8.3%. In 1999 there was an increase, when a 29.9% increase in TB mortality rate was registered. The growth rate of this indicator decreased by just 1.0% in 2000.

Quite similar tendencies were revealed while studying the changes in TB mortality rates in both groups of the population. The changes in TB mortality rates are closely connected to three factors: real deterioration of the epidemiological situation, alteration in the principles of registering/recording new TB cases, and information about TB cases.

Like the indicator of TB mortality, the growth of the rate of TB morbidity was first registered in 1993. The increase of TB incidence in 1993 was caused by a dramatic deterioration of the epidemiological situation in the whole country during this period. It was manifested in a significant growth of TB morbidity rates among the permanent population, a slight growth among the rest of population, and a dramatic growth among children registered in 1993 (by 12.7%) and 1994 (by 14.3%). In this period TB morbidity rates were calculated in accordance with regulations issued in the 1950s.

The second leap forward in TB incidence happened in 1995. This increase was mainly caused by an alteration in new TB case registration that came about when we proposed that all TB cases should be registered at the place of their detection including those at detention centers and prisons. The significant increase in TB incidence occurring in 1995 was mainly the result of inclusion of cases from detention centers and prisons, which were not included in earlier indicators of TB incidence.

The third TB morbidity growth, which was registered in 1999, was caused by two factors. First, there was a real deterioration of the epidemiological situation. Second, the year of 1999 marked the end of training courses for managers and statisticians of the TB service aimed at correcting the TB morbidity indicator. Therefore, in 1999 almost all areas of the RF included the data on TB incidence among occupants of penitentiary institutions, immigrants, homeless people, and other persons who were not covered earlier in their annual reports. Thus, having studied the rates of TB mortality and TB morbidity growth we came to the conclusion that the real peaks of epidemiological deterioration happened in Russia in 1993 and 1999.

The level of TB incidence greatly depends on the results of active TB case detection and on the methods of detection used. Of all new cases of lung TB registered in 2000, 64.1% were detected actively, that is, by self-referral to the medical service with a respiratory complaint. It is important to mention that if radiographic screening had not been carried out, about 45,000 patients would have remained undiagnosed. Microscopy of sputum smears revealed just 21,000 patients. Tuberculin skin testing revealed tuberculosis in 34,000 children, which was 75.4% of all new TB cases among children.

Although the indicator of TB incidence has been calculated more accurately in recent years, it still does not fully reveal the actual level of TB prevalence. The reason is that one group of sick people remains unknown to the medical service, because the TB morbidity rate reflects detected cases only. What is the prevalence of undetected cases? We have developed a range of criteria to consider undetected cases of TB. Our proposal is based on the assumption that the prevailing majority of patients will be detected sooner or later. The number of undetected patients is directly related to the number of cases in which TB was not diagnosed in a reasonable length of time. Cases in which TB was not diagnosed in a timely manner include the following:

- *Patients with chronic forms of TB.* In 2000 2521 patients were registered with fibrous-cavernous forms of TB. This represented 3.1% of all new TB cases.

- *Newly diagnosed adult patients with spontaneous resolution of TB having moderate and mild residual signs in the lungs.* A total of 8455 cases were recorded in this group in 2000. These patients are not considered to be carrying active forms of TB, and they have never been included in the indicator of TB incidence. They represent 8.9% of all new TB cases.

- *Newly diagnosed children and teenagers with spontaneous resolution of TB having residual signs of tuberculosis.* These children and teenagers are not considered to be active TB cases either and are recorded in a separate risk group. This group represents 23.3% of all first-time recorded children and teenagers and 1.6% of all new TB cases. There were 1571 cases like this in total.

Some indicators of fatal outcomes can be criteria of late detection of TB cases as well, such us:

- *Patients who died during the first year of observation and treatment.* These numbered 3934 of all new cases or 4.1%.

- *Patients with a postmortem diagnosis of TB.* These numbered 1663 cases or 1.7%.

- TB patients who were sputum smear–positive diagnosed by direct Z-N microscopy of a sputum smear should be included the cases of late TB detection. These patients made up 19,882 (20.9%) cases.

Thus, 37,996 cases of late TB detection were registered in 2000, which made up 39.9% of all new TB cases.

It is possible that these patients caught tuberculosis in 1999 or even earlier, but TB was only diagnosed in 2000; thus, the data were included in the indicator of TB incidence of 2000. It is very likely that a similar situation happens every year. The above data show that information about some groups of TB patients will be included in the reports on new TB cases sooner or later. These patients include those with chronic fibrous-cavernous forms of lung TB, patients who died of TB, and those with profuse sputum smear–positive disease. Therefore, every year 27,970 (29.3%) of all new cases are not detected in a timely manner. These patients were freely disseminating TB infection during the years preceding the time of detection and were at risk of developing severe forms of TB, the treatment for which is problematic and expensive, and which quite often results in death.

Another group of patients, however, the 10,026 cases in whom tuberculosis was treated without medical intervention (spontaneous resolution), was also not reflected in the indicator of TB incidence. Thus we can suppose that each year the official indicator of TB morbidity is 10.5% less than the real rate of incidence. At present, these patients do not need any treatment and are not dangerous from the epidemiological point of view. When their TB was active, however, no treatment was given to them, and no preventive measures were taken regarding their contacts. Thus, these people were disseminating TB infection, and neither they themselves nor their contacts (at home, at work, etc.) knew about the disease.

As far as reliability of TB morbidity rate figures among the population is concerned, it is necessary to note that these figures are about 10% lower than the real situation because complete information about all new cases is lacking. Up until now, state statistics do not completely cover the patients from other departments (e.g., Ministry of Defence and other structures), and these amount to about 1.5–2% in additional cases. In this respect we can forecast the growth of TB morbidity rates in the near future that reflects better coverage of patients from other departments. But to study the real level of TB prevalence, one should take into account the indicator of TB incidence among the population with permanent residence, and the basic figures of this indicator have not been altered greatly within recent years.

To assess the reliability of TB morbidity rate figures among children, it is necessary to consider the rate of primary infection among children. We have compared childhood TB incidence among different territories of Russia, ranging from the minimum to the maximum level using the primary infection indicator in the same territories. The indicators are not synchronized, and therefore we can suppose that they are not sufficiently reliable. It is important to study the reasons why they do not correspond. It is very likely that different territories have different diagnositic skills, causing us either to over- or underdiagnose TB among children. There is a great need for improvement of clinical and x-ray diagnostics of TB in children.[2]

Comparison of some other indicators proves that they are controversial as well. Higher death rates among new TB cases should correspond to a higher percentage of patients with fibrocavernous lung TB, but we could trace no correlation between these two indicators. Neither could we find any correlation between death rate and the indicator of treatment effectiveness of new TB cases (sputum conversion).

Thus, Russian statistical reporting presents an opportunity to undertake comprehensive and detailed analysis of the epidemiological situation and performance of TB institutions. Analysis of the statistics enables detection of defects in reporting and points us in the direction of what should be done for its improvement.

The increase of TB incidence among groups of the population with weakened immunity demonstrates the growing role of exogenous infection. TB incidence among children is gradually growing as well and has more than doubled since 1989 (from 7.5 to 17.9 per 100,000).[3]

One of the characteristic features of tuberculosis epidemiology in Russia in recent years is the prevailing growth of TB incidence among young persons compared

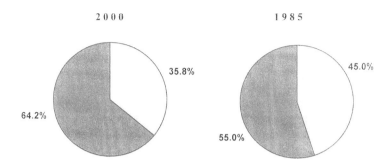

FIGURE 2. Percent of MBT-positive and MBT-negative TB patients among newly identified cases in Russia, by all methods of bacteriological analysis of sputum. *White area*: (positive). *Shaded area*: (negative).

to the elderly. In 1960, when the epidemiological situation was very unfavorable, the highest TB morbidity rate fell on the age group from 20 to 39. In 1965–1992, during the relatively favorable period, the peak of TB incidence was transferred to older persons aged 40–59 years. With deterioration of the epidemiological situation since 1992, the highest TB incidence is again registered in the younger age group. Within last six years, the TB incidence in people aged 15–19 years has increased 2.8 times, in people aged 20–39 years 2.6 times, in those aged 40–59 years 1.8 times, and in those aged 60 years and over 1.5 times.[4]

Men and women demonstrate different tendencies in the dynamics of age indicators of TB morbidity. In 1960–1996 the highest TB incidence in men was registered in the group aged 40–59 years of age, whereas after 1997 the peak of TB incidence was transferred to the younger group. From 1960 until now, the peak of TB incidence among women remains in the same age group of 20–39 years. This is evidence of young women having a predisposition to TB infection. A high level of mortality from tuberculosis among small children, especialy children in the first year of life, is further evidence of an exogenous infection increase.

The rate of TB incidence depends greatly on the quality of TB diagnostics. The decreasing percentage of sputum smear–positive patients among all new cases in recent years is evidence of a poor quality of bacteriologic diagnostics (FIG. 2). Dynamic comparison of the rates of sputum smear–positive and smear-negative TB proves the same. On the one hand, an increase in smear-negative forms of tuberculosis is evidence of worsening performance on the part of bacteriologic laboratories; on the other hand, it may indicate improved diagnosis of minor TB forms.

Is there any correlation between TB incidence in the population and patient treatment outcomes? The comparison of indicators of TB incidence among the population and effectiveness of treatment of new TB cases based on the sputum conversion criterion (by culture) reveals an inverse correlation between these two indicators, which might be producing an effect on each other. On the one hand, deterioration of socioeconomic conditions and worsening of TB service provisions result in TB incidence growth and a decrease in treatment effectiveness. On the other hand, worsening of treatment effectiveness leads to the growth of the infection reservoir because untreated patients lead to infection spreading within the community.

Multidrug resistance cannot produce a great effect on the effectiveness of treatment of new TB cases because they make up only 2.9% of the total. The evidence of this is the lack of correlation between the number of patients with sputum conversion and the number of patients with MDR TB.

CONCLUSIONS

The present-day TB epidemiological situation in Russia is characterized by growing exogenous infection. Peaks of epidemiological deterioration were registered in 1993 and 1999. A remarkable worsening of the epidemiological situation in 1999 was caused by the economic crisis in August 1999 and the dramatic deterioration of the living conditions of the population.

In the 1990s the tendencies of the epidemiologic development have changed. The spread of TB infection is subject to trends similar to those at the beginning of the 20th century. At that time the people who were not TB infected and had no immunity to tuberculosis, such as children, young men, and young women, had the highest TB mortality risk. The year 2000 demonstrated some stabilization of the rates of TB incidence among the population, childhood TB morbidity rates, and death rates among TB patients.

The official indicator of TB incidence among the population does not fully reflect the real level of TB morbidity because of undetected cases (approx. 10%). About 1.5% of cases are not included in state statistical reporting because they are patients of other departments. At the same time, some overdiagnosis of tuberculosis occurs (15%).

To control the spread of TB infection and to reduce the TB infection reservoir, it is necessary to detect TB patients before they become profuse bacillary excretors, to consider high-risk population groups as a first priority, to improve diagnostics, and to provide adequate treatment of TB patients. The procedure of recording/reporting cases needs further improvement as well.

REFERENCES

1. SHILOVA, M.V. 1993. Informative aspects of different indicators for assessment of TB prevalence. Tuberculosis and ecology. RIPh Guardian N1: 29 –33.
2. SHILOVA, M.V. 1999. Tuberculosis in Russia in 1999. Research Institute of Phthisiopulmonology, Moscow Medical Academy. Moscow.
3. AKSYONOVA, V.A., L.V. LEBEDEVA & A.F. MEISLER. 1999. Children's TB in Russia and the objectives of medical service aiming at its prevention and early detection. RIPh Guardian. N1: 23–27.
4. COMSTOCK, W. 2000. Epidemiology of tuberculosis. In Tuberculosis: a Comprehensive International Approach. B. Reichman & E.S. Hershfield, Eds.: 129–156. Marcel Dekker. New York.

Tuberculosis in Russia and the Problem of Multiple Drug Resistance

V.V. YEROKHIN, V.V. PUNGA, AND L.N. RYBKA

Central Tuberculosis Research Institute (CTRI), Russian Academy of Medical Science, Moscow, Russia

ABSTRACT: Tuberculosis cases in Russia doubled from 1991 to 2000, when the incidence reached 90 per 100,000; and Russian TB mortality rates are the highest in Europe. Implementation of WHO-recommended DOTS strategy is in the preliminary stages. The epidemiological data are presented as is the implementation strategy for stabilizing the epidemic.

KEYWORDS: tuberculosis; Russia; prisons: multidrug-resistant TB; epidemiology; DOTS

EPIDEMIOLOGY

Russia still shows high rates of TB morbidity and mortality. There was a doubling in the number of newly detected TB cases in 2000 compared to 1991, with a TB incidence of 90 per 100,000 population. The TB mortality rate has gone up as well, reaching 20.4 per 100,000 in 2000, the highest rate in Europe. More than 40,000 patients with contagious forms of TB are detected in Russia annually. More than 60,000 patients with chronic forms of tuberculosis excreting TB mycobacteria continuously are registered at TB clinics. At present, about 20–25% of new cases of lung TB with bacillary excretion are resistant to TB drugs (DR); in 6.7% of patients, TB mycobacteria are resistant to isoniazid and rifampicin, that is, they are multidrug resistant (MDR). In 1999 the following territories of Russia demonstrated the following rates of primary DR and MDR: Ivanovo Oblast—22% and 1.3%, respectively; Oryol Oblast—30% and 3%; Leningrad Oblast—27% and 5%; Tomsk Oblast—27% and 5%; Maryi-El Republic—20% and 4.3%. The treatment of these cases is extremely difficult, very expensive, and not quite effective.

TUBERCULOSIS IN PRISONS

The TB problem is even more dramatic in the penitentiary system. Here, the TB incidence and rates of TB mortality are 10 times higher than those of the nonincarcerated population. According to the data provided by the Medical Committee of the Penitentiary Department of the Russian Federation (RF) Ministry of Justice in 2000, the incidence of TB was 3,174 per 100,000 prisoners, whereas the TB mortality rate was 171 per 100,000. At penitentiary institutions of pilot regions, the proportion of TB mycobacteria with primary drug resistance to one or more drugs is much higher than that in civil institutions and ranges from 35% to 44%, including 15% to 22% of MDR forms.

THE REASONS FOR A WORSENING TUBERCULOSIS PICTURE

The causes of the present-day epidemiological situation are the following:
(1) Social and economic factors (deterioration of living conditions of a large proportion of the population, migration, unemployment, and resettlement.
(2) Inadequate management of TB services and the existence of a large reservoir of TB infection. There has been a marked reduction in the number of routine check-ups for tuberculosis by fluorographic screening. There has been an increase of TB cases detected as self-referrals to primary medical institutions, which are traditionally not very good at identifying TB cases because of the existence of specialized services.
(3) A shortage of TB drugs.
(4) A lack of strict and effective monitoring of sputum smear–positive patient detection and treatment, coupled with the noncompliant attitude of many patients toward treatment, resulting in the development of drug-resistant (DR) tuberculosis.
(5) The spread of HIV infection.
(6) An underestimate of the existing problem by the Russian Federal Government (RFG) and associated underfunding of the TB service.

The period during which the spread of TB increased coincided with the worsening of treatment effectiveness. Thus, in 1999 sputum smear conversion and cavity closure were reduced by 20% and 24.6%, respectively.

NEW COUNTERMEASURES

Under these circumstances, there is an urgent need for immediate tuberculosis control measures, because TB infection might take epidemic form. In 1998 the RFG adopted a Targeted Federal Program on TB Control, but it was not funded properly, especially during its first two years.

Directly Observed Treatment (Short Course)

WHO has declared that tuberculosis is a global problem and there is a pressing need to change the strategy of its control. The DOTS program is now the recommended system of anti-epidemic measures aimed at the prevention of TB infection spread and the most rational and effective approach in unfavorable socioeconomic circumstances. The major objective of the program is to detect not less than 70% of sputum smear–positive patients, to carry out observed chemotherapy with an optimal combination of TB drugs, and to cure 85% of newly detected cases.

At present, WHO strategy implementation and restructuring of TB services in different territories of Russia is in a preliminary stage. There is now agreement among WHO, the staff of the Central Tuberculosis Research Institute (CTRI), and TB specialists in the regions who have started to implement WHO recommendations. The RFG Ministry of Public Health and administration of the regions adopted mutually agreed-upon programs and action plans, arranged training for the staff, developed essential documents, supplied the necessary quantity of drugs for chemotherapy, and upgraded diagnostic laboratories with binocular microscopes. Implementation of the program started in Ivanovo Oblast in 1994; in Tomsk Oblast and Maryi-El Republic in 1995; in Leningrad, Murmansk, and Arkhangelsk Oblasts in 1998; and in Oryol Oblast in 1999. Since January 4, 2000, it has been started in Novgorod, Novosibirsk, and Vladimir Oblasts; in Altai Krai; and in the Republics of Karelia and Buryatia. Alongside the civil TB service, the program has been in place in the penitentiary service in Ivanovo and Tomsk Oblasts since 1997 and in Nizhny Novgorod, Vladimir, Arkhangelsk, and Kemerovo Oblasts and in the Maryi-El Republic since 1998. The CTRI acts as the methodological center with the WHO Cooperating Center on TB Training and the Coordinating Group based in it.

Implementation of WHO recommendations is now taking place in pilot regions of Russia with WHO participation, active support from CTRI, and sponsorship of nongovernmental organizations (NGOs) from Finland, Norway, the United States, England, and Germany. It has been suggested that some preliminary conclusions be reached to improve this pilot experience before extending the program in Russia.

LESSONS LEARNED

The following lessons have been learned so far from the implementation of WHO recommendations:

First, WHO recommendations on diagnostics, treatment, registration, reporting, and follow-up are quite simple; but their implementation requires great administrative input and the provision of ample time for staff training and the upgrading of laboratories.

Second, there is an obvious improvement in bacteriologic diagnostics of lung TB. The detection of patients with sputum smear–positive disease by the medical service of Ivanovo Oblast increased from 0.04% in 1992 to 46.6% in 1999, and it represented more than a half (52%) of all registered culture-positive patients.

Third, indicators of treatment effectiveness (cured, treatment completed) have not yet reached the level of 85% in the regions implementing WHO recommendations. The two reasons for this are poor patient management and a high incidence of TB mycobacteria resistance to TB drugs. The proportion of unfavorable outcomes (death, treatment failure, relapse) is about 20–25%, which is twice the usual acceptable figure. It is extremely difficult to perform observed treatment of outpatients, and this aim will not be achieved by TB services without the involvement of primary medical institutions. GP nurses as well as Red Cross nurses have been involved in observing patients take TB drugs. A system of incentives has been introduced for patients visiting medical institutions on a regular basis (reimbursement of transport costs and the provision of food), and treatment at home has been arranged as well. Identified rates of TB mycobacterial drug resistance and continuation of sputum smear positivity have resulted in discontinuation of standard treatment and adjustment of drug regimens.

The fourth important component of successful implementation of the program is reliable supplies of both first- and second-line TB drugs. TB spread cannot be controlled without the simultaneous solution of two problems: the treatment of new and relapse cases with mycobacteria sensitive to TB drugs and the treatment of MDR forms of TB and chronic cases.

EXPANDING THE PROGRAM

An expanded program of TB control and treatment of MDR forms has been implemented recently in Tomsk Oblast. At present preliminary measures for its implementation are being undertaken in civil and penitentiary medical institutions of Ivanovo and Oryol Oblasts. Successful implementation of the program is impossible without thorough monitoring of all the other components of the DOTS regime: detection, diagnosis, and treatment.

Both general medical institutions and specialized TB services are involved in microbiological diagnostics of TB in pilot regions. GP clinical diagnostic laboratories perform microscopy of sputum smears for TB mycobacteria on all suspected TB patients, examining not fewer than three specimens within two days.

The CTRI Reference Laboratory performs quality control on bacteriologic examinatons carried out in pilot regions. It controls the quality of first- and second-line drugs; provides sensitivity testing performed by Oblast (Republican) laboratories; and is responsible for administration, implementation, and management of the system of external quality control of TB microbiological diagnostics on the Oblast and Raion levels. Recently, the forms of registration and reporting have been amended in the RF to approximate international standards. Dispensary grouping is being reconsidered as well.

DRUG TREATMENT

The following are the first-line drugs for TB chemotherapy: isoniazid (H), rifampicin (R), pyrazinamide (Z), and ethambutol (E). Data obtained in different regions of Russia confirm high rates of resistance to streptomycin, which is why this antibiotic is not given to treat new cases. There are four categories of patients on different treatment regimens, which are prioritized as follows:

Category I consists of new TB cases with smutum smear–positive pulmonary disease and other seriously ill patients with severe forms of TB (meningitis, pericarditis, peritonitis, bilateral or extensive pleurisy, TB spondilitis, intestinal TB, urine genital TB, and smear-negative pulmonary TB with diffuse lesions of the parenchyma). The treatment regimen followed is $2HRZE$ or $4H_3R_3$, followed by $6HE$. (Large numbers indicate the number of months treatment is given, and the subscripts indicate the number of days per week. Where no subscript is given, a daily regimen is used.)

Category III consists of cases of sputum smear–negative pulmonary TB or other new cases not included in Category I. The treatment regimen for these cases is $2HRZE/4HR$ or $4H3R3/6HE$, similar to Category I.

Category II consists of cases involving relapse and failure of treatment (defaulter). This category is further subdivided into the following two subcategories: Category IIA consists of relapses for which the treatment regimen is $2HRZES/1HRZE/5HRE$ or $5H3R3E3$. Category IIB consists of those cases involving failure of treatment (exacerbation). Treatment regimens are decided individually, depending on the results of DST with obligatory inclusion of not less than two to three second-line drugs.

CONCLUSIONS

It is intended that strategic components of the program will be equally implemented in the regions of Russia (i.e., detection, treatment, registration and reporting), but such specific regional features such as geography, demography, and economic status will affect implementation. The assessment of treatment results is based on sputum smears, cultures, and clinical dynamics revealed by x-ray examination of lungs and other organs. The treatment regimen for TB patients who are sputum smear–positive with MDR bacilli consists of anticollapse therapy, surgery, and the administration of two or three second-line drugs. Obtained data demonstrate that this approach is sufficiently effective in reducing the number of TB patients excreting MDR bacilli.

Implementation of WHO recommendations in the form adapted to Russia is very likely to stabilize the TB epidemiological situation and to reduce TB mortality and morbidity rates. Implementation will also reduce the rates of TB mycobacterial drug resistance including MDR. At least we hope for that. Much will depend on socioeconomic conditions.

Molecular Techniques in the Diagnosis of *Mycobacterium tuberculosis* and the Detection of Drug Resistance

M. CAWS AND F.A. DROBNIEWSKI

PHLS Mycobacterium Reference Unit, Guy's, King's and St Thomas' School of Medicine, King's College Hospital (Dulwich), London SE22 8QF, UK

ABSTRACT: Early diagnosis of *Mycobacterium tuberculosis* disease is crucial in initiating treatment and interrupting the train of transmission. The increasing incidence of MDR TB worldwide has also placed emphasis on the need for early detection of drug resistance, particularly to isoniazid and rifampicin. Molecular diagnostic techniques and automated culture systems have reduced turn-around times in the modern mycobacteriology laboratory, and the continuing evaluation and development of such techniques is increasing the use of molecular technology in developed nations. Simple phenotypic methods for the detection of resistance to first-line drugs and genotypic kit-form assays for detection of rifampicin resistance have been developed that have become key tools in the containment of MDR TB.

KEYWORDS: *Mycobacterium tuberculosis*; drug resistance; multidrug-resistant tuberculosis; TB microbiology

INTRODUCTION

The World Health Organization (WHO) has estimated that one-third of the world's population is infected with *Mycobacterium tuberculosis* (*M.tb*)—two billion people.[1–3] It is the infectious disease with the greatest mortality, with 8 million new cases causing between two and three million deaths annually. Ninety-five percent of the disease burden is borne by developing nations. Tuberculosis is exacerbated by the human immunodeficiency virus (HIV) pandemic, with 6 million people estimated be coinfected worldwide.[4] The incidence of tuberculosis (TB) in many industrialized nations has also risen over the last two decades and is likely to continue to do so. In England and Wales, the incidence of new TB notifications rose from 8.4 per 100,000 in 1993 to 9.2 per 100,000 in 1998,[5] and provisional data show a further rise from 6,144 notifications in 1999 to 6,797 in 2000, an increase of 11% occurring mostly in the capital city, London.

The principal aims of TB microbiology are, first, the detection of mycobacteria, either by microscopy or molecular techniques; second, the isolation and identification by culture, using solid or liquid media; and third, the susceptibility testing of

Address for correspondence: M. Caws, PHLS Mycobacterium Reference Unit, Guy's, King's and St Thomas' School of Medicine, King's College Hospital (Dulwich), East Dulwich Grove, London SE22 8QF, U.K. Voice: 0208 693 1312.

mcaws@hotmail.com

138

cultures and the identification of drug-resistant, particularly multiple drug resistant (MDR TB) isolates. The laboratory is at the core of our understanding of the epidemiology of TB transmission and surveillance of drug-resistance patterns.

Since the development of acid-fast staining techniques in 1882 by Robert Koch, the principles of TB microscopic diagnosis have changed little, and acid-fast smear is still the rapidest method for the detection of *M.tb*. The sensitivity is only around 5×10^3 per ml, and microscopy must be supplemented with culture, which while sensitive is slow, taking 4–6 weeks to produce a positive result on most solid-culture media, such as LJ slopes. Recent development of automated liquid-culture systems, such as the Mycobacterial Growth Indicator Tubes (MGIT Bactec 960, Becton Dickinson, Franklin Lakes, USA) and the MB BacT Alert systems (Organon Technika, Boxtel, The Netherlands), have improved time to detection to 12–18 days and reduced hands-on time compared to their semiautomated predecessor, the Bactec 460TB. For optimal results these systems should be used in conjunction with solid-media-based culture. Safety of liquid culture systems is an important issue, because handling of liquid cultures carries an increased risk of potential microbial contamination of the laboratory from culture vials.

MOLECULAR DIAGNOSTIC TECHNIQUES

The advent of molecular technology has led to the development and implementation of tests that are both rapid and sensitive for the detection and identification of mycobacteria. They can be used in several ways: for the detection of mycobacteria, for the specific detection of *M.tb* complex, for the differentiation of *M.tb* complex and MOTT (mycobacteria other than tuberculosis), and for the detection of drug resistance.

Molecular detection methods utilize a series of common steps, starting with the amplification of nucleic acid sequences, which can be achieved using several techniques. The best known and most widely employed is the polymerase chain reaction (PCR). Other techniques include transcription-mediated amplification (Amplified MTD-2, Gen-probe, San-Diego, USA),[6] strand displacement amplification (Probe-Tec ET, Becton Dickinson, Franklin Lakes, USA),[7] ligase chain reaction (LCX MTB, Abbott, Illinois, USA),[8] and QB replicase Galileo system (Gene-Trak/Vysis, Illinois, USA).[9,10] These alternative techniques have shown performance comparable to PCR. Although some have been withdrawn at the clinical trial stage (Vitros, Johnson & Johnson, Rochester, USA and QB Replicase Galileo System, Gene-Trak/Vysis, Illinois, USA), many are now on the market with sensitivity and specificity consistently evaluated at over 90%. Detection systems can be colorimetric, such as in the Line probe assay, or LiPA (Innogenetics, Zwijndrecht, Belgium), and Amplicor TB (Roche Diagnostics, Indianapolis, USA) or through chemiluminescent or fluorescent tagging of probes.[11]

A major problem for these molecular techniques is cost. While it is relatively easy to scale up production of kits of molecular detection methods, once they have been developed, their execution requires skilled laboratory personnel, the concurrent performance of multiple controls, several dedicated laboratory areas, and the use of relatively expensive consumable reagents. All of these factors make the costs prohibitive for laboratories in developing nations. Furthermore, in developing nations, where perhaps 95% of mycobacterial disease is due to the MTB complex, the use of molecular techniques to differentiate MOTT is of little benefit, as appropriate therapy for MOTT disease is usually unattainable. Therefore, kits such as the Accuprobe system for the identification of a small number of pathogenic mycobacteria, which was introduced commercially on a wide scale in 1987 (Gen-Probe, San-Diego), would be of questionable value in these settings. A similar argument applies to molecular amplification–based methods.

Performance

The performance of molecular techniques in routine clinical use is hard to determine. While tests are being evaluated, they are performed by expert technicians under "ideal" conditions. Often, when these techniques are translated inappropriately to ill-equipped laboratories, performance will markedly decrease, and contamination will generate many false-positive results. Without appropriate, rigorous quality control, this may go undetected. The lack of a perfect gold standard for evaluation further complicates the issue. Discrepancies between culture data and molecular data are reevaluated with reference to presumptive clinical diagnosis; however, where agreement is found, the flawed gold standard is taken to be correct and to validate the result.

Similarly, the sensitivity of such tests is hard to determine. It is sometimes claimed that sensitivity will be theoretically as low as one bacillus, or genome equivalent; however, this is not generally borne out by experimental data. It is likely that organisms will be lost during sample preparation and, in the particular case of mycobacteria, clumping leads to uneven distribution of bacteria throughout the sample, so that duplicate tests often give discrepant results, which can be hard to interpret. The presence of inhibitors, such as drug metabolites or hemoglobin, in the sample can further reduce the sensitivity of the tests on individual samples.

The expense of commercially available molecular diagnostic kits has led many laboratories to develop their own "in-house" assays that, when suitably controlled, have similar sensitivity and specificity to those of commercial systems.

Limitations

Although molecular diagnostic tests provide rapid results, they have several drawbacks. They cannot replace conventional culture techniques and must be used in conjunction with culture to ensure optimal isolation rates and to establish archive cultures for further studies. Multiple negative, positive, and inhibition controls must be performed with each assay, to assure quality and reliability, elevating costs and the time required. Tests should only be carried out by staff with an adequate level of training and skill in molecular testing. Due to the high cost of these tests in routine use, samples should be prioritized rather than tested universally. For example, areas that should receive high priority include the differentiation of *M.tb* complex and *Mycobacterium avium* complex (MAC) or other MOTT in HIV patients, the identification of drug resistance in cases in which there is a high index of suspicion, samples from patients on drug therapy, or "precious" samples such as CSF in which the likelihood of a positive culture is reduced.

MOLECULAR TESTING FOR DRUG RESISTANCE

Mycobacteria spontaneously develop drug resistance, and the rates of mutation are different for each drug. For *M.tb* these have been shown to be approximately 10^8 to 10^9 for isoniazid and streptomycin, 10^{10} for rifampicin, 10^7 for ethambutol, and 10^9 for cycloserine.[12] It has been known almost since the inception of TB chemotherapy, when the first relapses following streptomycin monotherapy were seen, that therapy with any single TB drug leads to the selection of a drug-resistant population. For example, monotherapy with streptomycin led to a rise from 1 in 88,750 drug-resistant mutant bacteria in sputum to 1 in 367 after 15 weeks of treatment.[13] Combination therapy must be used, therefore, to reduce the probability of drug-resistant strains emerging. Multiple drug–resistant TB (MDR TB) is defined as resistance to at least isoniazid and rifampicin. In the United Kingdom, drug resistance has been monitored by the laboratory-based system MYCOBNET since 1994. MDR TB prevalence in initial isolates for the U.K. rose from 0.6% to 1.7% between 1993 and 1996, and then fell to 1.1% in 1999. In 1999, 6.3% of initial TB cases were resistant to one or more first-line TB drugs: 5.9% were resistant to isoniazid, 0.9% were resistant to rifampicin, 0.5% to ethambutol, 0.4% to pyrazinamide, and 1.1% were MDR TB.[14]

Traditional determination of drug resistance is by resistance ratio, minimum inhibitory concentration (MIC), or the proportion methods. These can be done in liquid media, such as Middlebrook 7H9, or solid media, such as Lowenstein-Jensen slopes or Middlebrook 7H10 agar. As with isolation techniques, faster susceptibility testing methods have been developed using the semiautomated Bactec system or automated systems such as MBBacT, MGIT, and Bactec.

The first stage in the development of molecular detection methods for drug resistance was the identification of the relevant genes and mutations involved in drug resistance. The simplest drug to analyze has been found to be rifampicin, for which approximately 95% of all clinical isolates resistant to rifampicin have a mutation in an 81–base pair region (codons 507–533) of the *rpoβ* gene encoding the beta chain of the DNA-dependent RNA polymerase.[15] This has made the development of genotypic methods for the detection of rifampicin resistance relatively straightforward. Because approximately 90% of all rifampicin-resistant isolates in the U.K. are also resistant to isoniazid, a positive result for rifampicin resistance can be taken as a strong indicator of MDR TB. Isoniazid resistance is much more complex, however, as at least four genes are known to be important. These are the *katG* gene, which encodes the catalse-peroxidase enzyme; *inhA/mabA*, which has a role in fatty acid elongation[16]; *ahpC*, which encodes the alkyl hydroperoxide reductase C[17]; and *oxyR*, which is the oxidative stress regulator.[18] Two genes have been identified that are important in streptomycin resistance: the *rrs* gene, which codes for the 16S rRNA, and *rpsL*, which codes for ribosomal protein S12. Similarly, ethambutol resistance involves mutations in the *embA, B,* and *C* genes,[19,20] encoding enzymes involved in lipoarabinomannan and arabinogalactan synthesis. Ciprofloxin resistance is conferred principally by mutations in the *gyrA, gyrB,* and *nor* genes, encoding DNA gyrase subunits A and B and an efflux protein, respectively. In a study by Sreevatsan *et al.*,[21] pyrazinamide resistance was found to be conferred by mutations in the *pncA* gene, which encodes pyrazinamidase. Although 72% of pyrazinamide-resistant isolates carried mutations in this region, there were many mutation sites throughout this gene, which makes the development of tests for pyrazinamide resistance far more complex than rifampicin.

Once genes such as these have been sequenced and the specific mutations identified, there are several options for the genotypic detection of drug resistance. The gold standard is DNA sequencing, but this is impractical in routine clinical use, due to the expense, skill, and time demands of the technique, although systems have become increasingly user-friendly. Alternative techniques that have been employed include PCR single-strand conformation polymorphism (PCR-SSCP) analysis,[22] heteroduplex analysis, mutation-specific priming, restriction enzyme analysis,[23] and solid-phase hybridization methods.[24]

PCR-SSCP relies on the difference in tertiary structure between two single strands of DNA that differ by a single mutation or more. The conformational change of the tertiary structure can be detected by a change in mobility when analyzed on a polyacrylamide gel.

Heteroduplex analysis involves mixing amplified DNA from the sample with that of reference drug–sensitive strains. The DNA is then denatured and cooled again to allow the DNA to hybridize into hybrid double-stranded DNA. The DNA is then analyzed on a denaturing electrophoresis gel. Where the sample DNA carries a drug-resistant mutation, there will be a mismatch in the complementary base-pairing, and the heteroduplex will have a different mobility than the homoduplex.

Solid-phase hybridization analysis involves the immobilization of DNA probes complementary to the most common mutations and to drug-sensitive patterns. Amplified DNA can then be hybridized to the probes and detected through fluorescence, radiolabel, or colorimetric reaction in the normal way. One such assay that is commercially available is the line-probe assay (LiPA, Innogenetics, Zwijndrecht, Belgium) for the detection of rifampicin resistance. One possible disadvantage of genotypic detection methods is that they give no indication of the susceptible-to-resistant ratio of organisms in a population and therefore may lead to the withdrawal of drugs from a regime when their therapeutic value is still high.

Other rapid detection systems have recently been developed based on phenotypic methods, which can be adapted for use as susceptibility tests. One such technique uses a mycobacteriophage such as phAE40 or phG518. Jacobs et al.[25,26] inserted the lux gene, which codes for luciferase, into the phage genome. This enzyme catalyzes the reaction of luciferin with ATP and emits light, which can then be detected. If the mycobacteria are grown in the presence of a drug, where the organism is susceptible, the mycobacteria will die; therefore the phage will fail to replicate, and no light will be emitted. Whereas this technique allows all types of resistant organisms to be detected, regardless of genotype, it requires expensive equipment and is therefore unsuitable for the developing world where rapid detection systems for drug resistance are most urgently required. The same group has addressed this problem by developing a simpler microtiter plate format with a film detection system.[27] A more economical approach is the PhaB (phage-amplified biologically) assay.[28] Mycobacteriophages are added to the test sample which then infect any mycobacteria present where they are protected from the subsequent addition of viricide, which kills all external phages. The viricide is then removed through wash steps, and the sample incubated until lysis of the bacteria releases the phage. The phage progeny are detected by plating onto a lawn of rapidly growing *Mycobacterium smegmatis* in which, following overnight incubation, they form plaques. The system has been adapted to allow susceptibility testing and showed 100% correlation with resistance ratio testing for rifampicin,[29] 94% for izoniazid, 96% for streptomycin, 100% for ciprofloxacin, 88% for ethambutol, and 87% for pyrazinamide.[30] This system is also relatively simple and cheap to perform. However, stringent precautions must be taken in a diagnostic or reference laboratory to avoid the contamination of reference strains and archive samples with mycobacteriophage. Other rapid phenotypic methods that have been investigated include flow cytometry,[31] which requires the provision of prohibitorily expensive equipment, and reverse transcriptase PCR (RT-PCR).

One such RT-PCR assay, which measured a reduction in inducible heat-shock protein *dnaK* mRNA levels in susceptible isolates exposed to rifampicin, showed 96% (46/48) correlation in susceptible isolates and 97% (35/36) correlation in resistant isolates.[29] Alternative RNA-based approaches have included measuring levels of pre-16S rRNA stem sequences through hybidization to specific radiolabeled probes for rifampicin and ciprofloxacin[32] and quantitative analysis of 85B mRNA for rifampicin and isoniazid.[33]

RAPID TESTS IN ROUTINE USE

The Public Health Laboratory Mycobacterium Reference Unit (PHLS MRU) offers a *Fastrack* diagnostic service for the detection of rifampicin resistance, using the commercially available LiPA kit (Innogenics, Zwijndrecht, UK).[34] Correlation with standard methods has been over 90%. Where *Fastrack* was performed on cultures, the correlation was 33/36 (91.7%); on primary specimens, 55/61 (90.2%); and on smear-positive sputum, 44/48 (91.7%). This rapid detection system allowed drug resistance to be detected on average 27.6 days earlier ($n = 56$) for smear-positive sputum specimens, 27.7 days earlier ($n = 61$) for all primary specimens, and 19.1 days ($n = 36$) when used for cultures.[35]

CONCLUSIONS

Molecular techniques have begun to revolutionize the mycobacteriology laboratory in developed nations, improving times for identification and drug susceptibility testing, where the basic methods have remained largely unchanged for nearly a century. Molecular diagnostic services have been introduced for identification from primary specimens, including CSF for the diagnosis of tuberculous meningitis, and drug susceptibility testing, where the greatest success has been with rifampicin-resistance detection and extrapolation to MDR TB presumptive diagnosis. It has been shown that, when rigorous quality control is implemented and staff fully trained in molecular diagnostics, performance can be maintained to trial levels. The great challenges that remain include bringing appropriate techniques to developing nations, where resources are limited. It has been estimated by the World Health Organization that worldwide case detection of sputum-smear positive is only around 35%.[36] The improvement of this figure is crucial to the containment and eventual elimination of tuberculosis worldwide. The spread of MDR TB threatens to undermine advances in TB control, and rapid and economically viable molecular diagnostic tests have a crucial role to play in the rapid diagnosis and treatment of drug-resistant *M.tb*, particularly MDR TB.

REFERENCES

1. DOLIN, P.J., M.C. RAVIGLIONE & A. KOCHI. 1994. Global tuberculosis incidence and mortality during 1990–2000. Bull. WHO **72:** 213–220.
2. DROBNIEWSKI, F.A., A. PABLOS-MÉNDEZ & M.C. RAVIGLIONE. 1997. Epidemiology of tuberculosis in the world. Seminars in respiratory and critical care medicine. **18:** 419–429.
3. RAVIGLIONE, M.C., D.E. SNIDER & A. KOCHI. 1995. Global epidemiology of tuberculosis—morbidity and mortality of a worldwide epidemic. JAMA **273:** 220–226.
4. COKER, R. & R. MILLER. 1997. HIV associated tuberculosis. Br. Med. J. **314:** 1847.
5. KUMAR, D., J.M. WATSON & J.H. DARBYSHIRE. 1997. Tuberculosis in England and Wales in 1993: results of a national survey. Thorax **52:** 1060.
6. MILLER, N., S.G. HERNANDEZ & T.J. CLEARY. 1994. Evaluation of Gen-Probe amplified *Mycobacterium tuberculosis* direct test and PCR for direct detection of *Mycobacterium tuberculosis* in clinical specimens. J. Clin. Microbiol. **32:** 393–397.
7. BERGMANN, J.S., W.E. KEATING & G.L. WOODS. 2000. Clinical evaluation of the BDProbeTec ET system for rapid detection of *Mycobacterium tuberculosis*. J. Clin. Microbiol. **38:** 863–865.
8. PIERSIMONI, C., A. CALLEGARO, C. SCARPARO, *et al.* 1998. Comparative evaluation of the new Gen-Probe *Mycobacterium tuberculosis* amplified direct test and the semi-automated Abbott LCx *Mycobacterium tuberculosis* assay for direct detection of *Mycobacterium tuberculosis* complex in respiratory and extrapulmonary specimens J. Clin. Microbiol. **36:** 3601–3604.
9. SMITH, J.H., G. RADCLIFFE, S. RIGBY, *et al.* 1997. Performance of an automated Q-beta replicase amplification assay for *Mycobacterium tuberculosis* in a clinical trial. J. Clin. Microbiol. **35:** 1484–1491.
10. DELLA-LATTA, P. 1999. The mycobacteriology milestones. Lab. Med. **30:** 408–417.
11. DROBNIEWSKI, F.A., P.G. MORE & G.S. HARRIS. 2000. Differentiation of *Mycobacterium tuberculosis* complex and nontuberculous mycobacterial liquid cultures by using peptide nucleic acid-fluorescence in situ hybridization Probes. J. Clin. Microbiol. **38:** 444–447.
12. GANGADHARAM, P.R.J. 1984. Drug resistance in mycobacteria. CRC Press. Boca Raton, FL.
13. HERBERT, J., J. WATSON & F.A. DROBNIEWSKI. 1999. The UK Mycobacterial Resistance Network Annual Report. Mycobnet Collaborating Group. CDSC. London.
14. TELENTI, A., P. IMBODEN & F. MARCHESI. 1993. Detection of rifampicin-resistance mutations in *Mycobacterium tuberculosis*. Lancet **341:** 647–649.
15. ZHANG, Y., B. HEYM, B. ALLEN, *et al.* 1992. The catalase-peroxidase gene and isoniazid resistance to *Mycobacterium tuberculosis*. Nature **358:** 591–593.
16. QUEMARD, A.J.C., A. SACCHETTINI, C. DESSEN, *et al.* 1995. Enzymatic characterisation of the target for isoniazid in *Mycobacterium tuberculosis*. Biochemistry **34:** 8235–8241.
17. SREEVATSAN, S., X. PAN & J. MUSSER. 1997. Analysis of the oxyR-ahpC region in isoniazid-resistant and -susceptible *Mycobacterium tuberculosis* complex organisms recovered from diseased humans and animals in diverse localities. Antimicrob. Agents Chemother. **41:** 600–606.
18. ALCAIDE, F., G. PFYFFER, A. TELENTI & I. AMALIO. 1997. Role of *embB* in natural and acquired resistance to ethambutol in mycobacteria. Antimicrob. Agents Chemother. **41:** 2270–2273.
19. SREEVATSAN, S., K. STOCKBAUER, X. PAN, *et al.* 1997. Ethambutol resistance in *Mycobacterium tuberculosis*: critical role of *embB* mutations. Antimicrob. Agents Chemother. **41:** 1677–1681.

20. SREEVATSAN, S., X. PAN, Y. ZHANG, *et al.* 1997. Mutations associated with pyrazinamide resistance in *pncA* of *Mycobacterium tuberculosis* complex organisms. **41:** 636–640.
21. TELENTI, A., P. IMBODEN & F. MARCHESI. 1993. Direct, automated detection of rifampin-resistant *Mycobacterium tuberculosis* by polymerase chain reaction and single-strand conformation polymorphism analysis. Antimicrob. Agents Chemother. **10:** 2054–2058.
22. TELENTI, A., F. MARCHESI & M. BALZ. 1993. Rapid identification of mycobacteria to species level by polymerase chain reaction and restriction enzyme analysis. J. Clin. Microbiol. **31:** 175–178.
23. ROSSAU, R., H. TRAORE, H. DE BEENHOUWER, *et al.* 1997. Evaluation of INNO-LiPA Rif. TB assay, a reverse hybridization assay for the simultaneous detection of Mycobacterium tuberclosis complex and its resistance to rifampin. Antimicrob. Agents Chemother. **41:** 2093–2098.
24. CARRIERE, C., P.F. RISKA, O. ZIMHONY, *et al.* 1997. Conditionally replicating luciferase reporter phages: improved sensitivity for rapid detection and assessment of drug susceptibility of *Mycobacterium tuberculosis.* J. Clin. Microbiol. **35:** 3232–3239.
25. JACOBS, W.R. 1993. Rapid assessment of drug susceptibilities of *Mycobacterium tuberculosis* by means of luciferase reporter phages. Science **260:** 819–822.
26. RISKA, P.F., Y. SU, S. BARDAROV, *et al.* 1999. Film-based determination of antibiotic susceptibilities of *Mycobacterium tuberculosis* strains by using a luciferase reporter phage and the bronx box. J. Clin. Microbiol. **37:** 1144–1149.
27. WILSON, S.M., Z. AL-SUWAIDI, R. MCNERNEY, *et al.* 1997. Evaluation of a new rapid bacteriophage-based method for the drug susceptibility testing of *Mycobacterium tuberculosis.* Nature Med. **3:** 465–468.
28. ELTRINGHAM, I.J., F.A. DROBNIEWSKI, J.A. MAGAN, *et al.* 1999. Evaluation of reverse transcription-PCR and a bacteriophage-based assay for rapid phenotypic detection of rifampin resistance in clinical isolates of *Mycobacterium tuberculosis.* J. Clin. Microbiol. **37:** 3524–3527.
29. ELTRINGHAM, I.J., S.M.WILSON & F.A. DROBNIEWSKI. 1999. Evaluation of a bacteriophage-based assay (Phage-amplified biologically assay) as a rapid screen for resistance to isoniazid, ethambutol, streptomycin, pyrazinamide and ciprofloxacin among clinical isolates of *Mycobacterium tuberculosis.* J. Clin. Microbiol. **37:** 3528–3532.
30. KIRK, S.M., G.H. MAZUREK, S.M. CALLISTER & A.V. MOORE. 1998. *Mycobacterium tuberculosis* susceptibility results in 24 hours by using flow cytommetry. Clin. Microbiol. Newslett. **20:** 83–87.
31. CANGELOSI, G.A., W.H. BRABANT, T.B. BRITSCHGI & C.K. WALLIS. 1996. Detection of rifampin and ciprofloxacin resistant *Mycobacterium tuberculosis* by using species-specific assays for precursor rRNA. Antimicrob. Agents Chemother. **40:** 1790–1795.
32. HELLYER, T.J., L.E. DESJARDIN, G.L. HEHMAN, *et al.* 1999. Quantitative analysis of mRNA as a marker for viability of *Mycobacterium tuberculosis.* J. Clin. Microbiol. **37:** 290–295.
33. WATTERSON, S.A., S.M. WILSON, M.D. YATES & F.A. DROBNIEWSKI. 1998. Comparison of three molecular assays for rapid detection of rifampin resistance in *Mycobacterium tuberculosis.* J. Clin. Microbiol. **36:** 1969–1973.
34. DROBNIEWSKI, F.A., S.A. WATTERSON, S.M. WILSON & G.S. HARRIS. 2000. A clinical, microbiological and economic analysis of a national service for the rapid molecular diagnosis of tuberculosis and rifampicin resisatnce in *Mycobacterium tuberculosis.* J. Med. Microbiol. **49:** 271–278.
35. RAVIGLIONE, M.C., C. DYE, S. SCHMIDT & A. KOCHI. 1997. Assessment of worldwide tuberculosis control for the WHO Global Surveillance Monitoring Project. Lancet **350:** 624–529.

Letting the Genome Out of the Bottle

Prospects for New Drug Development

DOUGLAS YOUNG

Department of Medical Microbiology, Centre for Molecular Microbiology and Infection, Imperial College, London SW7 2AZ, UK

ABSTRACT: Use of the information gained from sequencing the *Mycobacterium tuberculosis* genome will enable scientists to accelerate the development of reagents for improved tuberculosis control. Cloning and expressing genes encoding the enzymes involved in cell-wall biosynthesis will provide the tools for screening millions of novel compounds. Cell wall inhibitors will be mainly useful in treating resistant disease, but cost factors are likely to limit the application of novel compounds in the design of new treatment regimens. More effective might be an approach to target metabolic processes that are essential even in nondividing bacteria. A third target for drug action is elimination of latent disease through a drug that acts in synergy with the immune response.

KEYWORDS: tuberculosis; genomic sequencing; drug discovery programs; cell wall enzymes; latent TB infection

Elucidation of the complete genome sequence of *Mycobacterium tuberculosis* provides access to an immense reservoir of fundamental information about the evolution and constitution of the organism.[1] Use of this information to enhance understanding of the biology of tuberculosis is the driving force for research in the post-genomic era.[2] In principle, the genome sequence includes information about all of the possible targets to which new antimycobacterial agents might be directed. At the most direct level, structural and functional information about a particular protein target can be deduced from the sequence of its encoding gene. Further analysis of interactions between individual gene products provides information about the biosynthesis of more complex molecular structures and about the flux of metabolites essential for bacterial viability. How can we use this new information resource to accelerate development of reagents for improved tuberculosis control?

BREACHING THE WALL OF FORTRESS MYCOBACTERIUM

The outer coat is commonly viewed as the defining characteristic of a mycobacterium, determining its microbiological staining properties and its relationships with

Address for correspondence: Prof. Douglas Young, Division of Investigative Science, Imperial College School of Medicine, Norfolk Place, London W2 1PG, U.K.

d.young@ic.ac.uk

external reality.[3] Many current antimycobacterials (isoniazid, ethambutol, ethiona-mide, and pyrazinamide) affect processes involved in cell-wall biosynthesis, and there is every likelihood that novel reagents targeted against similar processes will have comparable efficacy. Many of these biosynthetic pathways are now understood at a genetic level. Knowledge built up through decades of traditional biochemistry allows identification of genes encoding enzymes that make up the pathways, and re-combinant DNA techniques have opened a new era of detailed structure–function analysis. One approach to exploiting this information in drug discovery programs is to clone and express genes encoding selected biosynthesis enzymes. The recombi-nant proteins can be used in functional assays to screen for inhibitors, and at the same time provide the opportunity to generate structural information for optimized drug design.[4] Following an alternative approach, changes induced in the bacteria as a result of the action of an existing drug—characteristic transcriptional signals, for example[5]—can be used to screen for novel compounds that exert an analogous in-hibitory mechanism. Both of these strategies are suitable for use in high-throughput screen formats, allowing testing of millions of novel compounds. Compounds for such screens are typically derived by combinatorial chemistry techniques that use simple building-block strategies to facilitate rapid generation of extensive libraries of structurally diverse small molecules. The principles and practice of modern high-throughput screening, and potential applications to tuberculosis, are comprehensive-ly described in the Scientific Blueprint recently developed by the Global Alliance for TB Drug Development.[6]

Drug discovery programs focused on cell-wall targets have a strong scientific foundation and a well-defined rationale; there are excellent prospects for identifica-tion of novel inhibitory compounds. This approach has the limitation, however, that new compounds are likely to have properties broadly similar to those of current drugs. It may be possible to select for some improvements in pharmacokinetic prop-erties and for avoidance of established resistance mechanisms, but it is hard to en-visage new cell-wall inhibitors driving major changes in the overall design of treatment regimens. They would clearly be drugs of choice for treatment of resistant disease, but cost factors are likely to argue against their routine replacement of ex-isting drugs. In that case, would a pharmaceutical company be able to recoup the considerable costs involved in taking a novel compound through the complex pro-cess of developing a promising "hit" into a clinically useful drug? This would seem to represent a significant economic risk, particularly in light of strong public oppo-sition to the practice of marketing drugs in low-income countries at prices that reflect research and development costs. This economic risk will have to be borne by the public sector; either by funding a guaranteed market for new drugs to treat multi-drug-resistant tuberculosis, or by carrying out at least parts of the development pro-cess within public or charitable institutions. The cost of development of a new drug is generally estimated to be on the order of half a billion dollars. Given the magni-tude of the effect of tuberculosis on global health and economy, this figure is well within the budget of institutions such as the World Bank, and mobilization of public–private financing to promote development of new cell-wall inhibitors warrants high priority in the battle to control tuberculosis.

IN VIVO PHENOTYPES: TARGETING PERSISTENT ORGANISMS

The economic case for drug development is much stronger for a compound that would significantly improve current therapy. A drug that reduced current treatment regimens from six months to six weeks would be likely to be adopted as standard therapy, for example, and would have widespread application even if unit costs were higher than existing drugs. The biological factors dictating the requirement for prolonged therapy in tuberculosis are the subject of extensive speculation.[7] A reasonable hypothesis is that a proportion of the bacteria persist in a form in which they are relatively resistant to the action of the drug. For example, in the case of a drug that acts by inhibition of cell-wall biosynthesis, bacteria will be immune to its effects if they don't happen to be engaged in construction of new cell-wall components. The presence of the drug must therefore be maintained until the persisting bacteria enter a renewed phase of cell division. Can this period be reduced by targeting some metabolic process that is essential even in nondividing bacteria?

It is widely recognized that all bacterial pathogens adapt to the environmental conditions they experience within the infected host and that the resulting biological properties of the organism—the *phenotype*—are therefore different from those seen in the microbiology laboratory. Many investigators are applying post-genomic tools to study the *in vivo* phenotype of *M. tuberculosis*; monitoring patterns of gene and protein expression, and constructing mutants with defects at individual genetic loci. An example of this approach in the context of potential drug discovery is the case of isocitrate lyase. McKinney and colleagues[8] demonstrated that this particular enzyme is essential if *M. tuberculosis* is to set up a chronic infection in mice. In contrast to enzymes required for cell-wall biosynthesis, isocitrate lyase is dispensable during the initial phase of active replication; it is thought to play a role in the lipid-based metabolism that prevails during the persistent phase of the infection. Inhibition of isocitrate lyase activity might therefore be a particularly effective route by which to attack persistent bacteria. The isocitrate lyase gene has been cloned and expressed, providing the basis for a novel drug discovery program.[9]

Targeting of *in vivo* phenotypes generates scientific excitement, but the corresponding drug screens present important practical problems. It can be anticipated that inhibitors of isocitrate lyase will have little or no effect on mycobacterial growth *in vitro*, for example, introducing a requirement for costly screening in animal models at an early stage in the drug discovery program. In an attempt to reproduce *in vivo* phenotypes in a simpler experimental system, we have developed an "*ex vivo*" screen. This involves infecting mice with luminescent reporter strains of *M. tuberculosis*,[10] sacrificing animals after several days or weeks, and establishing cell cultures from spleen or lung cells. Mycobacteria maintained in these cultures resemble those in intact animals in being held under the control of the host immune response and display a drug-susceptibility profile resembling that seen *in vivo*. Establishment of cultures in 24- or 96-well plate formats allows testing of dose–response relationships for multiple compounds from only a small number of animals.

LATENT TUBERCULOSIS

Elimination of latent tuberculosis presents a third target for drug action. It is well established that conventional drug treatment can reduce the risk of development of clinical disease in persons recently infected with *M. tuberculosis*: Can we imagine expanding this approach to prevent tuberculosis in the one-third of the global population estimated to be harboring latent infection? For 90% of infected individuals, the immune response provides a level of protection sufficient to avoid development of active disease, and it is attractive to consider development of drugs or vaccination protocols that might add to this protection. In contrast to the cell-wall targets discussed above, the scientific platform for a rational drug discovery program in this area has yet to be established. Latent infection is dependent on the presence of an effective immune response, but could be explained as an equilibrium reached by actively replicating mycobacteria together with coincident immune killing, the existence of a nonreplicating "dormant" form of mycobacteria (perhaps analogous to the persistent phenotype invoked above), or some intermediate between these two extremes. Understanding how a pathogen can be so aggressive during active disease and yet can maintain a stable and apparently harmless interaction for years or decades within the infected host remains a fundamental challenge for tuberculosis research.

In a recent study, we have investigated the effect of manipulation of antigen expression on *M. tuberculosis* infection in a murine model.[11] By interfering with regulatory circuits involved in control of gene expression, we constructed a mutant strain of mycobacteria characterized by constitutive overexpression of a set of heat-shock proteins. These proteins protect cells during exposure to harsh environments, but also provide an important signal by which the immune system recognizes the presence of an infection. The mutant strain was able to initiate an infection but—like the isocitrate lyase mutant described above—was defective in the chronic phase that develops subsequent to immune recognition. One possible explanation for these observations is that the higher level of antigen expression attracts a stronger immune response, stimulating a greater effort to clear the infection. Induction of antigen expression during latent infection might similarly trigger enhanced immune activity against the persisting organisms. An intervention of this type—a drug acting in synergy with the immune response—would be complementary to the current control strategies based on antibacterial therapy of active disease and prophylactic vaccination before infection.

CONCLUDING COMMENTS

Translation of information from the genome sequence into new tuberculosis drugs is limited by science and by economics. This article outlines a series of opportunities, ranging from scientifically highly tractable targets such as the cell-wall enzymes, to concepts of latent infection that stretch the limits of our conceptual understanding. Judicial investment of money and imagination in these areas will have an important influence on the prospects for improved tuberculosis control in the coming decades.

REFERENCES

1. COLE, S.T., R. BROSCH, J. PARKHILL, *et al.* 1998. Deciphering the biology of *Mycobacterium tuberculosis* from the complete genome sequence. Nature **393:** 537–544.

The Genetics of Host Resistance and Susceptibility to Tuberculosis

PETER DAVIES[a] AND JOHN GRANGE[b]

[a]*Consultant Respiratory Physician, Cardiothoracic Centre, Liverpool L14 3PE, U.K.*

[b]*Department of Microbiology, University College, London, UK*

ABSTRACT: The study of human genomics has the potential to aid our understanding of the interindividual and interpopulation differences in susceptibility to tuberculosis. Resistance to infection is affected by the ability of macrophages to phagocytose and destroy the bacilli. Several genes are involved in this process, and two have been the focus of recent interest: the natural resistance-associated protein (*NRAMP1*) gene and the genes coding for the vitamin D receptor. Susceptibility genes have also been discovered—for example, one on the X chromosome that may explain the increased susceptibility of males to tuberculosis. Studies have also focused on the variations in virulence of the bacillus in both its drug-susceptible and drug-resistant forms. These mechanisms must be understood in order to prevent, or combat, the emergence of a virulent, multidrug-resistant form of the bacillus that would be uncontrollable by means of today's treatment strategies.

KEYWORDS: tuberculosis; human genomics; vitamin D; X chromosome; multidrug-resistant tuberculosis; immune function

INTRODUCTION

One of the great mysteries of tuberculosis is that 90% of people infected with the organism never develop the disease. If even part of the reason for this is attributable to the genetic characteristics of these "resistant" individuals, then a careful study of the human genome should provide important information to help control and even eliminate this disease in the individual human host and the human population.

Within the group of people susceptible to disease, those least able to control growth of bacteria within their tissues run the highest risk of developing acquired drug-resistant disease, because the numbers of bacteria undergoing natural mutation to drug resistance will potentially be greater. The study of the genetic control of tuberculosis, to understand how we resist tuberculosis, is therefore relevant to the understanding of why drug resistance may arise in a human population.

Address for correspondence: Dr. Peter Davies, Cardiothoracic Centre, Thomas Drive, Liverpool L14 3PE, U.K.Voice: 44 151 293 2392; fax: 44 151 228 7688.
P.D.O.Davies@liverpool.ac.uk

GENETIC BASIS OF VARIATIONS IN RESISTANCE

Many studies, notably those on monozygotic and dizygotic twins, indicate that inherited genetic factors play a key role in determining susceptibility and resistance to overt tuberculosis following infection.[1] The immune interactions between the host and the highly complex molecular structure of the tubercle bacillus is multifactorial. From the standpoint of the host, resistance to infection is affected by the ability of macrophages to phagocytose and destroy the bacilli; and this, in turn, is affected by class II HLA-determined antigen presentation, the activation of macrophages by T-cell-derived cytokines and vitamin D,[2,3] and granuloma formation. Several of the genes involved in these processes have been identified, notably the HLA-DR2 and HLA-DQB1 loci, that determine which mycobacterial antigens are presented to helper T cells.[4,5] Non-HLA genes are also involved, and two in particular have been the focus of recent interest. One of these is the so-called natural resistance-associated macrophage protein (*NRAMP1*) gene.[6] This is the human equivalent of a well-described gene in the mouse responsible for resistance to intracellular parasites including *Leishmania*, *Salmonella*, and bacille Calmette-Guérin (BCG). Its function in determining human resistance to tuberculosis is unknown, although there is some evidence that it regulates the concentration of iron and other cations in the phagosomes of the macrophage.

The other non-HLA gene that appears to be involved in resistance to tuberculosis are those coding for the vitamin D receptor.[2] The importance of vitamin D in resistance to tuberculosis has been known since the 18th century, and cod liver oil and exposure to sunlight were once widely used treatments for this disease, with apparent benefit.[7] Interest reemerged during investigations on the cause, previously inadequately explained, of the relatively high incidence of nonrespiratory manifestations of tuberculosis in patients of Indian subcontinent ethnic origin living in the United Kingdom. The fact that a relatively high incidence of nonrespiratory tuberculosis occurs in AIDS patients led to the hypothesis that immigration might be associated with some form of acquired immunodeficiency.[8] A likely cause of this is a lowering, up to a 10-fold lowering in some cases, of serum vitamin D (25 hydroxycholecalciferol) levels in immigrants from tropical countries after arrival in the cold and cloudy United Kingdom.[9] This vitamin is essential for the full expression of macrophage activation, a key component of protective immunity in tuberculosis.[10] It is therefore postulated that people may be infected and develop latent tuberculosis in their countries of origin and proceed to active disease after their vitamin D levels fall in their new home country.

The ability of vitamin D to activate macrophages, and thereby to affect the outcome of infection by the tubercle bacillus, is genetically determined. Studies on a predominantly vegetarian population of Gujarati Asians living in west London suggested that the expression of genetically determined differences in vitamin D function are accentuated under conditions causing a deficiency of this vitamin. Thus the combination of the TT/Tt VDR genotype and vitamin D deficiency, and of the ff genotype and undetectable serum vitamin D levels, strongly predisposed these persons to active tuberculosis.[3]

A number of other genes affecting immune function have been associated with resistance to tuberculosis,[11] including genes determining the allotypes of the *Km*1 light chain immunoglobulin,[12] and of haptoglobin.[13,14] Whether these genes are of

TABLE 1. Factors involved in susceptibility or resistance to tuberculosis and subject to genetically determined variation

Factor or gene	Function or mode of action
Natural resistance-associated macrophage protein (NRAMP 1)	? Regulation of phagosome cation levels
HLA Class II	Antigen presentation
Vitamin D receptor	Macrophage activation
Locus on chromosome 15	Unknown
Locus on X chromosome	Unknown: may account for higher rates of tuberculosis in males
Haptoglobin	? Regulator of lymphocyte function
Km1 immunoglobulin allotypes	? Related to autoimmune tissue damage
Various cytokines	T-cell maturation and patterns of immune reactivity

direct functional importance or are merely linked to resistance-determining genes remains to be determined. Other genes of putative relevance are those determining the function of various cytokines involved in protective immunity.[15] Such specific genetic defects are rare; and, in general, susceptibility and resistance to tuberculosis is the result of a large number of genes inherited in a complex way, as clearly demonstrated in family-based linkage studies and population-based case-control studies.[11] The principal determinants of susceptibility and resistance to tuberculosis that have been shown to be affected by genotypic variation are listed in TABLE 1.

SUSCEPTIBILITY GENES

Resistance to tuberculosis is, at least in part, determined by genetic factors: certain genes are responsible for susceptibility to the disease. A major susceptibility allele may arbitrarily be defined as one with prevalent susceptibility variants determining a relative risk of disease of greater than threefold. A high prevalence of this allele within the disease population, usually of greater than 10%, will also be required to show susceptibility. In general, a genetic effect of a particular size may result from a large number of minor susceptibility genes (polygenes) or from a few major genes with polygenes. A large number of candidate genes, for example those affecting the synthesis of the cytokines tumor necrosis factor (TNFα) and INF-γ, that might have been expected to show association with tuberculosis have not done so.

TECHNIQUES OF GENE DETECTION

There are two methods for identifying susceptibility genes, and each has its merits and weaknesses. Linkage studies are family based, and data collection may prove difficult. They also tend to have a low power, so that moderate effects can be missed. On the other hand, as they are systematic and comprehensive, they are able to detect all major genes. Data is easier to collect in case-control association studies; and, because of their higher power, they can detect moderate effects. As they are based on the candidate gene approach, however, they can miss major genes. Some 300 markers are required to screen the entire human genome by linkage analysis compared to approximately 100,000 markers required to screen the human genome by association. There are about 200 genes in the region of a linkage.

An extensive genome-wide study in the Gambia and South Africa, based on families with two or more siblings developing tuberculosis, revealed two chromosomal regions that linked to susceptibility to clinical tuberculosis.[11] An independent association-based analysis using microsatellite markers supported the presence of susceptibility genes on chromosome 15 and the X chromosome. The finding of a susceptibility locus on the X chromosome may explain the widely documented increased susceptibility of males to tuberculosis. In the Gambian study, 70% of the tuberculosis patients were male.

THE MULTIFACTORIAL NATURE OF SUSCEPTIBILITY TO TUBERCULOSIS

It may therefore be concluded that the genetically determined components of the immune responses to tuberculosis and leprosy[16] are principally the results of the cumulative impact of a very large number of minor genes, but some major loci exist and may be mapped by linkage analysis of affected sibling pairs. From this it may be concluded that the outcome of infection depends on a highly complex interaction between the host immune system and the numerous molecules comprising the tubercle bacillus. Just as the innate and acquired host determinants of resistance and susceptibility are complex and multifactorial, so are the determinants of virulence of the tubercle bacillus. Many putative determinants of mycobacterial virulence have been described, and these interact with various components of the immune system. These include factors facilitating uptake of bacilli by macrophages and other cells and survival within macrophages and more recently discovered factors affecting bacterial dormancy and the phenomenon of latency.

Mycobacterial virulence factors determine the chance that an infection will proceed to a recognizable change in immune function, an *immunologically effective contact*, usually detected as the development of tuberculin positivity, and the chance of infection progressing to clinically overt disease—the *disease ratio*. Determination of both in humans is notoriously difficult, because there is no way of detecting infection that does not lead to immunological changes, and the nature of the infecting bacillus leading to the development of tuberculin positivity but not overt disease cannot be determined. In this context, it has been suggested that the serial mutations causing a drug-susceptible tubercle bacillus to become multidrug resistant would affect, possibly reduce, its "fitness" or virulence.[17] If this is indeed the case, a low disease ratio would lead to the eventual decline in prevalence of initial cases of multidrug-resistant tuberculosis, provided that the emergence of new cases of acquired resistance were prevented by strict application of the World Health Organization DOTS (directly observed treastment, short term) strategy. If, on the other hand, multidrug-resistant bacilli retain full virulence, then specific, albeit very costly, control measures such as the "DOTS-plus" strategy would be essential. One recent study suggests that the transmissibility and disease ratio of drug-susceptible and multidrug-resistant tuberculosis is of a similar order.[18] (In this respect, early findings that isoniazid-resistant strains were of low virulence for the guinea pig led to the dangerously false assumption that virulence for humans was likewise reduced. The ensuing use of isoniazid monotherapy, notably in India, for cases of overt tuberculosis generated a problem of isoniazid resistance that is with us today.) Clearly, further epidemiological and molecular microbiological work on this important issue is required in order that optimum disease control strategies may be planned.

CONCLUSIONS

The study of human genomics has a great potential to aid our understanding of the interindividual and interpopulation differences in susceptibility to tuberculosis. It can also be used to identify the effects of millennia of contact with *M. tuberculosis* on the evolution of our genome. The genomes of both *Homo sapiens* and *M. tuberculosis* have been mapped, and both remarkable achievements should help us to identify all the immunological, molecular, and biochemical pathways involved in susceptibility and resistance to tuberculosis and thereby aid the development of novel vaccines, diagnostic tests and therapies—both drugs and immunotherapeutic agents.

Over millennia, the human genome has evolved to afford variable though generally good protection against a fairly homogeneous population of tubercle bacilli. Only for the last few decades have genetically altered multidrug-resistant bacilli been selected for, producing unpredictable interactions with our immune systems. Animal and *in vitro* cell systems, despite inherent weaknesses and dubious relevance to human disease, suggest that tubercle bacilli are divisible into "wimpy" and "burly" variants.[19] Are those that have mutated to multidrug resistance, of genetic necessity, always among the "wimps," or could "burly" resistant variants arise and cause serious, spreading epidemics uncontrollable by the strategies in place today? Answers to these questions are urgently required, before a potential human health disaster strikes.

ACKNOWLEDGMENT

We would like to thank Professor Adrian Hill, who gave the original talk at the meeting, for his helpful suggestions in compiling this paper.

REFERENCES

1. COMSTOCK, G.W. 1978. Tuberculosis in twins: a re-analysis of the Prophit survey. Am. Rev. Respir. Dis. **117:** 621–624.
2. BELLAMY, R., C. RUWENDE, T. CORRAH, *et al.* 1999. Tuberculosis and chronic hepatitis B virus infection in Africans and variation in the vitamin D receptor gene. J. Infect. Dis. **179:** 721–724.
3. WILKINSON, R.J., M. LLEWELYM, Z. TOOSSI, *et al.* 2000. Influence of vitamin D deficiency and vitamin D receptor polymorphisms on tuberculosis among Gujarati Asians in west London: a case-control study. Lancet **355:** 618–521.

4. BOTHAMLEY, G.H., J.S. BECK, G.M. SCHREUDER, *et al.* 1989. Association of tuberculosis and *M. tuberculosis*-specific antibody levels with HLA. J. Infect. Dis. **159:** 549–55.

5. GOLDFELD, A.E., J.C. DELGADO, S. THIM, *et al.* 1998. Association of an HLA-DQ allele with clinical tuberculosis. J. Am. Med. Assoc. **279:** 226–228.

6. BELLAMY, R., C.R. RUWENDE, T. CORRAH, *et al.* 1998. Variations in the NRAMP-1 gene and susceptibility to tuberculosis in West Africans. N. Engl. J. Med. **338:** 640–444.

7. 1849. Report: Cod-liver oil treatment of tuberculosis. Brompton Hospital Records **1849:** 38.

8. DAVIES, P.D.O. 1985. A possible link between vitamin D deficiency and impaired host defence to *Mycobacterium tuberculosis*. Tubercle **66:** 301–306.

9. DAVIES, P.D.O. 1989. Vitamin D and tuberculosis. Am. Rev. Respir. Dis. **139:** 1571.

10. ROOK, G.A.W. 1988. The role of vitamin D in tuberculosis. Am. Rev. Respir. Dis. **138:** 768–770.

11. BELLAMY, R., N. BEYERS, K.P. MCADAM, *et al.* 2000. Genetic susceptibility to tuberculosis in Africans: a genome-wide scan. Proc. Natl. Acad. Sci. USA **97:** 8005–8009.

12. GIBSON, J.A., J.M. GRANGE, J.S. BECK & T. KARDJITO. 1987. An association between Km1 immunoglobulin allotype and pulmonary tuberculosis in Indonesia. Exp. Clin. Immunogenet. **4:** 129–135.

13. SHENDEROVA, R.J. & N.A. OSINA. 1991. Syvorotochenye sistemy krovi u bol'nykh tuberkulezom [The blood serum systems in patients with tuberculosis]. Probl. Tuberk. **3:** 54–56. (In Russian with English summary)

14. GRANGE, J.M., T. KARDJITO, J.S. BECK, *et al.* 1985. Haptoglobin: an immunoregulatory role in tuberculosis? Tubercle **66:** 41–47.

15. BELLAMY, R., C. RUWENDE, T. CORRAH, *et al.* 1998. Assessment of the interleukin 1 gene cluster and other candidate gene polymorphisms in host susceptibility to tuberculosis. Tuberc. Lung Dis. **79:** 83–89.

16. SIDDIQUI, M.R., S. MELSNER, K. TOSH, *et al.* 2001. A major susceptibility locus for leprosy in India maps to chromosome 10p13. (letter) Nature Genet. **27:** 439–441.

17. REMUS, N., J. REICHENBACH, C. PICARD, *et al.* 2001. Impaired interferon gamma-mediated immunity and susceptibility to mycobacterial infection in childhood. Paediatr. Res. **50:** 8–13.

18. DYE, C. & B.G. WILLIAMS. 2000. Criteria for the control of drug-resistant tuberculosis. Proc. Natl. Acad. Sci. USA **97:** 8180–8185.

19. SMALL, P.M. 1999. Tuberculosis in the 21st century: DOTS and SPOTS. Int. J. Tuberc. Lung Dis. **3:** 949–955.

Pharmacological Issues in the Treatment of Tuberculosis

CHARLES A. PELOQUIN

Department of Medicine, National Jewish Medical and Research Center, Denver, Colorado 80206, USA

Schools of Pharmacy and Medicine, University of Colorado, Denver, Colorado 80206, USA

ABSTRACT: A thorough review of the clinical trial data combined with new *in vitro* experimental information may make the optimization of dosages of TB drugs possible. Several factors can affect the selection and dosage of TB drugs including hepatic and renal impairment, pregnancy, duration of disease before treatment, and extent of debilitation. Drug interactions and pharmacodynamics must be considered, and their roles are discussed.

KEYWORDS: pharmacology; tuberculosis; dosing regimen; cycloserine; toxicity; therapeutic drug monitoring

INTRODUCTION

The topic of the pharmacology of the tuberculosis (TB) drugs is sufficiently large that only selected topics will be presented here. The first part of the discussion will be on general pharmacokinetic and pharmacodynamic principles and how they may relate to the TB drugs.[1] Data regarding these relationships generally can be derived in one of three ways. First, *in vitro* models can be used to simulate animal or human pharmacokinetics, once some knowledge of the *in vivo* system is acquired. Then, various techniques can be tried in which the organism (*M. tuberculosis*, in this case) is exposed to varying concentrations of the drugs. One can vary the peak concentration (C_{max}) and the duration that the organism is exposed to the drug (TIME), and one can integrate the concentration-versus-time curve to define an area under the curve (AUC).[2] All of these parameters can be compared to the minimal inhibitory concentration (MIC) determined *in vitro*, and calculations can be made for the relationships C_{max}/MIC, AUC > MIC, and TIME > MIC. For gram-positive and gram-negative infections, we have come to learn that for intracellular poisons such as the quinolones, the aminoglycosides, and probably the rifamycins, maximizing the C_{max}/MIC is desirable.[3,4] High C_{max}/MIC ratios tend to improve bacterial killing and may limit adaptive resistance and the selection of resistant subpopulations. For cell-wall-active agents such as the penicillins and the cephalosporins, TIME > MIC should be maximized when treating gram-positive and gram-negative infections.[5]

Address for correspondence: Charles A. Peloquin, Pharm.D., Pharmacokinetics Laboratory, Room D-106, National Jewish Medical and Research Center, 1400 Jackson Street, Denver, CO 80206. Voice: 303-398-1427; fax: 303-270-2229.

peloquinc@njc.org

MYCOBACTERIUM TUBERCULOSIS

These relationships work well for rapidly multiplying aerobic cocci and bacilli during logarithmic-phase growth. A similar state exists for most of the tubercle bacilli early in the treatment of TB. *In vitro*, it is more difficult to perform similar tests for the slow-growing *M. tuberculosis* than for bacteria, so less data are available.[6] Further, *M. tuberculosis* can achieve a poorly understood "latent" state *in vivo*, which is most likely to affect these relationships adversely. Organisms that are multiplying very slowly, or only intermittently, will be less susceptible to the actions of the drugs. Research efforts continue to try to define the key parameters for the TB drugs. In the author's opinion, C_{max} is likely to remain the most important parameter for drugs such as levofloxacin, streptomycin, amikacin, rifampin, rifabutin, and rifapentine, at least early in the treatment of a patient. For cycloserine, which has a mechanism of action that parallels that of penicillin, TIME > MIC is likely to be the most important. For the other agents that affect steps leading up to cell-wall construction, such as isoniazid, ethionamide, and ethambutol, an argument can be made either way. Only refined *in vitro* and *in vivo* testing will define the key pharmacodynamic parameters for these drugs. The advantage of acquiring such information is that we may rethink our dosing strategies. By combining a thorough review of the clinical trial data with new experimental information, it may be possible to optimize the dosing of these drugs. The results of such a new approach could include fewer failures and fewer relapses during treatment. A more distant goal would be shorter durations of treatment.

DOSING REGIMENS

When considering "optimized" dosing regimens, it is important to bear in mind factors inside the patient that can affect the relationships between the drugs and the organisms. The calculations of C_{max}/MIC, AUC > MIC, and TIME > MIC are based on what occurs in the blood or extracellular fluid. It does not directly address the issue of intracellular activity of the drugs. It is known that some drugs, such as the quinolones and the rifamycins, accumulate within white blood cells, including macrophages. That does not necessarily mean, however, that high concentrations of the active form of these drugs are present within the same intracellular compartment as *M. tuberculosis*. Therefore, enhanced intracellular penetration may not be synonymous with enhanced intracellular activity.

Other factors may weaken the relationships between the calculated pharmacodynamic parameters and *in vivo* activity in selected clinical cases. If the organisms are in areas where some of the drugs do not penetrate well, such as in the cerebrospinal fluid, aqueous humor, or bone, then the pharmacodynamic relationships may not hold up. Also, in selected areas of infection, such as abscesses and empyemas, the pH may decrease, or the oxygen content may decrease. These factors could reduce the activity of certain drugs, including the aminoglycosides. Finally, although it is infrequently an issue in the treatment of tuberculosis, foreign bodies can prevent the drugs and host cells from clearing the organisms. These various situations may require different dosing strategies than typically employed in "garden variety" cases.

DRUGS IN THE TREATMENT OF TUBERCULOSIS

If one examines the pharmacodynamic parameters for the TB drugs, it is clear that rifampin and isoniazid are considerably more potent than the other TB drugs, especially in regard to C_{max}/MIC. Loss of these two drugs cannot be offset. Clinical data prove that multidrug-resistant tuberculosis (MDR TB) takes far longer to cure, if cure can be achieved at all.[7] The other drugs perform best in supporting roles when given concurrently with rifampin and isoniazid. When these drugs are forced into the leading roles, the results for the patient are generally worse.

Unique among the "second-line" TB drugs is cycloserine.[8] This drug, which is also active against selected bacteria, has a long serum half-life. With the usual daily doses of 250 to 500 mg given twice daily, TIME > MIC can reach 100%. Given its cell-wall-focused mechanism of action, cycloserine is a drug that can be dosed in a manner that optimizes its activity. In contrast, ethionamide barely achieves C_{max}/MIC ratios in excess of 1, and with its short half-life, these inhibitory concentrations cannot be sustained.[9] Therefore, ethionamide may be considered the weakest of the TB drugs. That, combined with its propensity to cause serious gastrointestinal irritation, generally leaves ethionamide as the last of the TB drugs to be used. It appears that the propyl derivative prothionamide offers little advantage over ethionamide in these areas.

Other factors may affect the selection of TB drugs. Pregnancy and lactation are situations in which toxicity to a "third party" must be considered.[10] Ethionamide is known to be teratogenic, and the aminoglycosides have been associated with decreased hearing in newborns. So, unless the mother's survival requires their use, these agents should be avoided during pregnancy. Although nursing mothers deliver drug to their infants through breast milk, the doses provided are small and generally are not believed to be significant.

HEPATIC AND RENAL IMPAIRMENT

Hepatic and renal dysfunction may force clinicians to alter their drug selection. Ethambutol, cycloserine, levofloxacin, and the aminoglycosides depend significantly upon renal clearance for removal from the body.[10] Further, certain metabolites, including pyrazinoic acid, 5-hydroxypyrazinoic acid, and acetyl-*para*-aminosalicylic acid also require renal clearance. The toxicity of these metabolites is not known, nor is their contribution to the toxicity profile in combination with their parent drugs, so these factors must be considered when dosing with these agents. In general, for patients with renal failure, we recommend giving standard doses (those typically given daily) no more than three times weekly for ethambutol, aminoglycosides, and pyrazinamide. Levofloxacin probably can be given daily or every other day, depending on the severity of the renal dysfunction.[11] Because we give once-daily doses of levofloxacin for our TB patients with normal renal function, this may not require much of a change. It is possible to substitute ciprofloxacin for levofloxacin, since the former is cleared hepatically as well as renally. Other drugs may be used. We have had some experience giving *para*-aminosalicylic acid (PAS) granules twice daily in patients with renal failure.[12] Because only PAS, and not acetyl-PAS, has antimycobacterial activity, we try to dose PAS in a way that keeps inhibitory concentrations in the blood for most of the dosing interval. Our review of the literature indicates that there does not appear to be a good reason to avoid PAS in patients with renal failure who require the drug.

Hepatic dysfunction, as measured by changes in AST, ALT, and bilirubin, does not produce predictable effects on the hepatic clearances of drugs. Rifampin, isoniazid, pyrazinamide, ethionamide, PAS, and, in part, ciprofloxacin require hepatic clearance for removal from the body.[10] These drugs must be used cautiously in patients with hepatic dysfunction. With several of the TB drugs, an additional concern is the extent to which the TB drugs are producing the hepatic dysfunction. In patients with either renal or hepatic dysfunction, there is a chance to either underdose or overdose the patient. Clinicians should consider the option of therapeutic drug monitoring (TDM) in such cases, so that the appropriate, individualized dose can be provided to each patient.[2]

THERAPEUTIC DRUG MONITORING

Therapeutic drug monitoring (TDM) is never a substitute for sound clinical judgment, nor is it a substitute for directly observed treatment, when indicated. Nevertheless, TDM is a useful tool in a variety of clinical situations. It allows one to determine the extent to which the failure to achieve the desired clinical and bacteriological outcomes can be attributed to the inadequate dosing of the drugs. It also can resolve issues of drug–drug interactions before the patient experiences failure, relapse, or toxicity. In these ways, TDM is a very powerful ally in the management of complex clinical cases.

Several studies have looked at the serum concentrations of the TB drugs in patients with TB.[2,13–15] The available data suggest that TB treatment failures or recurrences result from a complex combination of factors, only one of which is inadequate drug doses. The other factors are not well defined and may include extent of disease, duration of disease before treatment, extent of debilitation, and possibly race. Further, additional patient-specific factors probably contribute to outcome. Therefore, it remains unlikely that small pharmacokinetic studies will provide definitive data regarding the role of TDM in the management of TB, and this topic is likely to remain controversial for years to come. Given the debates that surround aminoglycoside, vancomycin, and HIV protease inhibitor monitoring, TB drug TDM is in good company as a topic for debate.[16–22]

Several general principles can be stated that may help to put this issue in perspective.[23] Clearly, patients require some drug concentration for effect. Based on the above considerations, no single value is the "right" value for all patients. Ideally, one doses a drug based on clinical judgments regarding the patient's need for the drug. The initial dosing regimen then can be tested in the patient, and the serum concentrations measured. Subsequently, doses can be adjusted as needed. For populations of patients, the target ranges need to be designed broadly enough to avoid underdosing the most vulnerable patients. Therefore, many patients with serum concentrations modestly below the ranges should still be adequately treated. This conservative approach to constructing "normal" ranges makes it difficult to use "below the range" as a simple cut-off for use in single and multivariate analyses. Such an approach likely will not define the contribution of TDM to the care of TB patients.

A further confounding factor is the fact that patients receive multiple antibiotics at the same time.[24] It is not known whether a patient can have adequate concentrations of two out of three drugs, or three out of four drugs, and still be adequately treated. Clearly, it would depend on the patient's condition and which drugs are being considered. I have seen many clinical cases where low concentrations directly contributed to a poor response to treatment. Further, adjustment of the doses has overcome this problem, ultimately leading to successful clinical outcomes.[25,26] However, it is very difficult to identify the candidates for TDM at the outset of treatment based solely on demographic characteristics.

PHARMACODYNAMIC RELATIONSHIPS

One way to conceptualize the pharmacodynamics of any drug, and of the TB drugs in particular, is to picture an "S"-shaped curve. Typically, these pharmacodynamic relationships between serum drug concentrations (X) and the probability of therapeutic response (Y) can be described mathematically by Hill equations (FIG. 1).[1] At the lower left end of the curve, there is insufficient drug present to produce

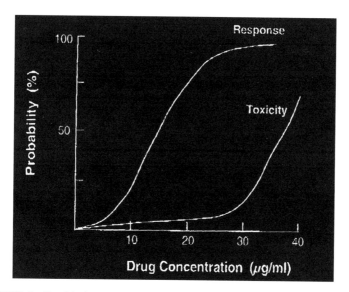

FIGURE 1. Graphical representation of concentration–response curves. "Response" represents the probability curve for therapeutic efficacy. "Toxicity" represents the probability curve for adverse drug reactions. In this example, concentrations between 20 and 30 µg/ml are likely to be effective, yet unlikely to be toxic. That forms the bases of a "therapeutic range." Note that some patients may respond, while others may be toxic, above or below that concentration range.

an observable response. Then, on the steep portion of the curve, modest changes in the serum concentrations produce relatively large changes in response. Such drugs are often termed "concentration-dependent" in regards to their activity. This appears to be the case with the quinolones, aminoglycosides, and rifamycins. Once the concentrations reach the plateau at the upper right portion of the curve, additional drug does not appear to produce further increases in response. Drugs operating in this portion of the curve are often termed "concentration-independent" in regards to their activity. Antibiotics in this category include penicillins, cephalosporins, and vancomycin.

Clearly, two factors greatly affect our perceptions of concentration–response relationships. One is the size of the steep portion of the curve. For some drugs, small increments in concentration complete the transition from no response to full response. For others, it may take large concentration increases to "saturate" the system. Second and most importantly, the toxicity profile of the drug dictates where on the curve we must operate. Aminoglycosides are "concentration-dependent" drugs in the clinical setting because toxicity prevents us from giving penicillin-sized doses to our patients. If we gave 4 grams of gentamicin per dose to our patients with gram-negative infections, for example, we might consider the drug "concentration-independent." In other words, we may have maximized its concentration response. For certain classes of drugs, however, the concentration (X) versus toxicity (Y) curve closely parallels the concentration–response curve. The separation between these two curves along the x-axis defines the "therapeutic range" of the drug. It is to be hoped that there are concentrations where a high probability of response is seen before there is an attendant high probability of toxicity. When a disease threatens the patient's life, it may be necessary to accept additional toxicity in order to cure the patient. These difficult decisions are best arrived at through discussions with the patient, whenever the clinical circumstances permit that.

SERUM CONCENTRATIONS

Once the decision is made to use an antibiotic, the targeted serum concentrations should be achieved as precisely as possible.[27] Carefully timed serum concentrations can be used to verify the doses or to allow calculation of new doses. It is important to consider that the decision to collect serum concentrations implies that the decision will be made to change the dose if necessary. It is not a good use of resources to acquire serum concentrations and then to ignore them. Some patients will require doses above the "usual" or "standard" doses, in spite of "absolute" terminology used in some dosing guidelines.[28] The "maximum" dose for any patient is the dose that produces the desired therapeutic effect with an acceptable degree of toxicity. Further, the extent of drug–drug interactions can be very difficult to predict in an individual patient. TDM may reveal that a particular patient needs far more than the usual dose of a drug because a second drug has increased its clearance. When such patients receive three or more interacting drugs, it is nearly impossible to predict the serum concentrations of each drug.[13] These clearly are situations where TDM is the preferred path for patient care.

INDICATIONS FOR SERUM CONCENTRATION MONITORING

When TB patients fail to respond appropriately to directly observed treatment, serum concentration monitoring and repeat susceptibility testing should be performed. Critically ill TB patients should receive drugs intravenously if possible. Injectable dosage forms are available for isoniazid, rifampin, streptomycin or amikacin, levofloxacin, and ciprofloxacin. The doses of drugs administered orally or by naso-gastric tube should be verified using TDM. In the treatment of MDR TB, the achievable serum concentrations of the "second-line" TB drugs are on the lower portion of the concentration–response curve. Therefore, it is reasonable to check the serum concentrations and adjust the doses of these weak drugs before embarking on many months of potentially toxic treatment. In conjunction with sound clinical judgment, TDM allows considerable flexibility in managing difficult cases of TB and MDR TB.

REFERENCES

1. BELLISSANT, E., et al. 1998. Methodological issues in pharmacokinetic–pharmaco-dynamic modeling. Clin. Pharmacokinet. **35:** 151–166.
2. PELOQUIN, C.A. 1997. Using therapeutic drug monitoring to dose the antimycobacterial drugs. Clin. Chest Med. **18:** 79–87.
3. LODE, H., et al. 1998 Pharmacodynamics of fluoroquinolones. Clin. Infect. Dis. **27:** 33–39.
4. LACY, M.K., et al. 1998. The pharmacodynamics of aminoglycosides. Clin. Infect. Dis. **27:** 23–27.
5. TURNIDGE, J.D., et al. 1998 The pharmacodynamics of β-lactams. Clin. Infect. Dis. **27:** 10–22.
6. BARTMANN, K. 1988. Antituberculosis Drugs. Springer-Verlag. Berlin.
7. GOBLE, M., et al. 1993. Treatment of 171 patients with pulmonary tuberculosis resistant to isoniazid and rifampin. N. Engl. J. Med. **328:** 527–532.
8. BERNING, S.E. & C.A. PELOQUIN. 1998. Antimycobacterial agents: cycloserine. In Antimicrobial Chemotherapy. V.L. Yu et al. Eds.: 638–642. Williams and Wilkins. Baltimore, MD.
9. BERNING, S.E. & C.A. PELOQUIN. 1998. Antimycobacterial agents: ethionamide. In Antimicrobial Chemotherapy. V.L. Yu et al. Eds.: 650–654. Williams and Wilkins. Baltimore, MD.
10. PELOQUIN, C.A. 1991. Antituberculosis drugs: pharmacokinetics. In Drug Susceptibility in the Chemotherapy of Mycobacterial Infections. L. Heifets, Ed.: 59–88. CRC Press. Boca Raton, FL.
11. MCEVOY, G.K., Ed. 2001. AHFS Drug Information. American Society of Hospital Pharmacists. Bethesda, MD.
12. MALONE, R.S., et al. 1999. The effect of hemodialysis on cycloserine, ethionamide, para-aminosalicylate, and clofazimine. Chest **116:** 984–990.
13. BURMAN, W.J. 1999. Therapeutic implications of drug interactions in the treatment of HIV-related tuberculosis. Clin. Infect. Dis. **28:** 419–430.
14. NARITA, M., et al. 2001. Tuberculosis recurrence: multivariate analysis of serum levels of tuberculosis drugs, human immunodeficiency virus status, and other risk factors. Clin. Infect. Dis. **32:** 515–517.

15. BURMAN, W.J. 2001. Comparative pharmacokinetics and pharmacodynamics of the rifamycin antibiotics. Clin. Pharmacokinet. **40:** 327–341.
16. BARZA, M. & M. LAUERMANN. 1978. Why monitor serum levels of gentamicin? Clin. Pharmacokinet. **3:** 202–215.
17. MCCORMACK, J.P. & P.J. JEWESSON. 1992. A critical reevaluation of the "therapeutic range" of aminoglycosides. Clin. Infect. Dis. **14:** 320–339.
18. BARCLAY, M.L., et al. 1999. Once daily aminoglycoside therapy. Is it less toxic than multiple daily doses and how should it be monitored? Clin. Pharmacokinet. **36:** 89–98.
19. SAYERS, J.F.B. 1988. Routine monitoring of serum vancomycin concentrations: the answer lies in the middle. Clin. Pharmocol. **7:** 18.
20. CANTU, T.G., et al. 1994. Serum vancomycin concentrations: reappraisal of their clinical value. Clin. Infect. Dis. **18:** 533–543.
21. MOELLERING, R.C. 1994. Editorial: monitoring serum vancomycin levels: climbing the mountain because it is there? Clin. Infect. Dis. **18:** 544–546.
22. PISCITELLI, S.C. 2001. The value of drug levels: the plot thickens. Medscape. http://id.medscape.com/Medscape/CNO/2001/RETRO/Story.cfm?story_id=2055
23. PELOQUIN, C.A. 2001. Tuberculosis drug serum levels (letter). Clin. Infect. Dis. **33:** 584–585.
24. MOUTON, J.W., et al. 1999. Use of pharmacodynamic indices to predict efficacy of combination therapy in vivo. Antimicrob. Agents Chemother. **43:** 2473–2478.
25. PELOQUIN, C.A., et al. 1993. Malabsorption of antimycobacterial medications. N. Engl. J. Med. **329:** 1122–1123.
26. PATEL, K.B., R. BELMONTE & H.M. CROWE. 1995. Drug malabsorption and resistant tuberculosis in HIV-infected patients (letter). N. Engl. J. Med. **332:** 336–337.
27. JELLIFFE, R. 2000. Goal-oriented, model-based drug regimens: setting individualized goals for each patient. Ther. Drug Monit. **22:** 325–329.
28. AMERICAN THORACIC SOCIETY. 1994. Treatment of tuberculosis and tuberculosis infection in adults and children. Am. J. Respir. Crit. Care. Med. **149:** 1359–1374.

DOTS and DOTS-Plus

Not the Only Answer

PAUL FARMER

Infectious Disease Division, Brigham and Women's Hospital and Department of Social Medicine, Harvard Medical School, Boston, Massachusetts 02115, USA

ABSTRACT: Multidrug-resistant tuberculosis is already a global pandemic, with focal "hot spots" of ongoing transmission. Although DOTS (directly observed treatment, short course) chemotherapy is the goal of global tuberculosis control, short-course chemotherapy will not cure multidrug-resistant tuberculosis. In settings of high transmission of multidrug-resistant tuberculosis, "DOTS plus" (a complementary DOTS-based strategy with provisions for treating multidrug-resistant tuberculosis) is warranted. DOTS-plus project implementation to date reveals important clinical, epidemiological, and economic lessons. Community-based strategies designed to enhance local capacity are cost effective and make it possible to meet new medical challenges.

KEYWORDS: multidrug-resistant tuberculosis; DOTS; DOTS-plus; public health; pan-resistant TB; transnational case finding

Tuberculosis remains the world's leading infectious cause of adult deaths, most of which are due not to multidrug-resistant tuberculosis (MDR TB), but to lack of access to effective treatment for drug-susceptible tuberculous disease.[1] New data suggest, however, that MDR TB is emerging as an increasingly important cause of morbidity and death. In the United States, Europe, and Latin America, highly resistant strains of tuberculosis have caused explosive institutional outbreaks (in hospitals, prisons, and homeless shelters) with high case fatality rates among immunosuppressed persons and high rates of transmission to other patients and to caregivers and their families.[2-8]

TRANSNATIONAL TUBERCULOSIS

As is often the case with emerging epidemics, it is most illustrative to begin with a "transnational" case. A 50-year-old U.S. citizen working in northern Lima as a relief worker came back to a well-known Boston teaching hospital with a two-month-long history of chronic enteropathy, fever, and cough. He was found to be HIV-positive, with a CD4 count of less than 50, an erythrocyte sedimentation rate of 68, and marked anemia. Acid-fast bacilli were present in sputum and stool. Although

Address for correspondence: Paul Farmer, M.D., Ph.D., Program in Infectious Disease and Social Change, Department of Social Medicine, Harvard Medical School, 641 Huntington Avenue, Boston, MA 02114. Voice: 617-432-3715; fax: 617-432-6045.
PIHPaul@aol.com

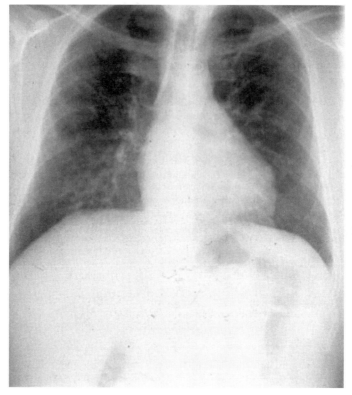

FIGURE 1. CXR, "transnational case."

HIV-associated systemic infection with atypical mycobacteria was suspected, the patient's chest x-ray showed scattered granulomas in both lungs (FIG. 1). Sputum and blood samples were sent to the Massachusetts State Laboratory Institute for mycobacterial culture. The patient was admitted to a common room initially and then, following consultation with the infectious disease service, placed in a room meeting requirements for respiratory precautions. In keeping with what is usually the prudent use of antibiotics and with standard practice, the patient was placed on an antituberculous regimen consisting of rifampin, isoniazid, ethambutol, and pyrazinamide. But in contrast to most patients with mycobacterial infections and HIV, this patient did not respond to therapy. He died of sepsis syndrome within two weeks of his presentation. When his sputum and blood cultures grew not atypical mycobacteria, but rather *M. tuberculosis*, his failure to respond to such powerful drugs was even more mysterious, since most patients with tuberculosis respond to these powerful agents whether HIV-infected or not. The mystery persisted until drug-susceptibility testing revealed that the patient died of disseminated TB resistant to all the first-line drugs. This is thus a very important case for several reasons, which I will explore in this chapter.

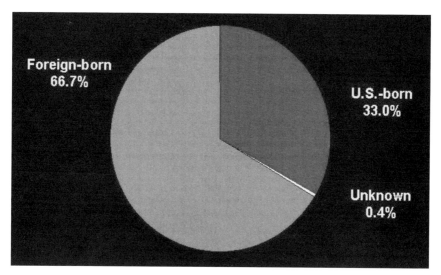

FIGURE 2. Reported TB cases, U.S. born and foreign-born persons, Massachusetts, 1998. Source: Centers for Disease Control and Prevention, 1998.

When confronted with a case of active pulmonary tuberculosis, the state of Massachusetts generally conducts active case finding. That is, contacts of patients are evaluated for active disease and for latent TB infection. But transnational case finding was not something in the state public health repertory. Yet in Massachusetts, some 70% of all TB cases are diagnosed in the foreign-born, so transnational thinking is most appropriate to this era (FIG. 2).[9] These are global problems, even if they call for local solutions.

TUBERCULOSIS CONTROL IN PERU

Given that the budget and activities of a public charity are sometimes less strict about changes in "line items," Partners In Health—a Boston-based organization I helped to found in 1987—decided to conduct our own active case finding. When in 1996 we met with Peruvian public health authorities, we were reminded that Peru has the best TB control program in the world. Upon close inspection, Peru probably *does* have the world's most successful TB control program, from a public health point of view.[10] The strategy that it has implemented is DOTS, and we knew from our own experience in central Haiti just how effective DOTS can be. But the "S" in DOTS means short-course chemotherapy, which is based on rifampin and isoniazid (FIG. 3). Since our transnational case was sick with a strain resistant to both of these drugs, we had to ask, Might there be other such cases in northern Lima? We discovered, of course, that a lot more was going on than met the eye. First of all, the prevalence of all forms of active TB among young adults (ages 15–44) was very high in Carabayllo: 800 per 100,000 in 1993 (FIG. 4).[11] This is not as high as some places in Haiti, but it is far higher than Peru's national average—less than 200 per

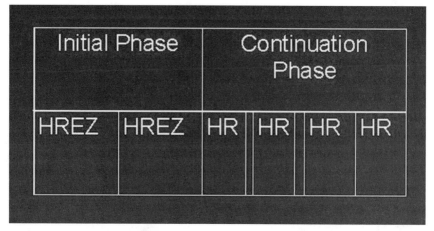

FIGURE 3. Short-course chemotherapy.

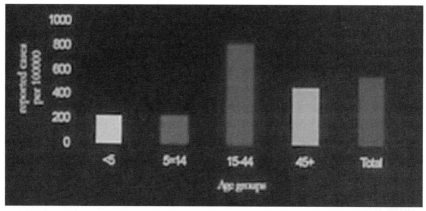

FIGURE 4. Estimated prevalence of all forms of active TB, Carabayllo, 1993. Source: Carabayllo TB Control Program data, 1993.

100,000[12]—and is an indicator of why someone who was vulnerable to an infectious disease would fall ill in a shantytown like Carabayllo (FIG. 5).

Second, we found many patients in northern Lima who had failed therapy, many of them several times (FIG. 6). Most of the time, TB patients fail therapy because they don't really complete therapy. With a good directly observed treatment (DOT) program, however, such an explanation becomes much less likely. Peru has, as I just mentioned, an excellent DOTS program. Who, then, are these patients who remain smear-positive throughout or at the end of therapy? Thanks to the Massachusetts State Laboratory Institute, we know that these patients have MDR TB. In our first survey of treatment failures, we found that more than 90% of patients in this region who failed one or several regimens of short-course chemotherapy had MDR TB.[13] What's

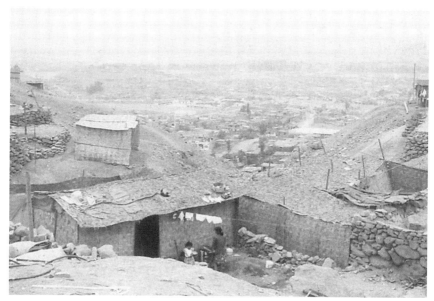

FIGURE 5. Carabayllo, Peru.

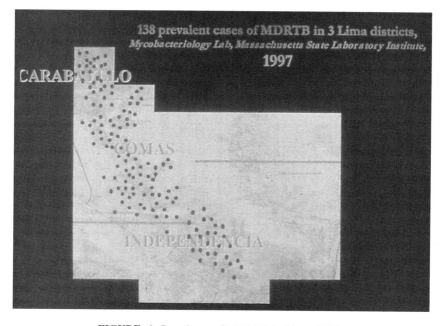

FIGURE 6. Prevalence of MDR TB in Lima, 1997.

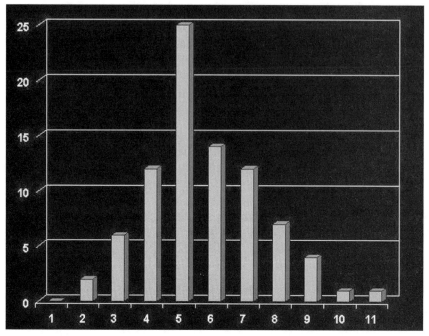

FIGURE 7. Mean number of drugs to which strains are resistant ($n = 84$); mean = 5.67.

worse, these patients were not sick with strains resistant to isoniazid and rifampin alone. Most were resistant to all four first-line drugs, and more than half of them were resistant to streptomycin as well. In this sample of the first 173 patients, most patients were sick with strains resistant to five drugs; some patients were resistant to as many as 11 drugs (FIG. 7). In subsequent samples, we have encountered patients who are sick with strains of *M. tuberculosis* resistant to 12 drugs (FIG. 8).[14] I would say there are probably six or seven good antituberculosis drugs.[15] Thus we discovered, before any therapeutic intervention on our part, pan-resistant tuberculosis.

PAN-RESISTANT TUBERCULOSIS

It is important, then, to take stock of this before proceeding: all those who raise the specter of pan-resistant tuberculosis as a reason to avoid using second-line drugs should acknowledge that such strains are already circulating. These patients are pushed back into the pre-antibiotic era. What is more, almost none of them—whether in northern Lima or in one of the MDR TB "hot spots" described in various WHO surveys[16]—is receiving therapy or is in respiratory isolation. Thus, this plague is already upon us.

What are the impacts of untreated MDR TB on this community, and why are such cases appearing in a country served by the best TB-control program in the world? We are working with our colleagues at the Massachusetts State Laboratory Institute

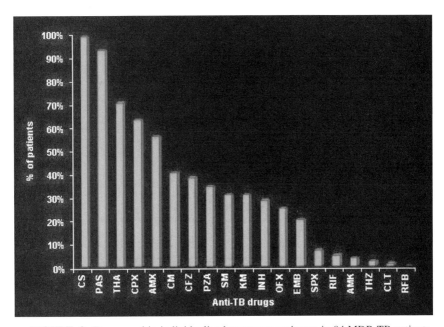

FIGURE 8. Drugs used in individualized treatment regimens in 84 MDR TB patients, Carabayllo, Peru. August 1996 to June 1999.

to complete RFLP (molecular fingerprinting) analyses of the hundreds of samples collected in northern Lima. In linking the molecular epidemiology of this outbreak to conventional epidemiology, clinical studies, and medical anthropology, we will advance a comprehensive study of a drug-resistant TB outbreak. We are examining the behavior of the patients, the providers, and the system in place to see how they come together to favor the emergence of drug-resistant tuberculosis in a setting in which most antituberculous agents are used prudently.

Although RFLP has not yet been completed, we have evidence of household clustering of MDR TB.[17] A single family in which at least eight young adults are sick or dead from MDR TB is shown in FIGURE 9. Within this family, molecular-level study shows the same mutation in the infecting strain of *M. tuberculosis*. That is, these are intrahousehold epidemics in which family members are passing drug-resistant strains one to the other. This should frighten members of the medical community because we have failed to keep up with the microbes: what prophylaxis do we offer to the PPD-positive close contacts of patients with MDR TB? Repeated calls for funding for such research have thus far failed to bring the unanswered question to the attention of funders. Even more troubling was the great difficulty we had in finding funds to treat patients with *active, infectious* MDR TB. The argument until recently, on the part of many international public health experts, was that the disease was too costly to treat.

When we started having difficulty finding the funds to treat patients with smear-positive pulmonary MDR TB on the grounds that it was not cost-effective to treat them, we countered with other logic as best we could. One reason that we think that

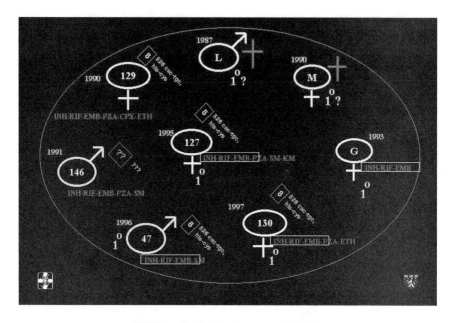

FIGURE 9. Family cluster of MDR TB.

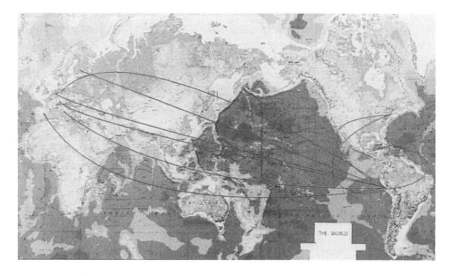

FIGURE 10. Known transnational cases of drug-resistant TB diagnosed among persons recently living in Peru.

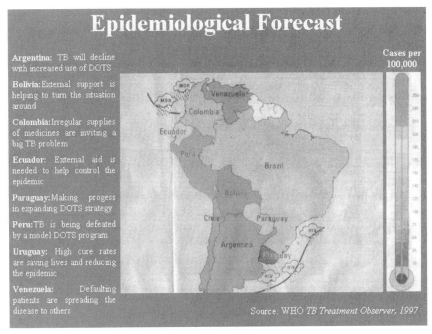

Epidemiological Forecast

Argentina: TB will decline with increased use of DOTS

Bolivia: External support is helping to turn the situation around

Colombia: Irregular supplies of medicines are inviting a big TB problem

Ecuador: External aid is needed to help control the epidemic

Paraguay: Making progress in expanding DOTS strategy

Peru: TB is being defeated by a model DOTS program

Uruguay: High cure rates are saving lives and reducing the epidemic

Venezuela: Defaulting patients are spreading the disease to others

Cases per 100,000

Source: WHO *TB Treatment Observer, 1997*

FIGURE 11. "Epidemiological Forecast," South America.

this is important is again revealed by epidemiology: In Massachusetts, as noted, most patients who have tuberculosis were not born in the United States; these are transnational cases in one sense or another. If reporting is correct, this is true throughout Western Europe and North America. Furthermore, there are cases all over Europe and North America that originate in Peru (FIG. 10).[18] The same can be said for other MDR TB "hot spots," the largest of which I will speak about later in this chapter.

In short, what is to be done about patients sick with MDR TB? Unfortunately, there wasn't a good program strategy in place. There was a great strategy in place to prevent the *emergence* of drug resistance—DOTS. The question is what happens in settings in which drug-resistant TB has already emerged? It is raining MDR TB over Colombia, according to a 1997 "epidemiological forecast" from the WHO (FIG. 11).[19] In Peru, however, TB is being defeated by a model DOTS program.[20] What about that subset who live with, and die from, a TB that is *not* defeated by a model DOTS program? Why does this question evince hostility from certain quarters? Are there scientific grounds that would have us believe that patients with MDR TB should not be treated?

Science? The anthropologist side of me starts to think there is something else going on. In fact, there was a significant epidemic of drug-resistant TB in northern Lima, and there was significant resistance to having it treated with anything outside the DOTS framework. When patients with primary MDR TB undergo short-course chemotherapy, they receive two months of ethambutol and pyrazinamide, followed by four months of something worse than placebo, because there are toxicities asso-

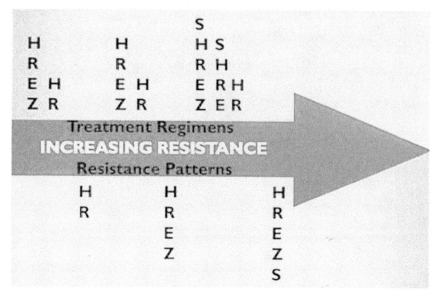

FIGURE 12. The amplifier effect of short-course chemotherapy. (From Farmer *et al.*, 1998 cited in Ref. 27; used with permission.)

ciated with even isoniazid and rifampin. Basically, two months of ethambutol and pyrazinamide is unlikely to cure a case of pulmonary MDR TB with a large bacillary load. The patients I describe here are not the majority of patients globally, but they are precisely the ones that we met in our work in northern Lima. In some local outbreaks—outside of Peru—they may well prove to be the majority of patients with active TB. As a result, you can have a great DOTS program that has beautiful documentation and careful quarterly reporting, and it would seem to be a great managerial success. Still, it would fail to cure the patients whose fates we discuss here. To most people, especially to patients and their families, clinical failure is just that—failure.

Let me pose a generic question: What happens when you administer drugs that can't cure, but you give the drugs anyway? One biologically salient possibility is what we've termed "the amplifier effect of short-course chemotherapy" (FIG. 12). In the example, the patient begins short-course chemotherapy sick with a strain of *M. tuberculosis* resistant only to isoniazid and rifampin. But as noted short-course chemotherapy usually consists of two months of four drugs, and four months of two drugs. In this instance, the patient is not cured, but the infecting strain does recruit new resistance to ethambutol and pyrazinamide. This is essentially iatrogenic amplification of drug resistance. Then, the patient often receives the recommended retreatment regimen, which, amazingly enough in my view, consists of the same four drugs plus one more: streptomycin. In many instances, the infecting strain acquires resistance to streptomycin. This is the reason why 67% of our patients in Lima are sick with strains resistant to all five first-line drugs. They have failed repeated courses of empiric therapy that were likely to fail.

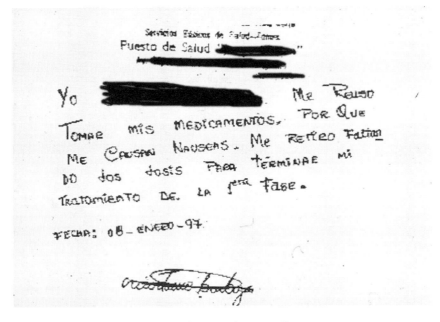

FIGURE 13. Note of noncompliance.

That is all very easy to say epidemiologically, but the impacts can be devastating clinically. In this local epidemic, the amplifier effect of short-course chemotherapy was the critical determinant of outcomes, and also of costs. Consider a young woman from what is locally called a "TB family." Eight adults in her family have MDR TB or are dead from it. She fell ill with MDR TB, and eventually responded to an individualized MDR TB regimen. But then, like everyone else in her family, her husband became ill. When her husband was shown to be smear-positive, we argued against giving him empiric short-course chemotherapy because chances were very high that he would have primary MDR TB. Sensible clinical recommendations were not in keeping with the reigning treatment strategies, however. As a result, when he received DOTS, he of course received the "S"—short-course chemotherapy. Every month he went in for an examination of his sputum with smear microscopy, and every month the result was positive, indicating he remained sick and infectious. So one day he refused the drugs. The public health officials said, "Well if you do that, you're going to have to sign a paper." (FIG. 13 shows the form.) So there it is in his medical record. He is a "noncompliant" patient with "acquired MDR TB." He belongs to a TB family, and these are problem people. They are smear-positive every month, and they are not responding to the drugs that they have been instructed to take. These people are caught in a bizarre trap related to what, in most instances, would be considered a prudent use of antibiotics. But it is a nightmare for them.

We began treating a cohort of these patients, most of whom were resistant to five or more drugs. Their chest x-rays showed more often than not extensive parenchymal

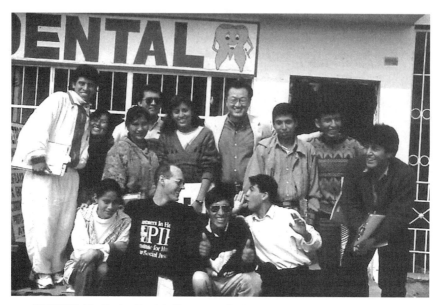

FIGURE 14. Socios En Salud's community health workers in Carabayllo, Peru.

destruction. We designed individualized treatment regimens for each of them, although most received a regimen based on an injectable, a fluoroquinolone, cyclo-serine, and PAS. We started calling it "the menu." At the outset of therapy, as we strug-gled to train DOT workers from this region, we received little encouragement from the public health community. We were told that these patients were "untreatable."[21] All sorts of words are used locally and internationally to describe such patients—"chronic" being the most common moniker. We were also told that they would not comply with therapy for MDR TB: there would be too many side effects, and they would abandon treatment.

There were also substantial logistic hurdles to overcome. Although a few of the drugs were donated to us, we had to buy almost all of them, at least initially. So this was our dilemma, in August of 1996, once we were sure that we had uncovered an epidemic of MDR TB: How are complex therapies delivered effectively in resource-poor settings? How well would they do, given they had, supposedly, an untreatable disease? We treated them by training a group of young people, many of whom were unemployed, as community health workers (FIG. 14). Furthermore, we worked hard to build a coalition involving Peru's national TB program, local public health facil-ities, and our TB laboratory (FIG. 15).

In contrast to predictions, the patients put up with side effects and with daily in-jections of drugs like capreomycin. Sometimes, these patients were loathe to stop any of the drugs, even when we recommended it, they were so pleased to be smear-negative each month. When we said, "you can stop your capreomycin now," some would reply, "Frankly, I don't want to. I'd rather continue it." Remember, these are people who'd been through repeated cycles of ineffective empiric therapy in order to survive. Their mean age was 29; most had children.

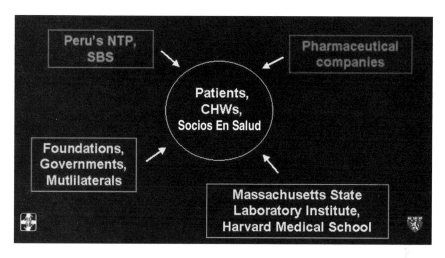

FIGURE 15. Components of a successful community-based MDR TB treatment program in Lima's northern cone.

Our group followed side effects closely, even though they were nowhere near as bad as we were told they would be.[22] We managed most of the side effects in the community. Of the initial 74 patients who were supposedly incurable, 85% were cured according to the most stringent criteria, which is culture, not smear (FIG. 16).[23] One patient who was HIV coinfected also did well and remains free of active tuberculosis two years after completion of therapy. In the end, then, we had succeeded in introducing evidence-based medicine into a Peruvian slum, relying heavily on local resources and also on the basic planks of the DOTS strategy.

A number of questions arise as a result of this project. The first question is whether it is really too expensive to treat MDR TB wherever it occurs, or whether it is too expensive not to treat it. This is an airborne pathogen, and one case of untreated pulmonary MDR TB can cause scores of new MDR TB infections. We should also ask whether different standards of care are appropriate to epidemic disease. The next question would be, Why is it so expensive, given that the medicines required have long been off patent?

A second question is whether MDR TB really "detracts attention and resources." That is not what happened in New York City, where a relatively small outbreak of MDR TB led to a massive change in TB control.[25] Resources were poured into the TB control infrastructure—appropriately, in my view. Although we do not have MDR TB in New York anymore, we still have what most would regard as robust funding for the TB program. Third, what of second-line drug prices? One of the drugs I mentioned, capreomycin, is made by only one company. On a certain day in 1997, one could buy a gram of capreomycin for about $30 at the Brigham and Women's Hospital in Boston; in Peru, for $21; and in Europe, for $8.80 (FIG. 17). One has to ask hard questions about why an off-patent drug made by the same company would be priced so differently in different countries. Working with colleagues at Médecins Sans Frontières and the WHO, we subsequently began a campaign to

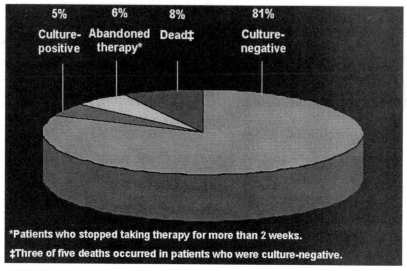

FIGURE 16. Multidrug-resistant tuberculosis cure rates have exceeded 80% in patients who are young, have no serious co-morbid disease (such as HIV infection), and have received individualized therapy based on results from drug susceptibility testing for 4 months or longer. This rate can be expected even among patients who are infected with strains of *Mycobacterium tuberculosis* that are highly resistant (to five or more drugs) and have significant parenchymal destruction as well as a history of prior antituberculosis treatments. (From Farmer *et al.*[33]; used with permission.)

lower the prices of some of these drugs. We learned that some companies do not want a TB indication to be found for their drug. We asked, "Well, why ever not?" The answer was clear enough: if drugs are proved to be effective against *M. tuberculosis*, they can be declared public health resources and taken off the market. TB remains, after HIV, the leading infectious killer of young adults in the world, at least in most of the world. This is a social disease par excellence, and the drugs ought to be managed as a societal resource. But the profit motive also undermines the prudent use of antibiotics.

DOTS-PLUS

We needed a name for our DOTS-based program to address MDR TB. Working with the World Health Organization, we came up with "DOTS-Plus."[26] The idea was to build on the managerial successes of DOTS without ignoring patients who would likely fail short-course chemotherapy because they were sick with drug-resistant TB. Over the course of the past couple of years, brisk debate is beginning to give way to consensus: DOTS is our best hope of preventing the emergence of resistance to antituberculous drugs, but once drug resistance is established in a population, DOTS alone will no longer suffice.[27]

In conclusion, I'd like to discuss what I regard as a major crucible for public health interventions in the future. I have already demonstrated that sometimes the

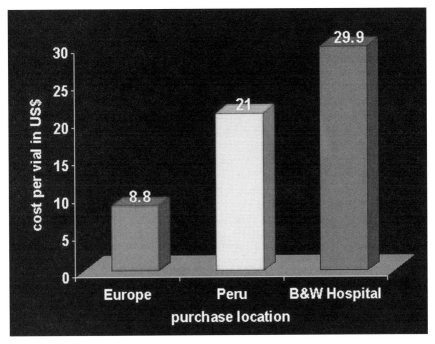

FIGURE 17. Cost comparison of capreomycin (1 g).

desire to control antibiotics and use them prudently can, in fact, lead to unanticipated effects. In the middle of an epidemic of drug-resistant tuberculosis, you don't want to rely on only the drugs to which patients have developed resistance. What is "prudent" in Haiti, say, may be imprudent within a neighborhood in northern Lima.

THE RUSSIAN CHALLENGE

Russia, the challenge to which I refer, offers the most dramatic example of just how bad things can get (FIG. 18). We have drug-susceptibility results, some of them from our own state lab in Massachusetts, which reveal that a minority of patients among a cohort of Siberian prisoners has pan-susceptible disease.[28] To a clinician, that spells disaster. When you lose isoniazid or rifampin, it is far more difficult to treat tuberculosis. The ugliest part of the story is not only that 20% to 25% of these prisoners have MDR TB, but also that tuberculosis is the leading cause of death of these young prisoners; it is also soon to be the leading cause of death for their jailors, doctors, and nurses. In FIGURE 19, you can see an image of these prisoners: mean age 29 and falling. FIGURE 20 presents the drug-susceptibility testing results in another prison in Western Siberia at the initiation of therapy. Note that only 25% of the patients had pan-susceptible disease and that the rest of them had drug-resistant disease. In this prison, at least 23% of the prisoners had MDR TB at the beginning of therapy. So, what would you recommend as empiric therapy for these young men?

Well, they received standardized short-course chemotherapy, but with one drug added to "reinforce" the regimen. And guess what that drug was: the very one to which most were already resistant, streptomycin. The treatment results using smear microscopy show, not surprisingly, that only 46% of these patients were cured.[29] In rural Haiti, in the face of famine, we chastise ourselves if we can't cure 95% of our TB patients.

TREATMENT OF MDR TB

There have been three chief objections to the treatment of MDR TB: that it is expensive, drawing resources away from the treatment of pan-susceptible disease; that it is technically difficult and yields low cure rates; and that treatment of drug-resistant strains, when improperly monitored, give rise to even more resistant organisms. Other claims include those about decreased virulence and transmissibility of MDR TB strains.

Each of these claims is open to critique. Although the treatment cost of a known MDR TB case is greater than that of a known pan-susceptible case, this observation is incorrectly applied to the treatment and, by extension, to the prevention costs of tuberculosis cases in general. If the drug-resistance pattern is unknown, the cost is not predictable. Available cost-effectiveness data do not address this specific question, and empiric data suggest that ineffective treatment of MDR TB with short-

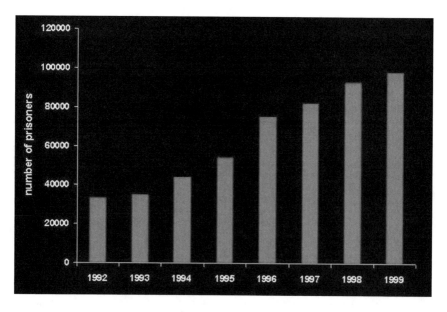

FIGURE 18. Prison prevalence of active pulmonary TB, Russian Federation, 1992–1999 [The Main Directorate of Corrections of the Ministry of Internal Affairs (GUIN), 1999].

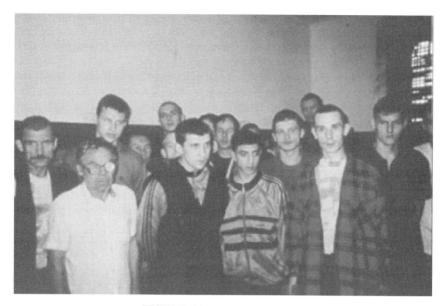

FIGURE 19. Prisoners in Russia.

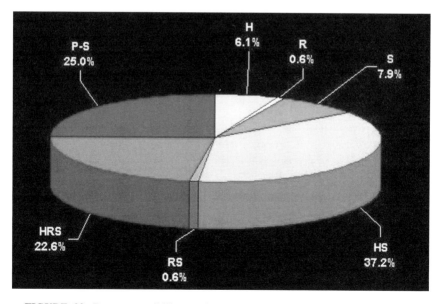

FIGURE 20. Drug-susceptibility results at treatment initiation, Marinsk prison, Ke-
nerovo, Russia (*n* = 164). Source: Kimerling, *et al.*[29]

course chemotherapy may increase the costs of tuberculosis treatment and prevention in the longer run.[30] In fact, many involved in advocacy for DOTS-Plus programs have argued that new resources must be brought to TB control in general and that the threat of MDR TB can serve as a means of bringing previously untapped public and private resources to TB control.[31] This proved true, certainly, of the outbreak of MDR TB in New York City.[32] Moreover, the specter of amplified resistance and of a growing proportion of drug-resistant TB exhorts us to act now before the costs of treating MDR TB increase even more dramatically.

THE FUTURE

The full characterization of the genome of *M. tuberculosis* reminds us that much has been accomplished, as does the decline of TB in much of the industrialized world. But the future of the global TB pandemic will be determined by the success of control measures in the high-prevalence areas in which resources are scarce. That TB could remain the world's leading infectious cause of adult deaths fully 50 years after the development of effective chemotherapy would no doubt surprise those who helped to develop these agents. The advent of HIV and of strains of *M. tuberculosis* resistant to all first-line drugs remind us of the need for new and more effective tools for the treatment and control of these persistent plagues. Applying these tools where the burden of disease is greatest will remain the central task of 21st century TB control.

ACKNOWLEDGMENTS

In giving a lecture, one can give the impression that the speaker, and not dozens of others, have done the work necessary to make a project succeed. The DOTS-Plus program in Peru would not have been possible without Dr. Jaime Bayona, the Socios En Salud team (especially the promotores and nurses), and the National TB Programme. We thank especially Thomas J. White and all those at Partners In Health, and also the Bill and Melinda Gates Foundation.

NOTES AND REFERENCES

1. WORLD HEALTH ORGANIZATION. 1997. WHO Report on the Tuberculosis Epidemic. WHO. Geneva.
2. VAILWAY, S., R. GREIFINGER, M. PAPANIA, *et al.* 1994. Multidrug-resistant tuberculosis in the New York state prison system, 1990–1991. J. Infect. Dis. **170:** 151–156.
3. NARDELL, E., B. MCINNIS, B. THOMAS & S. WIDHASS. 1986. Exogenous reinfection with tuberculosis in a shelter for the homeless. N. Engl. J. Med. **315:** 1570–1573.
4. BECK-SAGUE, C., S. DOOLEY, M. HOTTON, *et al.* 1992. Hospital outbreak of multidrug-resistant *Mycobacterium tuberculosis* infections: factors in transmission to staff and HIV-infected patients. JAMA **268:** 1280–1286.
5. BARNES, P., H. EL-HAJJ, S. PRESTON-MARTIN, *et al.* 1996. Transmission of tuberculosis among the urban homeless. JAMA **275:** 305–307.
6. PABLOS-MENDEZ, A., M. RAVIGLIONE, R. BATTAN & R. RAMOS-ZUNIGA. 1990. Drug resistant tuberculosis among the homeless in New York City. N.Y. State J. Med. **90:** 351–355.

7. KRITSKI, A., M.J. MARQUES, M.F. RABAHI, et al. 1996. Transmission of tuberculosis to
    close contacts of patients with multidrug-resistant tuberculosis. Am. J. Respir. Crit.
    Care Med. **153:** 331–335.
8. RULLÁN, J., D. HERRERA, R. CANO, et al. 1996. Nosocomial transmission of multidrug-
    resistant tuberculosis in Spain. Emerg. Infect. Dis. **2:** 125–129.
9. CENTERS FOR DISEASE CONTROL AND PREVENTION. 2000. Reported Tuberculosis in the
    United States, 1999. CDC. Atlanta, GA. The national rate stands at 41.6% for 1998,
    an increase of more than 10% since 1993, with six states reporting greater than 70%
    of foreign-born cases. See also TALBOT, E.A., M. MOORE, E. MCCRAY, et al. 2000.
    Tuberculosis among foreign-born persons in the United States, 1993–1998. JAMA
    284(22): 2894–2900.
10. For a concise overview of Peru's model National Tuberculosis Program, refer to
    Chapter 4 of The Global Impact of Drug-Resistant Tuberculosis: BECERRA, M.C., J.
    BAYONA, P.E. FARMER, et al. 1999. Defusing a time-bomb: the challenge of antitu-
    berculosis drug resistance in Peru. In Program in Infectious Disease and Social
    Change. The Global Impact of Drug-Resistant Tuberculosis. Harvard Medical
    School and the Open Society Institute. Boston, MA. 107–126.
11. This estimate is based on case notifications from the public clinics in Carabayllo
    (Estadistica e Informatica SRS Lima Norte. Tuberculosis control program regis-
    ters: district of Carabayllo. 1993). Our own active case finding between 1996 and
    1997 found total TB incidence among all residents to be 525 per 100,000, a 20%
    increase over that revealed by passive case-finding, and a figure twice as high as
    the national average See BECERRA, MC. 1999. Epidemiology of tuberculosis in the
    northern shantytowns of Lima, Peru. Sc.D. thesis, Harvard University, Boston,
    MA. See also SANGHAVI, D.M., R.H. GILMAN, A.G. LESCANO-GUEVARA, et al.
    Hyperendemic pulmonary tuberculosis in a Peruvian shantytown. Am. J. Epide-
    miol. **148(4):** 384–389.
12. MINISTERIO DE SALUD. 1998. Tuberculosis en el Peru—Informe 1997. Ministerio de
    Salud. Lima, Peru.
13. BECERRA, M.C., J. FREEMAN, J. BAYONA, et al. 2000. Using treatment failure under
    effective directly observed short-course chemotherapy programs to identify
    patients with multidrug-resistant tuberculosis. Int. J. Tuberc. Lung Dis. **4(2):** 108–
    114.
14. FARMER, P.E., E. PALACIOS, S.S. SHIN, et al. 2000. Innovative community-based treat-
    ment for multidrug resistant TB in a resource-poor setting. Oral presentation at the
    American Public Health Association Annual Meeting. Boston, MA, November 15,
    2000.
15. Drugs cidal against M. tuberculosis include isoniazid, rifampin, pyrazinamide,
    ethambutol, streptomycin (and other aminoglycosides as a class), capreomycin,
    and the fluoroquinolones. Other drugs are weakly cidal or mycobacteriostatic.
16. WORLD HEALTH ORGANIZATION. 2000. Anti-Tuberculosis Drug Resistance in the
    World, Report No. 2: The WHO/IUATLD Global Project on Anti-Tuberculosis
    Drug Resistance Surveillance 2000. WHO/CDS/TB/2000.278. World Health Orga-
    nization. Geneva.
17. FURIN, J.J., M.C. BECERRA, S.S. SHIN, et al. 2000. Amplifying resistance? Effect of
    administering short-course standardized resistance regimens in individuals
    infected with drug-resistant Mycobacterium tuberculosis strains. Eur. J. Clin.
    Microbiol. Infect. Dis. **2000:** 132–136. See also BECERRA, M.C. 1999. Epidemiol-
    ogy of tuberculosis in the northern shantytowns of Lima, Peru. Sc.D. thesis, Har-
    vard University, Boston, MA.
18. BECERRA, M.C., P.E. FARMER & J.Y. KIM. 1999. The problem of drug-resistant tuber-
    culosis: an overview. In Program in Infectious Disease and Social Change. The
    Global Impact of Drug-Resistant Tuberculosis. Harvard Medical School and the
    Open Society Institute. Boston, MA. 1–38.
19. WORLD HEALTH ORGANIZATION. 1997. TB Treatment Observer. March 24. WHO.
    Geneva.
20. WORLD HEALTH ORGANIZATION. 1997. TB Treatment Observer. March 24. WHO.
    Geneva.

21. WORLD HEALTH ORGANIZATION. 1998. WHO Fact Sheet No. 104, "Tuberculosis," revised February 1998. "There is no cure affordable to developing countries for some multidrug-resistant (MDR) strains." p. 2. WHO. Geneva.
22. FURIN, J.J., C.D. MITNICK, S.S. SHIN, et al. 2001. Occurrence of serious adverse effects in patients receiving community-based therapy for multidrug-resistant tuberculosis. Int. J. Tuberc. Lung Dis. 5(7): 648–656.
23. FARMER, P.E., J.Y. KIM, C. MITNICK, et al. 1999. Responding to outbreaks of MDRTB: introducing "DOTS-Plus." In Tuberculosis: A Comprehensive International Approach. 2nd ed. L.B. Reichman & E.S. Hershfield, Eds.: 447–469. Marcel Dekker. New York.
24. WORLD HEALTH ORGANIZATION. 1997. TB Treatment Observer. March 24, p. 2. WHO. Geneva.
25. For a summary of New York's TB outbreak, see GARRETT, L. 1994. The Coming Plague. Farrar, Straus, and Giroux. New York. See also FRIEDEN, T., E. FUJIWARA, R. WASHKO, et al. 1995. Tuberculosis in New York City: turning the tide. N. Engl. J. Med. 333(4): 229–233. For a critical commentary on the relative contribution of DOTS, see FARMER, P.E. & E. NARDELL. 1998. Nihilism and pragmatism in tuberculosis control. Am. J. Pub. Health 88(7): 4–5; and BAYER, R., C. STAYTON, M. DESVARIEUX, et al. 1998. Directly observed therapy and treatment completion for tuberculosis in the United States: is universal supervised therapy necessary? Am. J. Pub. Health 88(7): 1052–1058.
26. FARMER, P.E. & J.Y. KIM. 1998. Community-based approaches to the control of multidrug-resistant tuberculosis: introducing "DOTS-plus." Br. Med. J. 317(7159): 671–574.
27. For a review of the debate, see the following exchanges: FARMER, P.E., J. BAYONA, M. BECERRA, et al. 1998. The dilemma of MDRTB in the global era. Int. J. Tuberc. Lung Dis. 2(11): 869–876; ESPINAL, M.A., C. DYE, M.C. RAVIGLIONE, et al. 1999. Rational "DOTS Plus" for the control of MDR-TB. Int. J. Tuberc. Lung Dis. 3(7): 561–563; FARMER, P.E., J.J. FURIN, J. BAYONA, et al. 1999. Management of MDR-TB in resource-poor countries. Int. J. Tuberc. Lung Dis. 3(8): 643–645; FARMER P.E., J. BAYONA, M. BECERRA, et al. 1999. DOTS plus strategy in resource-poor countries. Int. J. Tuberc. Lung Dis. 3(9): 844.
28. FARMER, P.E., A.S. KONONETS, S.E. BORISOV, et al. 1999. Recrudescent tuberculosis in the Russian Federation. In Program in Infectious Disease and Social Change. The Global Impact of Drug-Resistant Tuberculosis. Harvard Medical School and the Open Society Institute, 1999; pp. 39–84. See also FARMER, P.E. 1999. Cruel and unusual: drug resistant tuberculosis as punishment. In Sentenced to Die? The Problem of TB in Prisons in East and Central Europe and Central Asia. V. Stern, Ed.: 70–80. International Centre for Prison Studies. London.
29. KIMERLING, M.E., H. KLUGE, N. VEZHNINA, et al. 1999. Inadequacy of the current WHO re-treatment regimen in a central Siberian prison: treatment failure and MDRTB. Int. J. Tuberc. Lung Dis. 3(5): 451–453. See also comment in: FARMER, P.E. 1999. Managerial successes, clinical failures. Int. J. Tuberc. Lung Dis. 3(5): 365–367.
30. HEIFETS, L.B. 1994. Antimycobacterial drugs. Sem. Respir. Infect. 9(2): 84–103.
31. FARMER, P., J. BAYONA, M. BECERRA, et al. 1998. The dilemma of MDR-TB in the global era. Int. J. Tuberc. Lung Dis. 2(11): 869–878.
32. FRIEDEN, T.R., P. FUJIWARA, R. WASHKO & M. HAMBURG. 1995. Tuberculosis in New York City—turning the tide. N. Engl. J. Med. 333(4): 229–233.
33. FARMER, P.E., J. FURIN & S. SHIN. 2000. Managing multidrug-resistant tuberculosis. J. Resp. Dis. 21(1): 53–56.

The Clinical Management of the Drug-Resistant Patient

PETER ORMEROD

Consultant Chest Physician, Blackburn Royal Infirmary, Blackburn, Lancashire, BB2 3LR, UK, and Department of Respiratory Medicine, Lancashire School of Postgraduate Medicine and Health, Preston, PR1 2HE, UK

ABSTRACT: The specific management of drug-resistant patients is only possible where facilities exist for both mycobacterial culture and for drug-susceptibility testing. Treatment guidelines in the United Kingdom and elsewhere are predicated on the drug-resistance data prevailing in the circumstances of their use. In developed countries, the inclusion of the fourth drug (ethambutol but occasionally streptomycin) depends on the level of isoniazid resistance expected or known in a given patient group. Most parts of the world do not have the capabilities to perform mycobacterial culture and drug-susceptibility testing. In these countries, therefore, the "standard" advised regimen has to cover the possibility of the commoner drug resistances. The view taken in the United Kingdom is that where drug-susceptibility tests are available, they should be followed, and treatment modified. The drug treatment of multidrug-resistant tuberculosis (MDR TB), defined as combined resistance to rifampicin and isoniazid, plus or minus other antituberculosis drugs, is complex, time consuming, and demanding on both patient and physician. In the United Kingdom the advice is that treatment should only be carried out by physicians with substantial experience in managing complex resistant cases, only in hospitals with appropriate isolation facilities, and in very close liaison with Mycobacteriology Reference Centres. Treatment should start with five or more drugs to which the organism is, or is likely to be, susceptible and continued until sputum cultures become negative. Treatment with three drugs should continue for at least an additional nine months.

KEYWORDS: clinical management; drug-resistant patient; drug susceptibility testing; multidrug-resistant tuberculosis; micobacterial culture

INTRODUCTION

The specific management of drug-resistant patients is only possible where facilities exist for both mycobacterial culture and for drug-susceptibility testing, which excludes most of the developing world. We are fortunate in the United Kingdom in having a relatively low incidence of drug resistance, with isoniazid resistance rates of approximately 6% in patients with no history of prior treatment and multidrug-resistant (MDR TB) rates of between 0.8 and 1.5% of isolates.[1] Rates of drug resis-

Address for correspondence: Professor Peter Ormerod, B.Sc., M.D., D.Sc.(Med), FRCP, Consultant Chest Physician, Blackburn Royal Infirmary, Blackburn, Lancashire, BB2 3LR, UK, pandpormerod@hotmail.com

tance are higher in many parts of the world, with rates of MDR TB of over 10% in patients with no prior treatment history in some of the Baltic republics and over 5% in Cote D'Ivoire, Dominican Republic, and Buenos Aires.[2] From a large database of positive cultures and epidemiological data held by the Public Health Laboratory Service Communicable Disease Surveillance Centre (Mycobnet) in the United Kingdom, we know that the odds ratio (OR) of drug resistance is increased in Indian subcontinent ethnic origin, OR 2.3 (1.3–4.1); Black-African ethnic origin, OR 2.2 (1.0–4.4); previous treatment, OR 3.1 (1.8–5.3); HIV-positivity, OR 4.3 (1.9–9.8); and residence in London, OR 1.7 (1.2–2.5).[3]

Treatment guidelines in the United Kingdom and elsewhere are predicated on the drug-resistance data prevailing in the circumstances of their use. In developed countries the inclusion of the fourth drug (ethambutol but occasionally streptomycin) depends on the level of isoniazid resistance expected or known in a given patient group. In the United Kingdom, the British Thoracic Society guidelines[4] recommend the omission of ethambutol in the initial phase only if the patient meets all the following criteria, based on the drug-resistance data held[1,3]:

- White ethnic origin
- Previously untreated for tuberculosis
- Known to be, or thought upon risk assessment likely to be, HIV-negative
- Not a known contact of drug-resistant disease

The European Respiratory Society[5] recommends the inclusion of ethambutol in the initial phase for those in WHO Treatment Group I, that is, new sputum smear-positive tuberculosis, new smear-negative tuberculosis with extensive parenchymal involvement, and new cases of severe extrapulmonary tuberculosis (not defined). A three-drug initial phase is recommended for those in WHO Category III, new smear-negative pulmonary tuberculosis (except in Category I) and new less severe forms of extrapulmonary tuberculosis. The American Thoracic Society[6] advises the inclusion of ethambutol or streptomycin in the initial phase of a daily regimen at an isoniazid-resistance prevalence of 4%.

Most parts of the world do not have the capabilities to perform mycobacterial culture and drug-susceptibility testing. In these countries, therefore, the "standard" advised regimen has to cover the possibility of the commoner drug resistances. Studies in Hong Kong using regimens of rifampicin, isoniazid, and pyrazinamide, with streptomycin or ethambutol and both streptomycin and ethambutol[7–9] and using rifampicin and isoniazid throughout with pyrazinamide for 2, 4, or 6 months,[10] showed that they were all effective in patients with initial isoniazid and/or streptomycin resistance. Treatment failures and relapse rates were low. If routine drug susceptibility tests are not available, these regimens can be assumed to be highly effective if such resistances are present. The results of these studies[7–10] provide the rationale for using four drugs in the initial phase, with rifampicin and isoniazid in the continuation phase, in areas or in population subgroups with significant incidences of isoniazid and/or streptomycin resistance.

An analysis of the influence of initial drug resistance on response to short-course regimens in the Medical Research Council (MRC) collaborative trials in Hong Kong, Singapore, and Africa was reported in 1986.[11] In those trials, patients with initial isoniazid and/or streptomycin resistance had a failure rate of 17% when given a six-month rifampicin and isoniazid regimen, and a failure rate of 12% in those given rifampicin in the two-month initial phase. As the number of drugs given in the regimen and the duration of rifampicin treatment increased, the failure rate fell, reaching only 2% of those receiving 4–5 drugs including rifampicin throughout a six-month regimen.

Relapse rates after chemotherapy were only slightly increased with initially resistant organisms. The key exception was that of rifampicin resistance, for which the outcome was much poorer (dicussed below).

Although this data applies to countries without drug-susceptibility testing, the view taken in the United Kingdom is that where drug susceptibility tests are available, they should be followed and treatment modified.[4] The strength of the scientific evidence to support various recommendations[12] is also given in the 1998 BTS treatment guidelines.[4]

MANAGEMENT OF NON-MDR RESISTANCE

Isolated Resistances

Streptomycin resistance. Some of the drug resistance reported, particularly in ethnic minority groups, is to streptomycin alone. This is not clinically important since streptomycin is not often used as a first-line drug in developed countries, and the efficacy of the regimen recommended for both respiratory and nonrespiratory tuberculosis is not affected.

Isoniazid resistance. It is important, as discussed earlier, to include ethambutol as a fourth drug in the initial phase for those known to be at higher risk of isoniazid resistance. If isoniazid resistance is known before treatment is started, a regimen of rifampicin, pyrazinamide, ethambutol, and streptomycin for two months, followed by rifampicin and ethambutol for seven months has been shown to give good results if fully supervised.[13] If definite pretreatment resistance to isoniazid is reported after the start of recommended chemotherapy,[4] isoniazid may be stopped, but ethambutol (15 mg/kg) and rifampicin should be given for a minimum of 12 months, together with pyrazinamide for two months.

Pyrazinamide resistance. M. bovis is naturally resistant to pyrazinamide. If the infecting organism is found to be *M. bovis* but is not resistant to other drugs, treatment should be with rifampicin and isoniazid for nine months, supplemented by two months of initial ethambutol. Isolated pyrazinamide resistance in *M. tuberculosis* is uncommon but should be treated with the same regimen as for *M. bovis*.

Ethambutol resistance. Isolated ethambutol resistance is also uncommon. If the organism is otherwise susceptible, the six-month regimen of rifampicin and isoniazid, supplemented by two months of initial pyrazinamide, is satisfactory.

Rifampicin resistance. Isolated rifampicin resistance is very uncommon, but does occur and requires modification and extension of treatment to a period of 18 months, that is, two months of treatment with isoniazid, ethambutol, and pyrazinamide plus isoniazid and ethambutol for an additional 16 months. In the substantial majority of cases (approximately 90%), however, rifampicin resistance is a marker for multidrug-resistant tuberculosis. The patient should therefore be treated and isolated as for multidrug-resistant tuberculosis until the full susceptibility pattern is available.

Rifampicin resistance in *M. tuberculosis* cultures can be successfully determined using molecular methods that allow the detection of rifampicin resistance in approximately 95% of those who are later proven to be resistant by conventional methods.[13–15] Techniques to determine rifampicin resistance in primary specimens such as sputum are becoming available,[16] but should only be used as a guide. Treatment with a rifampicin-based regimen should therefore continue, but with two or three additional drugs added to standard therapy until full susceptibilities are known.

Combined Resistances

Streptomycin and isoniazid resistance. Combined streptomycin and isoniazid resistance is the commonest dual resistance in the United Kingdom. Management should be as for isoniazid resistance found after treatment is commenced but with treatment fully supervised throughout.

Other combinations. Other combinations of non-MDR TB resistance are uncommon. Treatment needs to be individualized depending on the combination involved and is best determined after discussion with a highly experienced clinician and mycobacterial services.

Patients with drug resistance (excluding isolated streptomycin resistance) should be followed up for 12 months after cessation of therapy.

MULTIDRUG-RESISTANT TUBERCULOSIS

The risk factors for MDR TB are those for ordinary drug resistance, but even more exaggerated. The United Kingdom data[3] shows that the odds ratios for risk factors were previous treatment, 11.7 (95% confidence interval 5.5–20), HIV-positivity 8.9 (2.1–30.7), birth in India 4.6 (1.2–6.1), residence in London 4.0 (1.7–9.3), and male sex 2.2 (1.1–4.3). In countries without drug susceptibility testing, a patient experiencing treatment failure should be considered to be at risk for MDR TB, and anyone failing a supervised retreatment with a WHO category II retreatment regimen should be assumed to have MDR TB.

Infection Control

Patients with suspected MDR TB should have molecular testing of samples with rifampicin resistance probes where possible. Those with clinical or microbiological suspicion/proof of MDR TB should be isolated in a negative-pressure room and have infection control and HIV assessments made.[17,18] Criteria for the removal from strict respiratory isolation are also given.[4,17]

Clinical Management

The drug treatment of MDR TB, defined as combined resistance to rifampicin and isoniazid plus or minus other antituberculosis drugs, is complex, time consuming, and demanding on both patient and physician. In the United Kingdom the advice is that treatment should only be carried out by physicians with substantial experience in managing complex resistant cases, only in hospitals with appropriate isolation fa-

TABLE 1. Reserve drugs: dosages and side-effects

Drug	Children	Adults	Main side-effects
Streptomycin	15 mg/kg	15 mg/kg	Tinnitus, ataxia, vertigo (max. dose 1gm) renal impairment
Amikacin	15 mg/kg	15 mg/kg	As for streptomycin
Kanamycin		15 mg/kg	As for streptomycin
Capreomycin		15 mg/kg	As for streptomycin
Ethionamide or Prothionamide	15–20 mg/kg	<50 kg 375 mg bd >50 kg 500 mg bd	Gastrointestinal, hepatitis, avoid in pregnancy
Cycloserine		250–500 mg bd	Depression: fits
Ofloxacin		400 mg bd	Abdominal distress, headache Tremulousness
Ciprofloxacin		750 mg bd	As for ofloxacin plus drug interactions
Azithromycin		500 mg od	Gastrointestinal upset
Clarithromycin		500 mg bd	as azithromycin
Rifabutin		300–450 mg	as for rifampicin: uveitis can occur with drug interactions, e.g., macrolides. Often cross-resistance with rifampicin.
Thiacetazone	4 mg/kg	150 mg od	Gastrointestinal, vertigo, rash, conjunctivitis. AVOID if HIV-positive (Stevens-Johnson syndrome)
Clofazimine		300 mg od	Headache, diarrhea, red skin discoloration
PAS sodium	300 mg/kg	10 gm od 5 gm bd	Gastrointestinal, hepatitis, rash, or fever

cilities, and in very close liaison with Mycobacteriology Reference Centres. This may require the transfer of patients to an appropriate unit where both criteria are met.

Treatment of such patients has to be planned on an individual basis[19,20] and needs to include reserve drugs (see TABLE 1). Such treatments must be closely monitored because of the increased toxicity; but, more importantly, full compliance is essential to prevent the emergence of further drug resistance. Therefore, all such treatment must be directly observed throughout, both on an inpatient and an outpatient basis.

Treatment should start with five or more drugs to which the organism is, or is likely to be, susceptible and continued until sputum cultures become negative. Drug treatment then has to be continued with at least three drugs to which the organism is susceptible on *in vitro* testing for a minimum of nine further months, and perhaps up to or beyond 24 months, depending on the *in vitro* drug-resistance profile, the available drugs,[20] and the patient's HIV status. Consideration may also have to be given to resection of pulmonary lesions under drug cover.[20]

The outcome in MDR TB depends on how rapidly the diagnosis is made, what treatment and facilities are available, and the patient's HIV status. Results in patients who are HIV-positive have been poor with high mortalities, often because of late diagnosis,[21,22] but the outcome in those who are HIV-negative can be much better where appropriate facilities exist[19] and where the drug-resistance profile is less extensive.[23] After treatment, all MDR TB patients require long-term follow-up.

Michael Iseman has "Ten Commandments" for the treatment of tuberculosis, the first being "Thou shalt not add a single drug to a failing regimen," the second to tenth commandments are to repeat the first nine times to make sure the message has been received. It can therefore be argued that to give a WHO retreatment regimen[24] (Category II), which adds only a single drug to the combination that has failed (Category I) regimen, breaks the commandments, and may actually be adding to the incidence of MDR TB. This question needs to be debated.

REFERENCES

1. PUBLIC HEALTH LABORATORY SERVICE COMMUNICABLE DISEASE SURVEILLANCE CENTRE. 1999 (December). Tuberculosis Update. London.
2. PABLOS-MENDEZ, A., M.C. RAVIGLIONE, A. LASZLO, et al. 1998. Global surveillance for antituberculosis drug resistance. N. Engl. J. Med. **338:** 1641–1649.
3. HAYWARD, A.C., D.E. BENNETT, J. HERBERT, et al. 1996. Risk factors for drug resistance in patients with tuberculosis in England and Wales 1993–4. Thorax **51(Suppl. 3):** S32.
4. JOINT TUBERCULOSIS COMMITTEE OF THE BRITISH THORACIC SOCIETY. 1998. Chemotherapy and management of tuberculosis in the United Kingdom: recommendations Thorax **53:** 536–548.
5. MIGLIORI, G.B., M.C. RAVIGLIONE, T. SCHABERG, et al. 1999. Tuberculosis management in Europe. Eur. Respir. J. **14:** 978–992.
6. AMERICAN THORACIC SOCIETY. 1994. Treatment of tuberculosis and tuberculosis infection in adults and children. Am. J. Respir. Crit. Care Med. **149:** 1359–1374.
7. HONG KONG CHEST SERVICE/BRITISH MEDICAL RESEARCH COUNCIL. 1981. First report: controlled trial of four thrice-weekly regimens and a daily regimen all given for 6 months for pulmonary tuberculosis. Lancet **1:** 171–174.
8. HONG KONG CHEST SERVICE/BRITISH MEDICAL RESEARCH COUNCIL. 1982. Second report: controlled trial of four thrice-weekly regimens and a daily regimen all given for 6 months. The results up to 24 months. Tubercle **63:** 89–98.
9. HONG KONG CHEST SERVICE/ BRITISH MEDICAL RESEARCH COUNCIL. 1987. Five-year follow-up of a controlled trial of five 6-month regimens of chemotherapy for pulmonary tuberculosis. Am. Rev. Resp. Dis. **136:** 1339–1342.
10. HONG KONG CHEST SERVICE/BRITISH MEDICAL RESEARCH COUNCIL. 1991. Controlled trial of 2, 4 and 6 months of pyrazinamide in 6 month, three-times weekly regimens for smear-positive tuberculosis, including an assessment of a combined preparation of isoniazid, rifampicin and pyrazinamide. Results at 30 months. Am. Rev. Resp. Dis. **143:** 700–706.
11. MITCHISON, D.A. & A.J. NUNN. 1986. Influence of initial resistance on the response to short-course chemotherapy of pulmonary tuberculosis. Am. Rev. Resp. Dis. **133:** 423–430.
12. PETRIE, J.G., E. BARNWELL & J. GRIMSHAW, on behalf of the Scottish InterCollegiate Guidelines Network. 1995. Clinical Guidelines: Criteria for Appraisal for National Use. Royal College of Physicians. Edinburgh.
13. TELENTI, A., P. IMBODEN, F. MARCHESI, et al. 1993. Detection of rifampicin-resistance mutation in *Mycobacterium tuberculosis*. Lancet **341:** 647–650.
14. DROBNIEWSKI, F.A., R.J. KENT, N.G. STOKER, et al. 1994. Molecular biology in the diagnosis and epidemiology of tuberculosis. J. Hosp. Infect. **28:** 249–263.
15. DROBNIEWSKI, F.A. & A.L. POZNIAK. 1996. Molecular diagnosis, detection of drug resistance and epidemiology of tuberculosis. Br. J. Hosp. Med. **56:** 204–208.

16. GOYAL, M., R.J. SHAW, D.K. BANERJEE, et al. 1997. Rapid detection of multidrug-resistant tuberculosis. Eur. Respir. J. **10:** 120–124.
17. THE INTERDEPARTMENTAL WORKING GROUP ON TUBERCULOSIS. 1998. The prevention and control of tuberculosis in the United Kingdom: UK guidance on the prevention and control of (1) HIV-related tuberculosis and (2) Drug resistant, including multiple drug resistant, tuberculosis. Department of Health, London; The Scottish Office, Edinburgh; The Welsh Office, Cardiff. September 1998.
18. JOINT TUBERCULOSIS COMMITTEE OF THE BRITISH THORACIC SOCIETY. 2000. Control and prevention of tuberculosis in the United Kingdom: code of practice 2000. Thorax **55:** 887–901.
19. GOBLE, M., M. ISEMAN, L.A. MADSEN, et al. 1993. Treatment of 171 patients with pulmonary tuberculosis resistant to isoniazid and rifampin. N. Engl. J. Med. **328:** 527–532.
20. ISEMAN, M. 1993. Treatment of multidrug resistant tuberculosis. N. Engl. J. Med. **329:** 784–790.
21. DROBNIEWSKI, F.A. 1997. Is death inevitable with multiresistant TB plus HIV infection? Lancet **349:** 71–72.
22. SMALL, P.M., R.W. SHAFER, P.C. HOPEWELL, et al. 1993. Exogenous re-infection with multi-drug resistant *Mycobacterium tuberculosis* in patients with advanced HIV infection. N. Engl. J. Med. **328:** 1137–1144.
23. TELZAK, E.E., K. SEPOWITZ, P. ALPERT, et al. 1995. Multidrug-resistant TB in patients without HIV infection. N. Engl. J. Med. **333:** 907–911.
24. WORLD HEALTH ORGANISATION TUBERCULOSIS UNIT. DIVISION OF COMMUNICABLE DISEASES. 1991. Guidelines for Tuberculosis Treatment in Adults and Children in National Tuberculosis Programmes. WHO/TB/91: 1–61. WHO. Geneva.

Multidrug-Resistant Tuberculosis and HIV Infection

ANTON POZNIAK

Department of HIV and Genitourinary Medicine, Chelsea and Westminster Hospital, London SW10 9NH, UK

ABSTRACT: In the 1990s, outbreaks of multidrug-resistant tuberculosis (MDR TB) among HIV-positive patients ultimately led to the establishment in the developed world of a comprehensive TB control strategy for these patients that is effective. The treatment regimen for HIV and MDR TB is complicated by the fact that most of the drugs used have not been studied for interactions with antivirals. Hence, overlapping toxicities require intensive management and monitoring of these patients. Good public health policy is essential to preventing MDR TB outbreaks among immunosuppressed patients.

KEYWORDS: tuberculosis; HIV; multidrug-resistant TB; drug interaction

INTRODUCTION

Outbreaks of multidrug-resistant tuberculosis (MDR TB) among HIV-positive patients in the early 1990s, especially in the United States, highlighted the need for improvement in public health and hospital control of infection policy, laboratory and clinical management, research, development, and education in tuberculosis. This new focus, together with an increase in financial investment, has led to many developed countries having a comprehensive tuberculosis control strategy for immunocompromized persons that is more robust.

HIV AND TB

The biggest single risk factor for developing tuberculosis is HIV infection. In some countries in the world, especially sub-Saharan Africa, the co-infection rate of HIV and TB is estimated to be over 1,000 per 100,000 of population. In spite of some excellent TB control programs, many of these countries are still experiencing increases in tuberculosis case rates because of HIV co-infection. Few countries have universal HIV testing or comprehensive TB culture and drug sensitivity reporting, and so the global epidemiology of MDR TB in HIV-positive patients is as yet mostly unmeasured.[1] In the United States in 1998, it was estimated that 20% of all patients with TB were HIV co-infected, but the proportion with MDR TB was not known.

Address for correspondence: Anton Pozniak, Department of HIV and Genitourinary Medicine, Chelsea and Westminster Hospital, 369 Fulham Road, London SW10 9NH, U.K.
Anton.pozniak@chelwest.nhs.uk

The reason that HIV is strongly associated with MDR TB is through outbreaks. These occur because HIV-positive patients have an increased risk of developing active tuberculous disease once infected with *Mycobacterium tuberculosis*. Among those not infected with HIV, for every 10 persons exposed and infected with TB (whether drug sensitive or resistant), only one will develop tuberculous disease during his/her lifetime. For those with HIV infection, this risk of around 10% in a whole lifetime is telescoped down to only 1 to 2 years. Highly active antiretroviral therapy does have an impact on rates of developing tuberculosis, however, and may reduce the rates of tuberculosis in countries where patients are offered anti-HIV treatment.

MDR TB OUTBREAKS

Outbreaks have occurred in hospitals in Europe[2–6] and U.S. clinics[7] for HIV-positive patients and for substance abusers in prisons and homeless shelters.[8,9] From 1990 to 1992 nine large outbreaks of MDR TB were reported from the United States: All organisms isolated were resistant to isoniazid and rifampicin (as this is a definition of MDR TB), and most also had streptomycin and ethambutol resistance. The HIV infection rate among these patients was from 20 to 100%, and the mortality rate was from 60 to 89%. The interval from TB diagnosis to death was between 4 and 16 weeks. Various strains of MDR TB were circulating during this time, especially the notorious "W" strain, which infected 199 patients in New York from 1991 to 1994 and involved 30 hospitals.[10] Other types, named "N2," "W1," and "AB," infected a large number of patients in 10 to 16 hospitals. The majority of these outbreaks were brought under control by means of public health administrative measures, including infection control policies for patients with HIV who have a cough, segregation of potentially infectious patients, the use of negative pressure rooms, and submicron masks.[11–13] Procedures such as nebulization of pentamidine for PCP prophylaxis, saline for induced sputa, or even salbutamol for those with obstructive airway disease were no longer performed in open areas but confined to negative pressure rooms.

TREATMENT

The drug treatment regimens used for outbreak patients have been based on drug sensitivity patterns (see TABLE 1). Most of them included an 8 quinolone, such as ofloxacin, together with amikacin and, if sensitive, pyrazinamide. Other drugs have been used, but the long-term efficacy is unknown. Recently, it has been shown that a combination of amikacin, sparfloxacin, and ethionamide was useful in patients who were sensitive to these drugs.

The optimum duration of treatment for MDR TB is still unknown, and many cases are treated for 2 years after cultures convert to negative.

ALTERNATIVE THERAPIES

Some patients with localized disease and those with good cardiac pulmonary reserve and low bacterial burden can be considered for either partial or total lung re-

TABLE 1. HIV-associated multidrug-resistant tuberculosis outbreaks January 1990 to August 1992 in the United States

Facility	Total cases	Resistance pattern	HIV infection (%)	Mortality	Median interval TB diagnosis to death
Hosp A	65	H, R, (E, Eth)	93	72	7
Hosp B	35	H,R, (R, E)	100	89	16
Hosp C	70	H, R, S, (E, Eth, Ka, B)	94	82	4
Hosp D	29	H, R, (E, Eth)	91	83	4
Hosp E	7	H, R, S, (E, Eth, Ka, RB)	20	60	4
Hosp F	16	H, R, S, (eth, Ka, RB)	82	82	4
Hosp G	13	HR (E)	100	85	4
Prison system	42	HR (S, E, Eth, Ka, RB)	91	74	4

section. Nebulized interferon has been used in rendering sputum smears negative in such patients before surgery. It has also been used as a method to prevent the spread of infection when all other drug treatments have failed in non-HIV-infected MDR TB cases. The use of the immunomodulation with *M. vaccae* has not yet been used in a formal trial of MDR TB.

CONTACTS

For close contacts of patients with MDR TB, no clear guidelines exist as to what to do. It is easier to decide on a chemoprophylaxis regime if the drug sensitivity patterns are known. It is still not known whether or not this type of prophylaxis would work. A "Delphi symposium" decided that if infection and disease progression was likely, then ethambutol and pyrazinamide or a quinolone plus pyrazinamide might be used.[14] The role of the BCG vaccine in adults is still unknown. During the New York outbreaks, it was reported that physicians had BCG vaccinations in the hope that this might protect them if exposed.

PROGNOSIS AND PREDICTORS

Prognosis in HIV patients who are HIV positive and have MDR TB has been very poor, with between 25 and 30% of people surviving to 6 months if they are severely immune suppressed.[15]

Most of the factors responsible for MDR TB outbreaks have now been addressed by government or federal policy, but awareness of these factors is still important and can provide the guiding principles for prevention. The factors include inadequate control programs for TB, inadequate adherence to medication, infection control procedure breakdown through putting all the immune-suppressed patients in one area such as an open hospital ward, having a low index for suspicion of tuberculosis lead-

TABLE 2. Outbreak 1 UK contact and case finding

- Index and 7 other cases all HIV+, 2 alive now
- 187 HIV+ contacts
- 60 staff contacts
- 57 community contacts

ing to patients' infectiousness being prolonged, and having poor laboratory communication with clinicians.

The major risk factors for MDR TB in HIV patients are the same as in the general population: a history of previous treatment, birth, travel, or work in an area endemic for MDR TB and a history of poor adherence, sputum positivity continuing after 2 months of treatment, or being culture positive after 3 months. In addition some factors in the HIV population have been recognized as predictors of MDR TB. Severely immune-suppressed, HIV-positive patients seem more likely to develop MDR TB, probably because of the high risk of progression to disease once infected. A failure to become apyrexial by 2 weeks of treatment and development of hilar lymph nodes are other factors pointing towards possible MDR TB.[16,17]

One of the best predictors that patients will survive is having started on at least two drugs to which the organism is susceptible within 2 weeks of diagnosis. This often means a patient is given multiple drugs before the drug sensitivity patterns become available.[18,19]

In Europe there have been at least six outbreaks involving around 225 patients, and these have major implications for resource utilization and public health. (See TABLES 2 and 3.) The outbreaks require that a large number of staff be used in contact tracing and case finding. It is interesting to note that in the second outbreak in the United Kingdom very few people took the prophylaxis and, of those who did, almost all of them had stopped by 2 weeks.

One of the largest outbreaks of MDR TB occurred in Argentina over a 15-month period.[20] A total of 101 patients had resistance to five drugs, and survival was approximately 10%. Most of these patients were in contact with an intravenous drug user who was poorly adherent to treatment and had developed resistance.

There have been outbreaks of multidrug-resistant *M. bovis* in HIV patients in Spain involving 19 cases over 15 months. Resistance to 11 drugs was found, and all the patients died with a median survival of only 44 days. Their risk factor was severe immune suppression.[21]

It was thought that poor drug absorption might increase the risk of HIV-positive patients in developing MDR TB, but one study of drug absorption in AIDS patients[22] showed there was no difference in the T_{max}, C_{max}, and median area under the curve (AUC) for AIDS patients compared with HIV-negative patients. In fact it appeared that the AIDS patients, even those with GI problems, were absorbing rifampicin better than HIV-negative matched controls. It has also been suggested that HIV-positive patients required longer treatment for their tuberculosis and that inadequate length of treatment might lead to MDR TB. No evidence exists to support this, however, with duration of treatment and relapse being the same whether HIV patients are given 6 or 9 months of treatment for initial, fully drug-susceptible disease.

TABLE 3. Outbreak 2 UK contact and case finding

- Index HIV– and 6 other HIV cases
- 1298 general medical patients exposed
- 169 recalled
- 898 staff contacts
- 64 HIV patient contacts
- 476 HIV outpatient contacts
- TB resistant to H,R,ANS, Clo,Cyclo±Z,Cla,Cip
- TB sensitive to Eth,CapStrep,Ethio,Amik
- Prophyaxis PAS + ETH offered to 400
- Only 12 on prophylaxis, 10 stopped most by 2 weeks

SPORADIC MDR TB IN HIV

In South Africa patients were examined to see whether they were more likely to develop MDR TB outside an outbreak event. It was found that 12% of the HIV-negative compared with 2% of HIV-positive patients developed MDR TB during the follow-up.[23] The reason for this is that good public health control can prevent outbreaks even in developing countries. Those HIV patients involved in outbreaks may have fewer cavities, more fevers, and be more immunosuppressed than those who develop sporadic MDR TB.[24] Data from the South African gold mines in 1993–1997, where the potential for outbreaks was great, helped shed more light on the association between HIV and MDR TB. Miners' hostels, accommodating 2,000–3,000 men, most living with other men in a room, showed an increased incidence of TB from 1174 to 2476 per 100,000 over a 6-year period from 1990 to 1996 with an associated increase in HIV rates. Despite an HIV positivity of 28%, the MDR TB in new patients was only 1% of the total and even in retreatment cases was only 2.8%. There was no association between MDR TB and HIV status. The reason for the low incidence seen in retreatment cases was that there was a very good directly observed therapy (DOTS) strategy with a 93% treatment completion rate.

CONCLUSIONS

A major concern for many is that HIV might cause global outbreaks of MDR TB as more and more patients receive antituberculosis therapy in an environment in which the political and financial situation is unstable and DOTS strategies are not implemented in full. The direct impact of this would be outbreak transmission to immunosuppressed patients and then onwards to immune-competent persons. As a result, the already fragile control programs would be swamped. There have been cases of immunosuppressed patients being treated for fully drug-sensitive TB and them being exposed and acquiring drug-resistant strains while on therapy for the fully sensitive strain.[26]

The treatment regimen for HIV and MDR TB can be complex. Most of the drugs used in MDR TB have not had drug/drug interaction studies performed with antiviral compounds, and so the potential for adverse interreactions is considerable. There are major overlapping toxicities, particularly those causing hepatic and cutaneous reactions. Each patient requires intensive management and monitoring, and a minimal estimate for the care of an MDR TB case is $100,000.[27] If they are also HIV infected, this cost may be doubled over a 2-year period of treatment. The impact outbreaks have on case finding and contact tracing is enormous. (See TABLES 2 and 3.) Without good public health policy implemented inside and outside institutions like hospitals, the potential for large MDR TB outbreaks among immunosuppressed patients remains a frightening reality.

REFERENCES

1. PUNNOTOK, J., N. SHAFFER, T. NAIWATANAKUL, et al. 2000. Human immunodeficiency virus-related tuberculosis and primary drug resistance in Bangkok, Thailand. Int. J. Tuberc. Lung Dis. 6: 537–543.
2. HANNAN, M.M., H. PERES, F. MALTEZ, et al. 2001. Investigation and control of a large outbreak of multi-drug resistant tuberculosis at a central Lisbon hospital. J. Hosp. Infect. 72: 91–97.
3. MORO, M.L., I. ERRANTE, A. INFUSO, et al. 2000. Effectiveness of infection control measures in controlling a nosocomial outbreak of multidrug-resistant tuberculosis among HIV patients in Italy. Int. J. Tuberc. Lung Dis. 41: 61–58.
4. BREATHNACH, A.S., A. DE RUITER, G.M. HOLDSWORTH, et al. 1998. An outbreak of multi-drug-resistant tuberculosis in a London teaching hospital. J. Hosp. Infect. 92: 111–117.
5. CORONADO, V.G., C.M. BECK-SAGUE, M.D. HUTTON, et al. 1993. Transmission of multidrug-resistant Mycobacterium tuberculosis among persons with human immunodeficiency virus infection in an urban hospital: epidemiologic and restriction fragment length polymorphism analysis. J. Infect. 1684: 1052–1055.
6. CENTERS FOR DISEASE CONTROL AND PREVENTION. 1993. Outbreak of multidrug-resistant tuberculosis at a hospital—New York City, 1991. Morbid. Mortal. Wkly. Rep. 4222: 427, 433–434.
7. PITCHENIK, A.E., J. BURR, M. LAUFER, et al. 1990. Outbreaks of drug-resistant tuberculosis at AIDS centre. Lancet 336: 440–441.
8. CONOVER, C., R. RIDZON, S. VALWAY, et al. 2001. Outbreak of multidrug-resistant tuberculosis at a methadone treatment program. Int. J. Tuberc. Lung Dis. 1: 59–64.
9. CENTERS FOR DISEASE CONTROL AND PREVENTION. 1992. Transmission of multidrug-resistant tuberculosis among immunocompromised persons in a correctional system—New York, 1991. Morbid. Mortal. Wkly. Rep. 4128: 507–509.
10. SHAFER, R.W., P.M. SMALL, C. LARKIN, et al. 1995. Temporal trends and transmission patterns during the emergence of multidrug-resistant tuberculosis in New York City: a molecular epidemiologic assessment: J. Infect. Dis. 171: 170–176.
11. MORO, M.L., A. GORI, I. ERRANTE, et al. 1998. An outbreak of multidrug-resistant tuberculosis involving HIV-infected patients of two hospitals in Milan, Italy. Italian Multidrug-Resistant Tuberculosis Outbreak Study Group. AIDS 129: 1095–102.
12. MALONEY, S.A., M.L. PEARSON, M.T. GORDON, et al. 1995. Efficacy of control measures in preventing nosocomial transmission of multidrug-resistant tuberculosis to patients and health care workers. Ann. Intern. Med. 122: 90–95.
13. STROUD, L.A., J.I. TOKARS, M.H. GRIECO, et al. 1995. Evaluation of infection control measures in preventing the nosocomial transmission of multidrug-resistant Myco-

bacterium tuberculosis in a New York City hospital. Infect. Control Hosp. Epidemiol. **3:** 141–147.

14. PASSANNANTE, M.R., C.T. GALLAGHER & L.B. REICHMAN. 1994. Preventive therapy for contacts of multidrug-resistant tuberculosis. A Delphi survey. Chest **1062:** 431–434.

15. FISCHL, M.A., G.L. DAIKOS, R.B. UTTAMCHANDANI, *et al.* 1992. Clinical presentation and outcome of patients with HIV infection and tuberculosis caused by multiple-drug-resistant bacilli. Ann. Intern. Med. **117:** 184–190.

16. TELZAK, E.E., K.D. CHIRGWIN, E.T. NELSON, *et al.* 1999. Predictors for multidrug-resistant tuberculosis among HIV-infected patients and response to specific drug regimens. Terry Beirn Community Programs for Clinical Research on AIDS CPCRA and the AIDS Clinical Trials Group ACTG, National Institutes for Health. Int. J. Tuberc. Lung Dis. **4:** 337–343.

17. SALOMON, N., D.C. PERLMAN, P. FRIEDMANN, *et al.* 1995. Predictors and outcome of multidrug-resistant tuberculosis. Clin. Infect. Dis. **215:** 1245–1252.

18. PARK, M.M., A.L. DAVIS, N.W. SCHLUGER, *et al.* 1996. Related articles outcome of MDR-TB patients, 1983–1993. Prolonged survival with appropriate therapy. Am. J. Respir. Crit. Care Med. **531:** 317–324.

19. TURETT, G.S., E.E. TELZAK, L.V. TORIAN, *et al.* 1995. Improved outcomes for patients with multidrug-resistant tuberculosis. Clin. Infect. Dis. **215:** 1238–1244.

20. RITACCO, V., M. DI LONARDO, A. RENIERO, *et al.* 1997. Nosocomial spread of human munodeficiency virus-related multidrug-resistant tuberculosis in Buenos Aires. J. Infect. Dis. **763:** 637–642.

21. COBO, J., A. ASENSIO, S. MORENO, *et al.* 2001. Risk factors for nosocomial transmission of multidrug-resistant tuberculosis due to *Mycobacterium bovis* among HIV-infected patients. Int. J. Tuberc. Lung Dis. **5:** 413–418.

22. TAYLOR, B. & P.J. SMITH. 1998. Does AIDS impair the absorption of antituberculosis agents? Int. J. Tuberc. Lung Dis. **2(8):** 670–75.

23. ANASTASIS, D., G. PILLAI, V. RAMBIRITCH, *et al.* 1997. Related articles: a retrospective study of human immunodeficiency virus infection and drug-resistant tuberculosis in Durban, South Africa. Int. J. Tuberc. Lung Dis. **3:** 220–224.

24. SACKS, L.V., S. PENDLE, D. ORLOVIC, *et al.* 1999. A comparison of outbreak- and non-outbreak-related multidrug-resistant tuberculosis among human immunodeficiency virus-infected patients in a South African hospital. Clin. Infect. Dis. **91:** 96–101.

25. CHURCHYARD, G.J., E.L. CORBETT, I. KLEINSCHMIDT, *et al.* 2000. Drug-resistant tuberculosis in South African gold miners: incidence and associated factors. Int. J. Tuberc. Lung Dis. **5:** 433–440.

26. SMALL, P.M., R.W. SHAFER, P.C. HOPEWELL, *et al.* 1993. Exogenous reinfection with multidrug-resistant *Mycobacterium tuberculosis* in patients with advanced HIV infection. N. Engl. J. Med. **328:** 1137–1144.

27. WHITE, V.L. & J. MOORE-GILLON. 2000. Resource implications of patients with multi-drug resistant tuberculosis. Thorax **511:** 962–963.

Holding the Patient

GINI WILLIAMS

City University, London E1 2EA, UK

ABSTRACT: **Successfully controlling tuberculosis will require that we fully understand all the factors involved in a patient's ability to comply with treatment as well as our assumptions about what compliance and noncompliance mean. Influences on patients' lives, such as poverty, conflict, political instability, and racial and gender inequalities, will have a great impact on the success or failure of treatment. TB services should be designed to provide the support that patients need to enable them to be cured.**

KEYWORDS: **DOTS; tuberculosis; noncompliance**

Despite effective treatment for the last 50 years, tuberculosis is still not under control. On the contrary, it is one of the world's leading infectious killers. Even though it has been acknowledged that TB control programs around the world suffer from inconsistent drug supplies[1] and that as many as half of all active TB cases are never even diagnosed,[2] noncompliance is often blamed when a TB service does not work, for drug resistance being on the increase, and even for TB itself being on the increase. The very term "noncompliance" implies blame and a level of personal and structural resources that allows a person to consciously refuse treatment when, in fact, a host of other barriers to compliance need to be considered.

It is of course essential for someone with fully sensitive TB to complete his or her treatment in order to make a full recovery and not develop resistance to any of the first-line drugs. Persons with resistant strains also need to take their prescribed medication, but the effort of supporting them will often be more intense because the regimen for resistant TB is likely to be difficult and prolonged.

This paper explores the issues that need to be considered in order to assist those of us involved in TB control in holding patients for the full course of their treatment. Although an exploration of these issues is relevant to everyone working with TB patients, I will emphasize here the role of the TB nurse or community health worker. This paper will explore the full meaning of "holding the patient," refer to literature relating to compliance, and consider some of the results from an ethnographic study of persons receiving treatment for TB.

Address for correspondence: Gini Williams, Lecturer, City University, Alexander Building, Philpot St., London E1 2EA, U.K. Voice: 444 207 040 5968.

ginig@ginig.co.uk

"HOLDING" DEFINED

What does "holding the patient" actually involve? Some important aspects of assisting patients to complete their treatment lie within the full meaning of this phrase. The verb "to hold" has a number of definitions:

(1) To "keep or detain" (someone): We can use the Public Health Act in England to section people, but this has been shown to be very difficult to administer with any success. People can only be detained for a short period of time and then usually only when infectious. There are no facilities for incarceration.

(2) To "remain secure, intact or in position without breaking or giving way": We must hold a patient's attention for the full course of treatment. It is difficult to maintain the patient's motivation without understanding his or her cultural, social, and economic context and offering ongoing, accessible support and appropriate information. This is particularly important with MDR TB patients who will be on more medication for longer periods and are likely to suffer more side effects, fear, and uncertainty.

(3) To "contain or be capable of containing": Realistic caseload sizes (i.e., staffing levels) are required so that each patient's case can be managed effectively. Staff members need to be properly supported and have sufficient space and equipment to ensure the best possible access for people who need to use the service. Prioritization is essential to make the most of scarce resources—for instance, DOT (directly observed treatment) is very time-consuming. Within a well-structured TB service, it is possible to achieve high cure rates offering DOT on a selective basis, that is, to those who may have problems adhering to treatment. Insisting on giving all patients DOT can lead to a situation in which the most vulnerable patients do not receive the care they so desperately need.[3] In some places, because of excessive workloads, treatment is only given to people who are able to attend a clinic in order that every dose can be supervised.[3] This immediately rules out those persons in the most difficult circumstances.

(4) To "have in one's possession": This implies the need to take responsibility, in this case for patients and their successful completion of treatment. We cannot assume that patients are always able to take responsibility for their own treatment, and the service has to take responsibility for achieving a positive outcome. Supportive partnerships with other agencies are needed in order to meet the full range of each individual patient's needs. Advocacy is vital at every level to ensure that the patient is receiving the correct treatment and has access to the support he or she needs from a variety of different agencies. Regular audits can highlight whether or not the service is effective in achieving its objectives and that the quality is maintained.

(5) To "carry, support with one's arms," that is, to care for: If we don't care for patients adequately, how can they be expected to care for themselves? Treatment is standardized, but care needs to be planned on an individual basis. Each patient may have a different reaction to the TB diagnosis, with different personal adjustments to make. The successful completion of treatment is paramount to those of us who are health care providers, but the patients may have other priorities. In order to achieve our goal, we need to work with them to achieve theirs. In this context DOT can be seen as a means to offer the patient additional support. The six-month treatment needed to cure TB can become a window of opportunity to address some of the problems that led them to fall prey to an opportunistic disease like TB in the first place.

In spite of effective treatment and ever-advancing diagnostic techniques, TB and drug-resistant TB continue to rise among the poorest groups around the world. It does not, however, require huge investments to make positive changes, even in the most difficult circumstances; careful funding to make effective treatment available on a consistent and well-supported basis can have dramatic results. "In rural Haiti... we learned that cure rates could increase from under 50% to nearly 100% if comprehensive supports, including financial and nutritional aid, are put in place while patients are being treated." People have also been shown to be much more likely to use services that are welcoming and convenient for them, both geographically and in their hours of operation. (Farmer,[4] p. 208, citing Farmer et al.[5])

THE DISCOURSE SURROUNDING COMPLIANCE

The Meaning of "Compliance"

There will always be a very small number of people who refuse to come on board for a treatment program. It would be unrealistic and soul-destroying to expect to achieve success 100% of the time, but our success rate shouldn't be far off that mark. If we are unsuccessful we should be able to give an account of what happened so we can learn where we need an alternative approach.

Clinicians often label patients who do not take their prescribed treatment as noncompliant, "...an almost abusive term, which implies at least ignorance and often also irresponsibility, irrationality and moral blameworthiness."[7] More objectively, to comply is to ".... act in accordance with a wish or command"[8]: In the health field, this means that a patient follows the doctor's instructions. I am not going to dwell on the definition of compliance, nor am I going to use a different word. I acknowledge the fact that the term "noncompliance" implies deviance and the need to be controlled, but agree with Lerner[9] that focusing on the negative connotations of the term itself can restrict our potential to explore wider issues such as why it is so strongly associated with the assumption that patients should obey doctors in the first place.

Lerner[9] cites anthropologists who recommended that there should be more negotiation between doctors and patients and an acknowledgment that they have different expectations of their contact.[10,11] "Rather than replacing the paternalistic word 'compliance' with a more benign term respectful of patient autonomy, we need to integrate the issue of compliance into a model that accepts both a degree of physician control and patient resistance."[9] (p. 1428)

This assumes that patient has sufficient agency to be able to resist in the first place. It needs to be understood that patients won't necessarily be able or willing to comply with the treatment, and work needs to be done to address whatever their concerns or needs might be. The nurse or doctor is likely to have just one issue, that is, the treatment and the patient's response to it; whereas the patient may have many other concerns, which need to be addressed in conjunction with his or her clinical treatment.

Compliance as the "Norm"

The overwhelming assumption, in both research and practice, is that compliance is the expected norm and noncompliance is deviant.[12] For some reason, the evidence from numerous studies demonstrating that from one-third to one-half of all patients do not follow medical instructions or prescriptions has not been used to challenge this point of view.[12] Donovan and Blake studied what rheumatology patients felt and thought about the drugs they were prescribed and found, consistently with other studies, that around 50% of their informants failed to follow their treatment regimens as instructed.[12] It would seem, therefore, that this cannot be viewed as deviant behavior, and the behavior is not as straightforward as, say, simply refusing to comply with instructions. It also suggests that this is a valuable area for social and behavioral scientists to explore, especially when the consequences of noncompliance are considered.

Consequences of Noncompliance

Even under noninfectious conditions, noncompliance has resource implications for the National Health Service, both in terms of waste and the preventable acute episodes requiring intervention, admission to hospital, and so forth.[13] TB adds another layer of concern, because a noncompliant patient may lead to additional patients requiring care and/or developing drug resistance, which is very expensive to treat. It is of even greater importance, then, that we accept the fact that patients do not necessarily follow instructions given to them by health care personnel and that this may be attributable to any number of reasons, many of which are beyond the patient's control.

Factors Associated with Compliance

A number of reviews have looked at compliance with TB treatment[14] as well as compliance in general.[15] Ogden[3] identifies two themes upon which social scientists have tended to focus in relation to compliance, the first being the nature of the doctor–patient relationship (e.g., Zola[16,17]) and the second being the impact of cultural factors such as health beliefs (e.g., Barnhoorn and Adriaanse[18] and Becker[19]).

Farmer would argue, however, that these approaches fail to recognize the wider influences on patients' lives such as poverty, conflict, political instability, racial and gender inequalities, and so on, which are beyond the control of individuals and yet preclude their ability to follow medical instructions. The problem is far more complex than simply the physician trying to convince patients to take their treatment for the good of themselves and others. Many issues are involved, including understanding, trust, personal world view, motivation, memory, economics, ability, and accessibility of health services.

According to Zola[17] "We, the health researchers and providers,…do not sufficiently appreciate what following a medical regimen means to an individual, nor do we fully acknowledge the role that health personnel have in contributing to the very noncompliance we seek to reverse." (p. 241) Apart from any indirect contribution to treatment failure, clinical error contributes directly to patients receiving inadequate medication. Mistakes made by physicians are well documented in relation to cases of MDR TB."In reviewing the histories of [MDR TB] patients in a leading hospital in Colorado, Mahmoudi and Iseman discovered an average of 3.9 physician-directed errors per patient." (Farmer,[4] p. 199, citing Mahmoudi and Iseman[20])

In spite of this and the fact that most TB deaths occur in the poorest areas with the poorest services, noncompliance continues to be given as one of the main explanations for the existence of MDR TB and the fact that the incidence of TB continues to rise despite the existance of an effective cure.[4]

The Patient's Experience of TB Treatment

Donovan and Blake[12] suggest that we are making a mistake in assuming that compliance is as much on the patients' minds as it is on ours. "For patients, compliance is not an issue: they do not perceive taking drugs entirely in terms of obeying the doctor's orders. Instead they weigh up the costs and benefits of taking particular medications as they perceive them within the contexts and constraints of their everyday lives and needs." (p. 512)

I have recently completed a dissertation for an M.Sc. degree in medical anthropology.[22] My aim was to find out about the experience of being on TB treatment. It involved repeated, unstructured in-depth interviews with six young people who were in the middle of their treatment for TB. The sample was small in comparison to most health or medical research but was appropriate for ethnographic purposes. "The outcome of [anthropologists'] work is not necessarily expected to be definitive in its individual own right. It must be consistent with earlier work in the field but it may be at once contradictory, enhancing and transcending without having, like clinical conclusions, to replace its predecessors."[7] (p. 7)

None of the informants involved in the study saw compliance as an issue and reported taking their medication as prescribed. A number of them were puzzled about why some people would not do so. This was reinforced throughout the study period by related comments and references to medication.

The fact that all the informants took their treatment as a matter of course allowed me to consider what it was about this group that enabled them to comply apparently so easily. Within the dissertation I explored the themes that arose from the fieldwork and that have been identified in the literature as having an impact on compliance, namely, lay beliefs and experiences, information-giving and support, issues of agency, and cost–benefit analysis. The main findings in relation to patient compliance are discussed briefly below.

FACTORS THAT ENABLE PATIENTS TO COMPLETE TREATMENT

No conflict with religious/cultural beliefs. The sample was culturally mixed, but all of the informants could be described as being from an ethnic minority group. A number of them had very strong religious beliefs, but all of them spoke of gaining support from their faith in a higher being and of feeling encouraged by this to take their treatment. Religious belief does not necessarily preclude compliance. Farmer's research "… explored adherence to therapy among a group of patients with active tuberculosis in a village in Haiti, where local conceptions of tuberculosis are often strikingly at odds with conventional biomedical understandings."[4] (p. 213) He found in his sample that belief in sorcery as a cause of TB had little effect on patient's motivation to comply with treatment.[4] (p. 221) (An overemphasis on cultural barriers to compliance can obscure other factors such as those discussed below. It is important to assess the sense made of TB or its treatment by each patient within his or her individual belief system and cultural context.)

Present/past experience: recovery with treatment/death without. The informants' attitudes toward diagnosis and the stigma attached to TB seemed to vary according to the their past experience or prior knowledge of the disease. A number of them had known people who had died from TB, having not received treatment. The informants reported different reactions to their diagnosis and reflected different attitudes toward the stigma they felt attached to the disease. Nearly all of them reported being reluctant to tell others about their disease but for different reasons. They all reported seeing signs of improvement and related this to a wish to continue treatment.

Availability of good information. According to Ley and Llewelyn, "...in general patients want more information about their condition and their treatment, but many feel they are not told enough, many do not understand what they are told, and many do not remember what is said.... It is...likely that patients' compliance with advice [is] adversely affected by the lack of information."[13] (p. 75) They argue, as Donovan and Blake[12] do, that the clinicians need to change their behavior to improve communication but suffer from the assumption that compliance is the norm and that as long as patients know, understand, and remember they will comply with instructions.

It was evident both from the interviews and from participant observation that concerted efforts were made by the TB team to give patients the information they needed throughout their treatment. All of the informants valued the fact that they could easily access support and advice from members of the TB team either by phone, during routine visits, or by coming to the chest clinic in person.

Good support from family and clinic staff. The lack of family support is rarely mentioned in the literature in relation to compliance, although Haynes did find family instability to be one of the few variables consistent with noncompliance.[23] The relationships the informants had with their families emerged as a strong theme in this study and appeared to be an important aspect in the informants' attitudes toward their treatment and their ability to continue with it.

Other sources of support described by the informants included the doctors and nurses at the chest clinic. Donovan and Blake's conclusion to their study of rheumatology is that "The key to improving rates of compliance...is the development of active, co-operative relationships between patients and doctors. For this to be successful, doctors will need to recognize patients' decision-making abilities, to try to understand patients' needs and constraints, and to work with patients in the development of treatment regimes."[12] (p. 512)

Benefits outweighing the costs. Donovan and Blake argue that the importance of developing a good relationship with patients has to go much deeper than being able to provide information in an appropriate and useful way. They believe that ". . . much of the work about noncompliance, suggesting that patients are too ignorant to understand medical instructions or that they forget large proportions of what they are told, is misplaced."[12] (p. 188) In their study of patients with rheumatoid arthritis, they found that "When they were offered treatment and advice in the clinics patients carried out what amounted to a cost–benefit analysis of each item."[12] (p. 510)

Becker and Rosenstock argue that "When an illness has been diagnosed and a course of treatment recommended, the individual's perception of the threat represented by symptoms or by the future course of the condition becomes central. It is in relation to this threat that possible actions and their costs can be evaluated when decisions are made."[24] Looking at the sample in this study, it was apparent that the patients felt they had a lot to lose if they did not take the treatment.

Lewis describes how important it is for people to see a physical benefit in taking treatment.[25] In the village in the West Sepik Province of Papua New Guinea, where he was doing his fieldwork, a number of people were reluctant to take treatment for leprosy. They told him that they did not feel that it was that serious a condition. When treatment became available for another condition that they felt was more severe, however, they were very keen to use medication that they could see was of benefit. Their reluctance was not simply, as the nurse had reported, because they were uncooperative and obstinate about not taking their treatment.

High levels of personal agency. According to Rapport and Overing, "The concepts of agent and agency, perhaps related most closely to that of power, are usually deployed in debates over the relationship between individuals and social structure. They also pertain to the nature of individual consciousness, its ability to constitute and reconstitute itself, and, ultimately, the extent of its freedom from exterior determination."[26] With low personal agency, cost–benefit analysis is heavily weighted against the patient being able to receive appropriate treatment, let alone to have the luxury to choose whether or not they should take it. In Haiti, Farmer describes people with TB, who have a choice between selling all of their family's possessions and going without treatment.[4]

Not all of the informants in this study would have had access to effective TB treatment had they not come to the United Kingdom, which in itself demonstrates their ability and opportunity to take some control over their lives. All of them could organize themselves, get jobs, study, access health care, and so forth. They were not only working, but also studying to improve their prospects in the future. All of their lives had been to a greater or lesser extent disrupted by the disease, but they had the wherewithall and the support to make the necessary adjustments.

CONCLUSION

We need to ask why people are not able to comply with treatment and eliminate all other possibilities before concluding that the patient is willfully refusing treatment. "Patient-dependent failure should be a 'diagnosis of exclusion'—invoked only after poor program design and lack of access are excluded."[4] (p. 227)

There is no doubt that we have to broaden the debate and recognize that housing, sanitation, and employment still have an impact on the vulnerability of people to fall prey to diseases such as tuberculosis; but there is also a need for pragmatism."Even if we lack the formulas necessary to 'cure' poverty and social inequalities, we do have at our disposal the cure for almost all cases of tuberculosis."[4] (p. 209)

When someone is diagnosed with TB and is prescribed treatment, the health service is in effect asking them to become part of the TB control program. This should place the patient in a partnership position rather than a culpable one. They didn't ask for this job; they are unlikely to have had any training or experience; and each will start with different resources.

TB services need to be set up to make the benefit of treatment outweigh the "cost" and to provide the relevant information and support needed by each individual patient to enable him or her to be successfully cured of TB. This can only be achieved when patients are seen as part of the solution rather than as part of the problem.

REFERENCES

1. WEIL, D. 1994. Drug supply—meeting a global need. *In* Tuberculosis: Back to the Future. J. Porter & K. McAdam, Eds.: 124–149. John Wiley. Chichester, U.K.
2. WORLD HEALTH ORGANISATION. 2001. Global TB Control. WHO Report 2000. World Health Organisation. Geneva.
3. OGDEN, J. 1999. Compliance versus adherence: just a matter of language? Chapter 9. *In* Tuberculosis: An Interdisciplinary Perspective. J. Grange & J. Porter, Eds. Imperial College Press. London.
4. FARMER, P. 1999. Infections and Inequality: The Modern Plagues. University of California Press. Berkeley, CA.
5. FARMER, P.E., S. ROBIN, S.L. RAMILUS & J.Y. KIM. 1991. Tuberculosis, poverty and "compliance": lessons from rural Haiti. Semin. Respir. Infect. **6:** 373–379.
6. FRIEDEN, T.P., P. FUJIWARA, R. WASHKO & M. HAMBURG. 1995. Tuberculosis in New York—turning the tide. N. Engl. J. Med. **333(4):** 229–233.
7. FRANKENBERG, R. 1994. Learning from AIDS: the future of anthropology. *In* The Future of Anthropology: Its Relevance to the Contemporary World. Akbar S. Ahmed & Cris N. Shore, Eds. Athlone. London/Atlantic Highlands, NJ.
8. 1998. New Oxford Dictionary of English. Oxford University Press. Oxford.
9. LERNER, B. 1997. From careless consumptives to recalcitrant patients: the historical construction of compliance. Soc. Sci. Med. **45:** 1423–1431.
10. GOOD, B. & M. DELVECCHIO GOOD. 1981. The meaning of symptoms: a cultural hermeneutic model for clinical practice *In* The Relevance of Social Science for Medicine. L. Eisenberg & A. Kleinman, Eds.: 165–196. Reidel. Dordrecht.
11. KATON, W. & A. KLEINMAN. 1981. Doctor–patient negotiation and other social science strategies in patient care. *In* The Relevance of Social Science for Medicine. L. Eisenberg & A. Kleinman, Eds.: 165–196. Reidel. Dordrecht.
12. DONOVAN, J. & R. BLAKE. 1992. Patient non-compliance: deviance or reasoned decision-making? Soc. Sci. Med. **34(5):** 507–513.
13. LEY, P. & S. LLEWELYN. 1995. Improving patients' understanding, recall, satisfaction and compliance, Chapter 5. *In* Health Psychology Processes and Applications. 2nd edit. A. Broome & C. Llewelyn, Eds. Chapman and Hall. London.
14. VOLMINK, J. & P. GARNER. 1997. Promoting adherence to tuberculosis treatment. *In* Infectious Diseases. Module of The Cochrane Database of Systematic Reviews. P. Garner, H. Gelband, P. Olliaro, *et al.*, Eds. The Cochrane Collaboration, Issue 2. Update Software. Updated quarterly. Oxford.
15. HOMEDES, N. & A. UGALDE. 1993. Review article: patients' compliance with medical treatments in the third world: what do we know? Hlth. Policy Plan. **8:** 291–314.
16. ZOLA, I.K. 1973. Pathways to the doctor—from person to patient. Soc. Sci. Med. **7:** 677–689.
17. ZOLA, I.K. 1980. Structural constraints in the doctor–patient relationship: the case of non-compliance. Chapter 11. *In* L. Eisenberg & A. Kleinman, Eds. The Relevance of Social Science for Medicine. Reidel. Dordrecht.
18. BARNHOORN, F. & H. ADRIAANSE. 1992. In search of factors responsible for noncompliance among tuberculosis patients in Wardha District, India. Soc. Sci. Med. **34:** 291–306.
19. BECKER, M.H. 1979. Patient perceptions and compliance: recent studies of the health belief model. *In* Compliance in Health Care. R.B. Haynes, D.W. Taylor, D. Sackett, Eds. John Hopkins University Press. Baltimore.
20. FARMER, P.E. 1997. Social scientists and the new turberculosis. Soc. Sci. Med. **44:** 347–358.

21. MAHMOUDI, A. & M.D. ISEMAN. 1993. Pittfalls in the care of patients with tuberculosis: common errors and their association with the acquisition of drug resistance. JAMA **270(1):** 65–68.
22. GLEISSBERG, V.G. 2001. Patient views on tuberculosis: is compliance with treatment the key to success or beside the point? Unpublished. M.Sc. dissertation.
23. HAYNES, R.B. 1976. A critical review of the "determinants" of patient compliance with therapeutic regimens. *In* Compliance with Therapeutic Regimens. D. Sackett & R. Haynes, Eds.: 26–39. John Hopkins University Press. Baltimore.
24. BECKER, M.H. & I. ROSENSTOCK. 1984. Compliance with medical advice. *In* Health Care and Human Behaviour. A. Steptoe & A. Matthews, Eds. Academic Press. London.
25. LEWIS, G. 1993. Double standards of treatment evaluation. Chapter 9. *In* Knowledge, Power and Practice: The Anthropology of Medicine and Everyday Life. S. Lindenbaum & Lock. University of California Press. Berkeley.
26. RAPPORT, N. & J. OVERING. 2000. Social and Cultural Anthropology: The Key Concepts. Routledge. London.

Moral Problems in the Use of Coercion in Dealing with Nonadherence in the Diagnosis and Treatment of Tuberculosis

LEN DOYAL

*Department of Human Science and Medical Ethics, St. Bartholomew's and
The Royal London School of Medicine and Dentistry, Queen Mary,
University of London, London E1 2AD, UK*

ABSTRACT: Coercion and detainment can be a morally acceptable strategy to fight the spread of tuberculosis, but these measures need to be placed into a much broader context than that of their short-term potential effectiveness. TB should be de-stigmatized by full acknowledgment that we all share the blame for its perpetuation. When coercion and detention are necessary, they should incorporate a strategy of optimum protection for minimum violation of autonomy. National and international health care programs should provide effective and nonthreatening treatments for TB and other related illnesses such as HIV and should develop policies to tackle the environmental causes of TB and provide support for vulnerable victims. Corporate pressures to continue world poverty must be undermined.

KEYWORDS: Nonadherence; tuberculosis; coercion; detention; moral problems; HIV

Tuberculosis (TB) is a global scourge that does untold damage to human potential. In the absence of effective treatment, those who contract the disease will not flourish and may even die as a result of the infection. If we believe that individuals have the right at least to try to optimize their personal potential, then TB can constitute a major constraint to the achievement of this and other widely recognized social rights.[1] The size of the current epidemic is alarming and continues to increase. According to the World Health Organisation (WHO), two million people die from TB every year, and approximately 35 million will perish by the year 2020. This means that TB has a higher mortality than AIDS and malaria combined. Between 10 and 15 persons will contract TB from each infected individual. TB kills more women than the combined causes of maternal mortality.[2–4] Finally, the spread of strains of TB that are resistant to multiple combinations of antibiotics (MDR TB), constitutes a further grave risk to public health. Were such strains to take hold in densely populated urban areas, the human costs would be incalculable.[5]

Address for correspondence: Professor Len Doyal, Department of Human Science and Medical Ethics, St. Bartholomew's and The Royal London School of Medicine and Dentistry, Queen Mary, University of London, Turner Street, London E1 2AD, U.K.
l.doyal@mds.qmw.ac.uk

The individual and collective threat of TB poses the moral problem explored in this paper. On the one hand, it is widely accepted that individual patients have rights and that health professionals have duties to respect these rights. On the other hand, some patients with TB may pose a serious risk of infection to others. If this is the case and if they resist curative treatment, what actions are morally appropriate? Should we go so far as resorting to coercion or even detainment in the name of protecting the public health? This paper will argue that coercion and detention in the treatment of TB can be morally justified. Strict controls should be placed, however, on the exercise of this threat to civil liberty. Moreover, those who are infected should not be blamed for the spread of the disease. Instead, the responsibility should be laid very clearly at the door of those who are in a position to control the epidemic through the instigation of social and economic change, but who fail to do so.

CLINICAL DUTIES OF CARE

The rights of individual patients are linked to the professional duties of clinical care. Three such duties are relevant here.[6] First, clinicians should protect the lives and health of their patients to an acceptable standard. Second, clinicians should respect the autonomy of their patients to the same standard. "Autonomy" should be taken to mean the general right of competent people to exercise choice over their lives when this is practically feasible—to be able to plan what they can of their future on the basis of relevant information and understanding. Within medicine, this translates into the duty to obtain informed consent to treatment and to respect the confidentiality of information communicated in relation to treatment. The third clinical duty is that of justice: patients should be treated fairly, and preference should not be shown on the basis of anything other than clinical need.

Why should health care professionals take these rights and duties seriously? There are two classic answers. The first is a common argument about the importance of trust in medicine, especially in the face of infectious disease. If patients believe that they will be given substandard medicine, will be forced to have treatments they don't want, and will be discriminated against because of their personal attributes, then they will not trust health professionals. If they don't have such trust, they may well not present themselves for treatment and will potentially spread their diseases to others, including to health professionals.

The second argument for taking the rights and duties of patients seriously is based on rational self-interest and logical consistency.[7] Youth and good health will not last forever—or even for very long. Financial resources can be even more transient. Any individual may contract a disease. Therefore, it is prudent for individuals and communities to plan rationally for health care. This will entail the support of provisions to ensure that the best treatment is available, that it is provided on the basis of informed choice and respect for confidentiality, and that it is not allocated on the basis of arbitrary discrimination.

Clinicians usually believe that patients should do their best to adhere to treatment that is in their best interests. Yet the imposition of such a duty logically entails that patients have the practical ability to respond positively. This in turn will depend on patients' already existing levels of physical health and autonomy. For example, those with poor levels of physical health may be unable to follow therapeutic instructions.

Patients with low levels of understanding about their clinical condition, with little self-confidence to do anything about it, and with little or no encouragement from those around them may also find adherence difficult. To be consistent, clinicians should therefore do all they can to preserve and improve the physical health and autonomy of their patients—to take the duties of care seriously.

MORAL TENSIONS IN RESPECTING INDIVIDUAL AUTONOMY

While there are good reasons for believing that health professionals should take very seriously all of their clinical duties toward patients unfortunate enough to have contracted TB, the duty to respect autonomy will be of particular importance. It is hard to overestimate how seriously people take what they perceive to be their right to self-determination. Nonconsensual and deliberate physical contact by others may produce a very strong reaction. What we allow others to do with our bodies is a matter for us and not for them to decide, and this includes any touching done by health professionals. Reflecting these deep moral feelings of bodily integrity, the law forbids such nonconsensual touching.[8] Most professional codes of good clinical practice do the same.[9–13]

The same argument applies to reasons for expecting health professionals to respect autonomy through protecting the confidentiality of patients. Privacy is taken very seriously as a human right because of the importance of secure intimacy in personal development and of the individual harm that confidential information can cause if it is made public. Often, such information is of a medical character and, again, it is for this reason that both the law and professional ethics dictate that the general right to confidentiality be respected.[14]

Yet there is also a wide consensus that the human rights under consideration are not absolute. On the one hand, a right is a claim on others that stipulates specific duties that they are expected, and should expect themselves, to take seriously. It follows, for example, from an acceptance of property rights that the property of others should not be intentionally damaged. A breach of this duty—a strict one in law—risks moral and judicial censure. Similarly, in ordinary circumstances, if health professionals treat patients without their consent or breach their confidentiality, they risk similar censure.

On the other hand, one thing that will entail restrictions on individual rights is the potential harm that respect for them may cause others.[15] For example, the owners of automobiles may drive them to any legal destination. Nevertheless, doing so dangerously risks a fine or loss of license.

There are many moral justifications for such constraints on the expression of individual rights. We have moral obligations to protect others from harm because we become who we are and achieve personal success through our social interaction with them—through their helping and not harming us.[16] To act in ways that will foreseeably lead to the harm of others is therefore an unacceptable form of moral free-riding, incurring potential benefit from the actions of others without reciprocating it. Not to do so may also lead to others refusing to help us when we are in need. It is hardly in anyone's rational self-interest to be regarded as being a public menace who cares little for the well-being of others. Further, logical consistency dictates that if we are committed to moral visions of the good and of good citizenship—of what types of actions are right and wrong and worthy of respect or censure—then we should want others to do their best to do what we believe to be good and right. We should want others to do their best be good citizens on our terms. Yet to inflict harm on them will make them unable to do so—to the degree that it makes them physically, mentally, or emotionally incapable of doing their best.

The law recognizes such moral arguments and commands respect for them. This is why it places limits on the clinical duty of care to respect confidentiality when to do so would place others at specific risk of harm.[17] In the context of infectious disease, most nations have public health legislation that sometimes holds the public safety to be of higher moral importance than respect for individual autonomy.[8] Such legislation, and supporting case law, justify breaches of confidentiality through demanding compulsory notification of serious infectious diseases to public health authorities by individual health professionals. Equally, testing for the presence of infection, treatment, and even quarantine or detainment in hospital can be done without the consent of infected patients when necessary.[18]

Now all of this might seem to be straightforward, if individuals have no inherent moral right to place others at serious risk of harm. However, there are important qualifications to this moral axiom. On the one hand, the risk to the public health must be significant. On the other hand, proposed restrictions on individual civil liberties must be practically capable of fairly achieving the goal of protecting the public health. Without the prospect of such success, the arguments in favor of respect for individual autonomy should take moral precedence over those of such protection.[19]

THE CASE OF TUBERCULOSIS

All of these arguments have particular resonance when dealing with TB. There can be little doubt that the use of directly observed treatment (DOT) as a strategy for dealing with the epidemic in many parts of the world has been successful in the treatment of large numbers of patients who would have otherwise been disabled or killed by TB.[2] DOT has also halted the course of many infections which may have evolved into MDR TB with its associated high mortality rates.

Yet there is a down side. It is relatively easy to make DOT compulsory for those patients deemed most likely not to adhere to it voluntarily. Although this can be morally and legally justified for reasons already outlined, it is a very short step from supervising treatment to insisting that patients receive such treatment and to then detaining them if they refuse or resist. This chain of events often occurs when professionals are concerned only with getting those who are infected to take their medication properly, irrespective of whether or not they pose any immediate risk to the public (e.g., through being infected but not infectious).[20]

It is precisely this pattern of thinking that led to the widespread use of detention in the United States as a means of forcing adherence to treatment for TB before its decline in the 50s and 60s.[21] The dramatic increase of infection in some North American cities in the 1980s and 90s witnessed this same willingness to sacrifice individual autonomy in the name of public good, although on a much lesser scale.[22–25] For example, New York City—where levels of infection and resistance to antibiotics reached their peak in the mid 1990s—became a showcase for compulsory DOT and detention policies. Because a drastic reduction in TB incidence occurred by the end of the millennium, this seemed to lend credibility to authoritarian strategies.[23,24]

However, research has confirmed that far from offering the public complete protection from infection, the threat of public disclosure and compulsory treatment may drive some infected persons underground where they still constitute a serious risk to others.[2] There are many reasons for this behavior. Even for patients who have some material security, the stigma of having TB is well known and can lead to devastating loss of social status and social mobility. This in turn can have an impact on the person's ability to make a living and to fulfil strongly felt family responsibilities. Lack of understanding about the causes and prevention of TB will add to such anxieties, making nonadherence to treatment all the more likely. Until the patient's illness becomes acute, denial may be the order of the day—by which time others will almost certainly have been infected as well.

When patients are already materially impoverished and socially marginalized, they will be even more unlikely to find enough order in their lives to adhere to treatment. For example, they may be so overwhelmed with immediate physical, emotional, and environmental problems that the development of any long-term perspective on their health is implausible. Equally, poor and indigent sufferers from TB may rightly believe that they are receiving little sympathy or community support and substandard clinical care—that the third duty of care of justice is not being observed toward them. To the degree that this is so, or believed to be so, they may well feel anger and little concern about the health of a public that they believe has shown so little interest in their basic welfare.[21,23]

These problems have all been magnified by the links between TB and HIV, which adds yet another layer to the personal price of disclosure.[25] At the same time, infection with HIV means that further infection with TB is more likely, along with possible further infection with MDR TB. Thus, without adequate assurance of material, emotional, and environmental support, the threat of coercion and detention may backfire. Only those whose whereabouts and infectious status are known can be coerced or detained for treatment. If patients go underground because of anxieties about the loss of autonomy, the potential value of coercion or detainment will be lost, and the interest of the public will not be served.[22]

WHAT SHOULD BE DONE?

Given the preceding arguments, nonadherence to treatment may justify denying patients their civil liberties. For many, just the threat of such a denial may encourage them to be more cooperative. In New York, for example, the actual rates of detention implemented to protect the public were small, and administrators did not appear to abuse the wide, draconian powers with which they were entrusted.[24] Nevertheless, there is wide agreement that such powers must be accompanied by procedures that guarantee detainees due process and a right to appeal. In particular, detention should only be for the protection of the public in ways that are immediate and documentable.[26,27] Where detainment is an option of control, it might not lead to the confinement of noninfectious patients simply because they are nonadherent or, even worse, the belief that their lifestyle might lead to nonadherence.

Further, the value of coercion and detention in preventing TB should not be exaggerated. Civil liberties—especially the duty of care to respect the autonomy of people suffering from TB—should only be curtailed to the degree that every effort has been made to optimize the success of treatment without it. Any coercion deployed in encouraging nonadherent patients to submit to DOT must be balanced with help to develop the self-respect and self-control necessary for them to optimize their own health in the future. Otherwise, short-term success may lead only to long-term reinfection.

Avoiding this consequence will necessitate greater expenditure on their education and other social resources. Success in minimizing the prevalence of TB will need to be focused on both effective treatment and improving the low levels of basic need satisfaction that lead to nonadherence and that have long been known to encourage the development and spread of infection.[28] It will be especially important to provide more material help for the developing world, where the inextricable links between TB and poverty are most evident.

It should be clear from this analysis that blame for the spread of TB cannot be laid at the door only of nonadherent victims. Although they must share some responsibility for their role in transmitting the disease, the net must be cast much wider to include those citizens of the developed world who indirectly benefit from world poverty, including that in their own nations. It would be wrong, however, to exaggerate their responsibility. Although some could make a small contribution to the alleviation of poverty, the direct link between them and the poverty from which they benefit is too remote.[16]

This argument, however, does not apply to physicians who knowingly deemphasize the importance of poor basic need satisfaction in the control of TB in favor of what they present as more immediately practical strategies such as DOT. However good the quality of their immediate care—and nothing in this paper should be interpreted as devaluing its importance—they cannot escape a moral responsibility to use their professional expertise and social status to further the political struggle against the poverty that fuels the spread of TB. How much they are able to do will vary, depending on the circumstances in which they find themselves. But what cannot be justified is doing nothing, or worse, using their professional positions as physicians to undermine the efforts of those who are taking their political/medical responsibilities seriously.[29]

In the final analysis, however, those who carry most responsibility are the corporate, national, and international leaders who benefit directly from such poverty and refuse to take practical steps to abolish it. They can foresee the damaging effects of both their actions and their inactions and yet do nothing to prevent them. Arguments that economic intervention of the sort required will only increase poverty in the long term have been shown to be without merit. In so many developing countries where TB is rampant, the cycle of poverty is such that no economic improvement is or can be in sight. Indeed, the burden of disease in such countries—fueled by the poverty in question—merely adds to the implausibility of such improvement. More specifically, the current G8 leaders have had the opportunity to relieve the burden of debt from many developing countries in order to free resources for better health care and the relief of poverty. They have shown gross irresponsibility in not taking more serious steps toward doing so.[30]

Ironically, therefore, if detainment is to be deemed a deterrent to irresponsible health behavior by nonadherent victims of TB who might harm others, the same moral logic should apparently apply to those corporate or national leaders whose own irresponsible behavior will most certainly harm them on a much *greater* scale. The fact that political contingencies dictate that such leaders will not be detained to prevent the continuation of such extensive harm only serves to highlight the vulnerability of those who may lose their freedom for causing much less harm.

CONCLUSION

In this paper, I have outlined the circumstances in which coercion and detainment can be a morally acceptable strategy to fight the spread of TB. I have argued, however, that a balance must be struck between the use of such policies and the devastating impact that they may have on the dignity and self-respect of those who are coerced and detained as a consequence. To obtain this balance:

- The best way to destigmatize TB is to make it clear that we all share the blame for its perpetuation. This should help to promote treatment adherence.

- When programs of coercion and detention are implemented to deal with potentially dangerous victims of TB, they should incorporate a "mini-opt" strategy of optimum protection for minimum violation of autonomy.

- National and international health care programs should be instituted that provide effective and nonthreatening treatments for TB and for other illnesses that increase the risk of contracting it—especially HIV.

- National and international policies need to be developed to tackle the environmental causes of TB and to provide educational, emotional, and social support for poor and vulnerable victims.

- We must struggle to undermine the corporate pressures to continue world poverty and to find ways of publicly blaming and punishing those individuals most responsible for it. Physicians have a special duty in this respect through constantly explaining that TB is controllable through environmental and economic policies and that it should be prevented as well as treated.

Finally, those who prefer not to think about such matters should be reminded that they might not avoid infection themselves. As the HIV epidemic has shown us, what goes around, comes around. TB and MDR TB do not require a passport. It is therefore not just moral sentiment but rational self-interest that dictates that we place the management and cure of TB into a much broader context than the short-term potential effectiveness and moral justifiability of coercion and detainment.

ACKNOWLEDGMENTS

Special thanks to Professor Lesley Doyal for heroic editing and Dr. John Moore-Gillon for being such an excellent colleague and clinician.

REFERENCES

1. ANNAS, G. 1998. Human rights and health—the Universal Declaration of Human Rights at 50. N. Engl. J. Med. **339:** 1778–1781.
2. WORLD HEALTH ORGANISATION. 1998. Report on the Global Tuberculosis Epidemic. WHO. Geneva. p. 27.
3. WORLD HEALTH ORGANISATION. 2000. Fact Sheet 104. (Revised April 2000): http://www.who.int/inf-fs/en/fact104.html
4. WORLD HEALTH ORGANISATION. 2001. Global Tuberculosis Control. WHO. Geneva.
5. ASPINAL, M.D., A. LASZLO, L. SIMONSEN, et al. 2001. Global trends in resistance to antituberculosis drugs. N. Engl. J. Med. **344:** 1294–1303.
6. DOYAL, L. with SIR CYRIL CHANTER. 2000. Medical ethics: the duties of care in principle and practice. In Clinical Negligence. M. Powers & N. Harris, Eds. Butterworths. London.
7. DOYAL, L. 2001. The moral foundations of the clinical duties of care: needs, duties and rights. Bioethics **15:** 520–535.
8. DE CRUZ, P. 2001. Comparative Health Care Law. Cavendish. London. pp. 3–46.
9. ROYAL COLLEGE OF SURGEONS. 1997. The Surgeons's Duty of Care. RCS. London.
10. BRITISH MEDICAL ASSOCIATION. 2001. Report of the Consent Working Party: Incorporating Consent Tool Kit. BMA. London.
11. DEPARTMENT OF HEALTH. 2001. Reference Guide to Consent for Examination or Treatment. Department of Health. London.
12. CANADIAN MEDICAL ASSOCIATION. 1996. Code of Ethics. CMA. Ottawa.
13. AMERICAN MEDICAL ASSOCIATION. 1997. Code of Medical Ethics. AMA. Chicago.
14. DOYAL, L. 1997. Human need and the right of patients to privacy. J. Contemp. Health Law Policy **14:** 1–21.
15. DOYAL, L. 1994. The limits of the duty of confidentiality in the treatment of HIV and AIDS. Br. J. Fam. Plan. **20:** 51–55.
16. DOYAL, L. & I. GOUGH. 1991. A Theory of Human Need. Macmillan. London.
17. McHALE, J. 1994. Medical Confidentiality and Legal Privilege. Routledge. London.
18. GOSTIN, L.O. 1993. Controlling the resurgent tuberculosis epidemic: a 50-state survey of TB statutes and proposals for reform. JAMA **269:** 255–261.
19. GOSTIN, L.O. 2000. Public Health Law. University of California Press. Berkely. pp. 85–112; 203–234.
20. COKER, R. 2001. Just coercion? Detention of nonadherent tuberculosis patients. Ann. N.Y. Acad. Sci. This volume.
21. LERNER, B. 1998. Contagion and Confinement. 1998. Johns Hopkins University Press. Baltimore, MD. pp. 87–138.
22. OSCHERWITZ, T., P. TULSKY, S. ROGER, et al. 1997. Detention of persistently nonadherent patients with tuberculosis. JAMA **278:** 843–846.
23. COKER, R. 2000. From Chaos to Coercion. St. Martin's Press. New York.
24. GASNER, M.R., K.L. MAW, G.E. FELDMAN, et al. 1999. The use of legal action in New York City to ensure treatment of tuberculosis. N. Engl. J. Med. **340:** 359–366.
25. SNIDER, D.E. & K.G. CASTRO. 1998. The global threat of drug-resistant tuberculosis. N. Engl. J. Med. **338:** 1689–1690.
26. CHAMPION, E.W. 1999. Liberty and the control of tuberculosis. N. Engl. J. Med. **340:** 385–386.
27. COKER, R. 1999. Public health, civil liberties and tuberculosis. Br. Med. J. **318:** 1434–1435.
28. DOYAL, L. 1979. The Political Economy of Health. Pluto Press. London. pp. 96–137.
29. McCALLY, M., A. HAINES, O. FEIN, et al. 1998. Poverty and ill health: physicians can, and should, make a difference. Ann. Int. Med. **129:** 726–733.
30. BRUGHA, R. & G. WALT. 2001. A global health fund: a leap of faith? Br. Med. J. **323:** 152–154.

Just Coercion? Detention of Nonadherent Tuberculosis Patients

RICHARD COKER

Department of Public Health and Policy, London School of Hygiene and Tropical Medicine, Keppel Street, London WC1E 7HT, United Kingdom

ABSTRACT: The need to balance the rights of individuals and to protect the public health will bring with it demands for the restriction of individuals' liberty. Three points should always be considered when these measures are adopted: (1) the lack of evidence that detention benefits the public health; (2) the risk that fundamental human rights may be overridden unnecessarily; and (3) that coercive practices may act as a smokescreen for improved, but more complex or more costly, public health responses to the causes of TB control failures. The policies of New York City and England are presented, and the argument is made that neither is just.

KEYWORDS: tuberculosis; coercion; detention; New York City; England; public health policy

Understanding national public health policies requires a nuanced appreciation of historical and cultural determinants of such approaches. A couple of years ago, I submitted a commentary on the use of coercion as a public health tool to a journal for publication. One reviewer suggested that "the author will be suggesting next that immunizations shouldn't be mandatory." There was an implicit assumption that, in order to be effective, such a sanction was a necessary, indeed a fundamental, component of an immunization program. Many colleagues from the United States have been surprised to learn that immunization is *not* mandatory in the United Kingdom. The country's framing and application of public health laws reflect contemporary balances between the state, society, and individuals, and also on historical and cultural mores.

The use of coercion in the pursuit of public health has a long history. We need only contemplate the burning alive of 1,000 Jews in response to plague in 14th century France; the consequences of the Contagious Diseases Acts of 19th century England, under which prostitutes were detained for treatment of venereal diseases for months; the treatment and incarceration of the mentally ill over the centuries; and the incarceration for more than 20 years of the notorious Typhoid Mary on New York's North Brother's Island, to name a just a few instances in which, in the name of public health, the use of coercion as a tool has been deemed necessary. Coercive measures have long been a feature of public health campaigns.[1–4]

Address for correspondence: Dr. Richard Coker, Research Fellow, Department of Public Health and Policy, London School of Hygiene and Tropical Medicine, Keppel Street, London WC1E 7HT, UK. Voice: +44 (0) 207 612 7810; fax: +44 (0) 207 612 7812.
Richard.coker@lshtm.ac.uk

COERCION

Public health historically, therefore, has constrained the rights of individuals and organizations to protect community interests in health. This paper highlights a number of issues that we should, I believe, contemplate if coercion is to be part of tuberculosis public health policy.

But first we should define what we mean by the term "coercion." Coercion can be defined as the act of compelling someone to do something by the use of power, intimidation, or threats. It is a complex concept that covers a spectrum of meanings, from the subtle to the overt, from friendly persuasion to the overt use of force.

Coercion is frequently used as a pejorative term: that, because it removes the autonomy of an individual, coercion always demeans the individual who is coerced. Yet, to take this view is to suggest that the use of coercion is never just. But this is not so. Many noncompliant patients with tuberculosis who ultimately ended up detained on New York's Roosevelt Island during the 1990s said they were grateful, in the end, to the city. For some, their health and life-expectancy improved immeasurably as a result. For others, the chaos of their lives had been transformed into a calm in which they could reflect upon their life's course. Others, however, felt the pain of coercion more than the benefit and remained angry at the removal of their liberty.[5]

Irrespective of the detainees' perspective, however, few would argue that given an explicit, defined threat, coercion is not justified in order to remove a public health threat. Indeed, most would say it would be unethical *not* to remove such a threat; that not to use coercion is ethically unjustifiable where public health is dependent on its use, proportional to the benefits gained, and where procedural due processes are observed. John Stewart Mill's utilitarian "harm principle" conveys this notion well: "One very simple principle [justifies state coercion]. That principle is, that the sole end for which mankind are warranted, individually or collectively, in interference with the liberty of action of any of their number, is self-protection. That the only purpose for which power can be rightfully exercised over any member of a civilised community, against his will, is to prevent harm to others ...."

So when, under what circumstances, is coercion justified? The 1984 Siracusa Principles, a set of principles under which departure from the 1966 International Covenant on Civil and Political Rights is recognized internationally, frame the just restriction or limitation of human rights. These principles determine that any restriction must be in accordance with the law, legitimate, and necessary. The action must be the least restrictive alternative that is reasonably available, and its application must not be discriminatory (TABLE 1).

TABLE 1. Siracusa Principles

The restriction is provided for and carried out in accordance with the law.
The restriction is in the interest of a legitimate objective of general interest.
The restriction is strictly necessary in a democratic society to achieve the objective.
There are no less intrusive and restrictive means available to reach the same goal.
The restriction is not imposed arbitrarily, that is, in an unreasonable or otherwise discriminatory manner.

Although only infrequently stated explicitly, underpinning the use of coercion as a tool is societal and policy-makers' understanding and perception of risk. Public health regulation is, in essence, an attempt to control risk. But risk is a complex notion. The nature of risk is important. If risk arises as a consequence of air-borne transmission, our perception is different than if it requires physical contact. Likewise, the duration of threat posed informs our response. If a threat exists over only days, our responses are different than if a threat persists over months or years. The severity of harm that might result also helps define our reaction. Public health and societal responses to gonorrhea are very different from sexually transmitted HIV, for example; anxiety regarding multidrug-resistant tuberculosis has prompted more drastic action than for drug-sensitive tuberculosis.

The social, cultural, and historical context in which threats occur determines professional and public reactions. Quarantine of persons infected with HIV in Cuba was introduced but has been deemed largely unacceptable in most other nation states. Legislative responses to control risk, such as legislation to make seatbelt wearing mandatory, has been complied with to varying degrees in different countries, suggesting that acceptance of such civil liberties restrictions is dependent on cultural context.[6] The detention of persons with tuberculosis was viewed as unacceptable in 19th century Britain despite the passage of laws enabling the detention of persons with other communicable diseases. By the 1930s detention of persons with tuberculosis was viewed as acceptable, but strict civil safeguards were introduced to safeguard such individuals from abuse.[7]

One critical issue that should inform rational policy-making in response to tuberculosis is objective evidence of risks posed. Yet, there is much that remains uncertain: considerable uncertainty continues to surround notions of infectiousness, virulence, and host susceptibility. And this is particularly so when it comes to understanding risks associated, or emanating from, individuals rather than populations. For any individual, the risks of disease development are difficult to predict, the impact of partial or erratic treatment makes any predictions very uncertain, and any assessment of the risks posed to others an inexact science.

Yet within these areas of uncertainty, judgments are, and must be, made. Public health law can, or rather should, help delineate the boundaries of these perennial tensions and uncertainties in any "trade-off between public goods and private rights, and the dilemma of whether to use coercive or voluntary public health measures."[8]

One way of examining societal approaches to those who pose a public health threat can be through an analysis of the evolution of laws and their application. Two examples illustrate some fundamental changes over recent years with the use of public health law, the use of coercive public health measures, in tuberculosis control. Both are in the area of the use of isolation or civil detention.

NEW YORK CITY

In New York, in the early 1990s, in response to rising rates of drug resistance, high rates of MDR TB, and a population of patients who were unable or unwilling to comply with treatment, the city authorities amended their public health regulations.[5,9,10] Two facilities house detainees. Bellevue Hospital houses a small detention unit for infectious (smear-positive) individuals, and in Roosevelt Island's

Goldwater Memorial Hospital noninfectious individuals are detained. Between 1993 and 1997 more than 200 noninfectious individuals were detained, representing approximately 1% of tuberculosis patients. Most of those detained on Roosevelt Island have been held for many months, many for the full duration of their treatment, including some for two years.[5,10]

Two clauses in the city's amended public health codes are important when we reflect upon legal shifts in approaches to "recalcitrant" persons with tuberculosis. Historically, the authority to detain individuals in New York City had been somewhat vague and, in practice, been limited to infectious individuals.[11] Therefore the city amended its health regulations and gave the Commissioner of Health the authority to "issue any orders he or she deems necessary to protect the public health."[12]

In addition, the provisions authorized the Commissioner to order the removal and detention of a person "where there is a substantial likelihood, based on such person's past or present behavior, that he or she cannot be relied upon to participate in and/or to complete an appropriate prescribed course of medication for tuberculosis...," whether or not their disease was infectious.[12]

The first clause expanded the authority of the state making, at their discretion, the broad application of these public health legal tools. The second clause represents a fundamental and significant shift in the law away from notion of *risk assessment* to notion of *compliance-assessment*.[5] In practice, in New York those who fail to comply with treatment can be detained, and the duration of their detention is explicitly dependent upon their compliance with antituberculosis treatment and *not* on any assessment of the threat they pose to public health. That is, there is an implicit assumption that poor patient compliance *automatically* and *always* conveys a risk to public health.

In New York, in order to protect individuals from unjustified, arbitrary legal decisions, several safeguards are provided. Persons issued with detention orders are provided, free of charge, with legal representation. Lawyers, independent of the Commissioner of Health and the Bureau of Tuberculosis Control but paid for by the city, provide legal advice to those threatened with detention. These lawyers also represent their clients at formally set, regular automatic court reviews of the judgments passed down.

ENGLAND

In England over recent years, there has been a steady increase in the issuance of detention orders for persons with tuberculosis.[13] Although no central records are kept on the number of orders for detention issued and as a consequence determining trends in the use of detention as a tool to protect public health has been uncertain, a recent survey suggests approximately 30 orders have been issued in recent years, nearly half from London. These 30 orders represent about 0.2% of pulmonary tuberculosis cases.[13,14] In addition, although when the law was first drafted it was considered that detention would only be applied for short periods of a few weeks, in recent years orders for detention periods of months—and on occasion six months—have become the norm.[13]

The 1984 Public Health Act, under which detention is authorized is, like the earlier New York City code, vague and provides few safeguards from abuse.[7] Detention can be authorized where a justice of the peace considers that proper precautions to prevent the spread of infection cannot be taken and that others are at serious risk of infection. Detention can theoretically be extended as frequently and for as long "as it appears to him [that is, the justice of the peace] to be necessary to do so."

There are, therefore, few protections for individuals in England and Wales from arbitrary detention. Although the detention of all persons so far may be justifiable, it is not *clear* that this is the case. For example, unlike in New York City, there is no codified review process, no limit to the duration of periods of detention ordered (nor their extensions), and no right to representation. Nor are cases subjected to detention open to public scrutiny. These safeguards had earlier existed: They were removed, somewhat ironically, at the height of the liberal era when concern for the welfare and protection from arbitrary abuse of those many of society's most vulnerable, including the mentally ill, was being (or had been) codified.[7] This is not to suggest that abuse occurs, simply that there is no evidence that it does not. Without legal protections and monitoring of trends, a veil obscures the use of an important public tool, and accusations of abuse are hard to refute.

A second issue of importance is whether the detention of persons beyond their period of "infectiousness" is legal. The law is unclear on this point. Under Section 38 of the 1984 Public Health Act a Justice of the Peace may extend the period of detention in hospital "as often as it appears to him to be necessary to do so." But the 1984 act relates to cases of "tuberculosis of the respiratory tract in an *infectious* state." It is unclear, therefore, whether persons receiving treatment who become noninfectious can be detained lawfully. This has not been tested in the courts.[15]

Recently, through the 1998 Human Rights Act, British law incorporated the European Convention on Human Rights. The European Court, under the European Convention on Human Rights, recognizes that detention becomes unlawful if it ceases to serve the purpose of the original order, that is, in the setting of tuberculosis, to protect the public health from an infectious risk. So if, for example, an individual with tuberculosis is detained and receives treatment for, say, four months, it might be argued that the original purpose of the order is now not being served in the sense that the risk posed to the public health has dwindled such that that lesser risk is now acceptable. It is this difficult judgment that the courts must make, a judgment that, as time passes, becomes increasingly difficult and favors release. Whatever the answer, each case should be judged on this "threat" basis alone and not, I would argue, because of the wishes of the medical team (or any other authority) to see an individual complete his or her course of treatment.

JUST COERCION?

It is unclear whether New York and England (no detention orders have been issued in Wales) represent a broad shift in the use of coercive public health tools to support tuberculosis control efforts. Certainly New York City is not unique in the United States in its approach but is simply the most prominent. Several states have modeled their tuberculosis regulations on the amended New York codes, and detention in facilities including jails is not infrequent in some states.[16–18] Concerns over tuberculosis control in Europe and Israel too have caused some to draft new regulations enabling mandatory treatment of noncompliant individuals in Norway and use of prisons to detain individuals.[19,20]

In both New York and England, and indeed elsewhere where detention of persons with tuberculosis is sanctioned, issues of uncertainty and risk are complex. Does a patient who has completed four months of treatment pose an "infectious risk" to the public if he defaults? And is that risk of such magnitude that the threat of detention is an appropriate sanction for the state to use? Should a detainee be released when he no longer poses a public health threat or should he be held until he has completed his treatment?

I would argue that, whereas for a prisoner convicted of a crime, early release from detention is a privilege, if a detainee no longer poses a threat (or *cannot* be predicted to pose a threat in the foreseeable future) release should be a right and not a privilege, and continued detention is fundamentally, therefore, unjust. The burden should be on the state to *justify* detention. It is not sufficient to justify detention when the courts are uncertain as to whether the detainee presents more than a minimal risk to the public. If this is not the case, the detainees may be detained on the basis simply of "irrational fears, speculation, stereotypes, or pernicious mythologies"[21] rather than on well-established scientific information.

Is the use of detention in the control of tuberculosis important given that it appears so few individuals end up detained? I would argue yes. Nation states and other lawmaking authorities are increasingly concerned about tuberculosis and, in particular, about the scourge of drug-resistant strains. One part of the international armamentarium in the DOTS strategy is the DOT component, the aim of which is to ensure treatment compliance. And, in support of measures to enhance compliance, many policymakers may (and indeed are) considering sanctions to support other efforts to ensure treatment compliance and protect the public health.

There will always be a need to balance the rights of individuals and the need to protect the public health, and there will always be demands for the restriction of individuals' liberty. But we should, I would argue, be cautious when we adopt these measures and consider the following points: First, that in the case of detention and the control of tuberculosis there is little evidence to show that this policy benefits the public health. Second, that there is a risk that fundamental human rights may be overridden unnecessarily. And third, that coercive practices may act as a smokescreen for improved, but more complex or more costly, public health responses to the root causes of tuberculosis control failures. These may include improving the lot of homeless people, removing the "causes of recalcitrance" (to echo Britain's Labour Government's mantra on crime), the wider use of incentives, the removal of structural service hurdles that hinder treatment adherence, and addressing issues of criminal justice, to name a few.

The title of this paper includes the phrase 'Just Coercion?' Coercion is likely to remain a tool in the armamentarium of public health officials. But we must be sure that its use is justified. Gostin has described a framework that reflects the Siracusa Principles mentioned earlier that tailors them for analysis of public health tools. He argues convincingly that, before coercion is justifiable, the risk posed should be demonstrable, the proposed interventions should be demonstrably effective, and the approach should be cost-effective. In addition, he argues that any sanctions should be the least restrictive necessary to achieve the purpose and that the policy should be fair and nondiscriminatory. If we scrutinize the policies of detention in New York

City and England using these human rights principles, I would argue they are not just.

ACKNOWLEDGMENTS

Much of the research that informs this paper was conducted while I was a Harkness fellow supported by the Commonwealth Fund of New York and subsequently a research associate at The Wellcome Trust supported by the Wellcome Trust. The views expressed are mine alone.

REFERENCES

1. KRAUT, A.M. 1994. Silent Travellers: Germs, Genes, and the "Immigrant Menace." Johns Hopkins University Press. Baltimore, MD.
2. KNAPP, V.J. 1989. Disease and Its Impact on Modern European History. Edwin Mellen Press. Lewiston, NY.
3. PORTER, D. & R. PORTER. 1988. The enforcement of health: the British debate. *In* AIDS: The Burdens of History. E. Fee & D.M. Fox, Eds.: 97–120. University of California Press. Berkeley/London.
4. GREENOUGH, P. 1995. Intimidation, coercion and resistance in the final stages of the South Asian smallpox eradication campaign, 1973–1975. Soc. Sci. Med. **41(5):** 633–645.
5. COKER, R.J. 2000. From Chaos to Coercion: Detention and the Control of Tuberculosis. St. Martin's Press. New York.
6. LEICHTER, H.M. 1991. Free to Be Foolish: Politics and Health Promotion in the United States and Great Britain. Princeton University Press. Princeton, NJ.
7. COKER, R.J. 1984. Civil liberties and public good: detention of tuberculous patients and the Public Health Act of 1984. Med. Hist. In press.
8. GOSTIN, L.O. 2000. Public Health Law: Power, Duty, Restraint. University of California Press. Berkeley/Los Angeles/London.
9. FRIEDEN, T.R., P.I. FUJIWARA, R.M. WASHKO & M.A. HAMBURG. 1995. Tuberculosis in New York City—turning the tide. N. Engl. J. Med. **333:** 229–233.
10. GASNER, M.R., K.L. MAW, G.E. FELDMAN, *et al.* 1998. The use of legal action in New York City to ensure treatment of tuberculosis. N. Engl. J. Med. **340:** 359–366.
11. BALL, C.A. & M. BARNES. 1994. Public health and individual rights: tuberculosis control and detention procedures in New York City. Yale Law Pol. Rev. **12(1):** 38–67.
12. DEPARTMENT OF HEALTH (NY). 1993. Notice of adoption of an amendment to section 11.47 of the New York City health code. Department of Health, Board of Health. New York.
13. COKER, R.J. 2001. National survey of detention and TB. Thorax **36:** 818.
14. — 1998. 306 c447-8W. Hansard.
15. COKER, R.J. 2000. The law, human rights, and the detention of individuals with tuberculosis in England and Wales. J. Publ. Hlth. Med. **6:** 12–16.
16. — 1996. Detaining Nonadherent Tuberculosis Patients until Cure: A 50-State Legal Survey. Policy and Legal Dilemmas Regarding Refractory Tuberculosis Patients. Conference proceedings at the Francis J. Curry National Tuberculosis Center, October 24 and 25, 1996. University of California, San Francisco, California.
17. GOSTIN, L.O. 1993. Controlling the resurgent tuberculosis epidemic: a 50-state survey of TB statutes and proposals for reform. JAMA **269 (2):** 255–261.
18. BURMAN, W.J., D.L. COHN, C.A. RIETMETJER, *et al.* 1997. Short-term incarceration for the management of noncompliance with tuberculosis treatment. Chest **112:** 57–62.
19. — 1994. Communicable Diseases Control Act, Norway.

20. WEILER-RAVELL, D., D. CHEMTOB, R.J. COKER & A. LEVENTHAL. 2001. Compulsory hospitalisation before and after the reorganisation of tuberculosis services in Israel. Submitted for publication.
21. School Board of Nassau County, FL v. Arline, 480 US 273, 288 (1987).

Missed Opportunities?

Coercion or Commitment: Policies of Prevention

JOHN D.H. PORTER[a,b] AND JESSICA A. OGDEN[b]

Departments of [a]Infectious and Tropical Diseases and [b]Public Health and Policy, London School of Hygiene and Tropical Medicine, London WC1E 7HT, UK

ABSTRACT: The DOTS strategy (directly observed therapy, short course) has been the cornerstone of international TB control policy since the early 1990s. This strategy has provided the international community with an advocacy tool to harness funds for TB as well as a method for helping country programs to achieve high cure rates for TB. But as much as the strategy is seen as successful by some, it is perceived as unsuccessful by others. This paper looks at the results of the introduction of DOTS into control programs and discusses research relating to direct observation of treatment. It asks how policies like DOTS are created, and how they are administered and transferred from the international to the national and finally to the local level. The discipline of public health policy is used to interrogate the creation and history of the DOTS strategy in order to find ways of aiding the transfer of the policy to national and local levels. Finally, the paper asks whether the concepts of "control" and "elimination" continue to be useful in the management of infectious diseases. We ask whether it is time to change the perspective to policies that focus more on the context of implementation and the importance of the development of care, integration, and flexibility rather than cure, targets, and short-term solutions.

KEYWORDS: tuberculosis; DOTS; public health; TB control programs; health policy

INTRODUCTION

The title of the paper "Missed Opportunities?" should be viewed from a positive perspective, stressing the question mark. Of course opportunities are missed, because it is never possible to see and understand the whole picture except, perhaps, in hindsight. An interrogation of a policy like DOTS is an opportunity to consider the positive and negative aspects of the policy and to find additional, perhaps more appropriate, ways of controlling a disease like TB. There is an international TB control strategy, but are there perspectives that are missing that are important? Can these perspectives be found by understanding how the policy was created, and if so, how can these perspectives be developed in future policy creation for the control of infectious diseases?

Address for correspondence: Dr. John Porter, M.D., FRCP, FFPHM, Reader in International Health, Departments of Infectious and Tropical Diseases and Public Health and Policy, London School of Hygiene and Tropical Medicine, Keppel Street, London WC1E 7HT, U.K. Voice: 020-7927-2298; fax: 020-7637-4314.

j.porter@lshtm.ac.uk

The DOTS strategy contains five elements: government commitment, case detection by sputum microscopy, standardized treatment regimes of 6–8 months with direct observation (DOT) for at least the initial two months, regular supply of anti-TB drugs, and a standardized recording and reporting system.[1] Contained within this strategy is both commitment, in the form of government commitment, and the potential for coercion in the form of direct observation of therapy, which is part of the standardized treatment regimen.

HEALTH POLICY

Health policy asks *how* we do things. How decisions are made and how they are acted upon. Walt, for example, suggests that health policy is "a broad statement of goals, objectives and means that creates the framework for activity."[2] Another definition is "a purposive course of action followed by an actor or set of actors in dealing with a problem or matter of concern."[3] Both definitions emphasize that policy is a process that creates frameworks, structures, and systems. Policy looks at the "macro level," at the power in the political system, at consensus and conflict; for example, what is political commitment to DOTS? It also looks at the "micro-level," at mechanisms within the system and the administrative routine of policy making; for example, how the standardized reporting system works for TB control.

A method for interrogating a policy like DOTS is to look at the "content," context, process, and actors around the creation and implementation of the policy.[2] The content is the DOTS strategy; the context relates to its implementation in different parts of the world; the process asks the question "How is it implemented in different settings; and the actors are the individuals and organizations involved in its creation and dissemination at the local, national, and international level.

The DOTS strategy has a structure that includes goals and objectives but does not contain information on *how* it should be implemented. The *process* of implementation is, of course, difficult and at the same time fascinating, because it involves many different human factors: managers, health care workers, patients, organizations, and government, to name a few. All of the human actors, and the processes they create, need to be able to interrelate in order to create a system that supports the care of a person with TB.

HISTORY OF DOTS

The historical perspective is important in looking at policy creation, and the last 10 years has been a fascinating period of time for people working in tuberculosis control. The DOTS story is fascinating and complex, and, because it is being published elsewhere,[4] we will provide here just a thumbnail sketch. In the 1970s and early 1980s, there was little interest in the disease internationally. Much of the process of administering TB treatment to patients was supposed to have been devolved to primary health care structures following the Declaration of Alma Ata in 1978.[5] The picture began to change in the mid 1980s with increasing numbers of TB cases reported from industrialized countries and the discovery of the association between HIV and TB. During this period, Karel Styblo continued to work on the support of TB control programs in sub-Saharan Africa, and this work caught the attention of the World Bank and the newly established Global Tuberculosis Programme (GTB). In 1990 an economist, Chris Murray, together with Styblo and others, published a paper declaring that Styblo's approach to TB control was cost-effective.[6] In 1992–1993 New York City experienced a serious outbreak of multidrug-resistant tuberculosis, and late in 1993 WHO declared tuberculosis to be a global emergency. The following year WHO's Global TB Programme published its "Framework for the Control of Tuberculosis," based on Styblo's African work, and the term (or brand name) "DOTS" was coined to represent the new approach. In 1996 the China DOTS story was published, indicating the success of the program, which was supported by funds from the World Bank.[7] The year 2000 saw the meeting of Ministers of Health and Finance in The Netherlands and the development of the Amsterdam Declaration to STOP TB.[8] The countries signing the document, which included the world's 20 high-burden countries, declared their understanding of the importance of TB mortality and their commitment to its control in their countries and, therefore, the world.

SYSTEMS FAILURE—ISSUES FOR DOTS

An aspect of the discipline of health policy is to look at the structures and systems created by policies. The historical perspective indicates that there are already many lessons for policymakers that have been created within the scientific paradigm that has been dominant since before Koch's discovery of the tubercle bacillus in 1882. Three aspects will be discussed: the creation of policy using "evidence-based research" and how it is too slow for the needs of policy makers; the importance of health care infrastructure in the delivery of TB services; and the need to support and care for health workers, as well as patients, in the process of delivery of a health system for TB. Policy can usefully be created at the international level; but if it does not link with the national and local levels, it will fail, because these are the levels that require the creation and maintenance of *systems*. These systems are both simply physical structures and, more importantly, systems that link groups of people and organizations. Policies that do not also create these systems where they are lacking, or that ignore/do not take adequate account of existing systems, will not make sense at local level, and thus may not be implementable.

The Creation of Policy Using Evidence-Based Research: "Current Evidence-Based Research Methods Are Too Slow for the Creation of Policy"

The DOTS strategy has been created in the international arena at a time when the concept of evidence-based research is an important perspective. Indeed, TB programs do have a large body of research from which to draw to answer questions about TB control activities. The Indian National Tuberculosis Programme (NTP), established in 1962, for example, was developed from a variety of clinical, epidemiological, and socioeconomic studies, which were used as "evidence" on which to base the structure and functioning of the program. These studies and others, published before and since, provide a strong body of evidence that can be used to strengthen existing programs and to develop new ones.

A problem with the current research methods for an evidence base, however, is that they are too slow; and the answers to the problems often appear a long time after policy has had to be created. This is true for the DOTS strategy—particularly the "direct observation of treatment" component—which some critics believed was not adequately researched before being released. Two reports on randomized, controlled trials published in *The Lancet* question the need for direct observation of patients (DOT),[9,10] and indeed both indicate that DOT confers no benefit over self-administration of therapy within the context of a strengthened TB program (i.e., DOTS). In addition, a systematic review of trials on adherence, published in 1997, indicates that almost any intervention (food, subsidies, observation, loans, etc.) will assist the TB patient to get better,[11] thus also questioning the need for DOT.

The Importance of the Health Care Infrastructure

The health care infrastructure has always been seen as an essential part of TB control. Work in India in preparation for the establishment of the National Programme in 1962 stated that the TB program could only function effectively within a strong health care infrastructure.[12] In the United States, many of the problems that arose in New York in the mid 1980s were due to the collapse of public health care infrastructures that had been developed to control diseases like TB.[13] Thus, however intriguing and innovative the new technological creations for TB control (e.g., improved drugs, vaccines, diagnostics) may be, they will continue to require a healthy and well-functioning implementation structure. "Magic bullets" need to be used to do their magic, and to be used they need a structure for their delivery that works and makes sense to those delivering them.

Support of Health Care Workers

Since 1996, the Tuberculosis Research Programme at the London School of Hygiene and Tropical Medicine has been working with colleagues in India on the effect of the introduction of the Revised National Tuberculosis Control Programme (RNTCP) into the country. Between 1996 and 1998, the LRS Institute in Delhi conducted a study in two TB clinics in Delhi. The main finding from this study, which was early in the implementation of the RNTCP, was that health care workers unofficially screened patients to determine those most likely to complete treatment with direct observation.[14,15] Patients who were not included were those with no ration card, who had recently moved to Delhi, who were migrants or daily wage earners, who were factory shift workers, or whose residences were difficult to reach. These patients could be considered vulnerable. It can be argued that the health care workers had developed this unofficial system because of the failure of the health system to support them: too large a patient load, too strong an emphasis on targets that were not obtainable without changing the system, and so forth. The studies stress the importance not only of the physical infrastructure of the health care system, but also of ensuring that health care staff are well supported within the system.

The messages from the Indian studies were the following: that an adequate health care infrastructure is essential; a regular drug supply produces confidence and draws people back to the clinics; that health care workers need to be supported within the system; and that TB patients want to get better, and if provided with a little support will try hard to complete their treatment. This is a similar finding to that reported by Volmink and Garner in their systematic review.

POLICY TRANSFER

Another aspect of policy interrogation is the aspect of *transfer*. Policy transfer is a process by which knowledge about policies, administrative arrangements, and institutions in one time and/or place is used in the development of policies, administrative arrangements, and institutions in another time and/or place.[16] DOTS was a policy that was created at the international level in the early 1990s and subsequently transferred to individual countries for implementation. A study being conducted at the London School of Hygiene and Tropical Medicine, in collaboration with the Centre for Health Policy in Johannesburg and Mondelane University in Mozambique, is exploring these processes.[c]

The study of the transfer of policy draws lessons and identifies factors that facilitate and constrain transfer. The following types of questions can be addressed: How far has policy transfer occurred? Under what conditions will policy transfer occur? What aspects of the policy are transferred? Methods include literature review, review of "grey material" (unpublished information from organizations and individuals), and interviews with key actors. One of the hypotheses informing this study was that the development of policies like DOTS for the control of infectious diseases is usually a linear and top-down process, being created at the international level and subsequently transferred down to national and local levels (FIG. 1).[14] An important question to ask is, Does this process facilitate effective policy? Would policies like

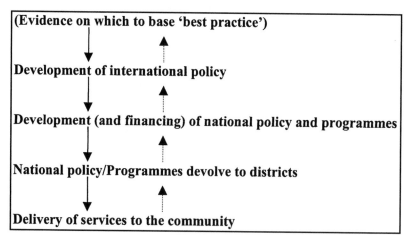

FIGURE 1. Flow of information and expertise as a linear process.

[c]We are grateful to our colleagues on this study, Gill Walt and Louisiana Lush at LSHTM, Helen Schneider at CHP, and Julie Cliff at Mondelane University for allowing us to draw on this study before its completion and publication.

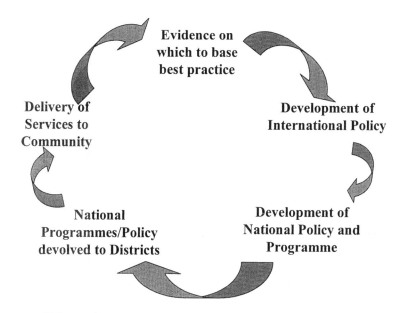

FIGURE 2. Flow of information and expertise as a cyclical process.

DOTS be more effective if a parallel flow of information from the local community level could be passed up the system to influence the creation of international policy, and, if so, how can this process be effected? Would a cyclical process be more effective (Fig. 2)?[14]

Preliminary results from phase one of this study indicate that DOTS was developed at the international level, largely on the basis of the context-specific Styblo studies, and aggressively promoted on the strength of the China results. Compelled by a concern to maintain the momentum of interest and funding being put toward TB, the Global TB Programme (GTB) adopted an essentially political approach to policy transfer. The effort was to "sell" DOTS to those who hold the purse strings and to those in power, to garner political commitment; and, judging from the number of signatories to the Amsterdam Declaration, they were extremely successful. Thus at least at this preliminary stage, it appears that DOTS *was* indeed developed and promoted in a top-down, linear fashion. The next phase of the study, currently under way, will help us understand whether this is how the process was perceived by bureaucrats, researchers, and clinicians at the national and local levels, and if so, whether and how the nature of the process has affected uptake and implementation. It will be interesting to discover whether the Delhi experience described above has been repeated in these other, very different kinds of settings.

ERADICATION AND CONTROL

This paper highlights the importance of systems within disease-control programs like those for TB. Although the past 100 years have produced a wealth of scientific information and important breakthroughs in the treatment of infectious diseases, there continues to be the necessity for implementation of policies. We argue that this requires an understanding of individuals and how they operate in groups and organizations, as shown in the Delhi study described above.[17] What systems need to be developed and established to provide a "healthy" infrastructure in which people can work effectively to combat diseases like TB?

Perspectives are changing in disease-control activities. These changes are being supported by scholars from disciplines outside of biomedicine that are now working in disease control. For example, anthropologists and other social scientists of medicine have been critical of the imbalances of power between the biomedical establishment and the communities in which they work. They have taken note of the "medical gaze" under which so many aspects of ordinary human life can be distorted and medicalized to meet the needs of those in power (cf. Foucault[18]). They have also tried to make these critiques useful for those in the business of public health, through looking at how these processes are inscribed in the doctrine of control, and to offer a way forward (e.g. Ogden[14]). Tyler, in his book on ethnography, states, "Scientific thought succumbed because it violated the first law of culture, which says that the more man controls anything, the more uncontrollable both become."[19]

A further development is that health is increasingly being included in other sectors. The fact that strong economies require healthy populations is increasingly becoming accepted wisdom, and this means that policy makers are increasingly interested in understanding what the links are between the health of communities, economic development, education, and political stability.

Disease control activists, like Donald Henderson of smallpox-eradication fame, are starting to say that the focus on eradication within public health is perhaps no longer appropriate. With the rise of the human rights agenda, there is increasing international pressure to abide by the Declaration of Human Rights and the need to allow individuals to be fully informed of disease control policy with an ability to state that they do not want to be included in a particular disease control policy. In a presentation at the Royal College of Physicians, London in 1998, Henderson said, "In the world of infectious diseases today, it is increasingly difficult to discover those who advocate simply the effective control of a disease as a practical objective. Rather, 'eradication' has become the popular lure with its implicit promise of permanency and ultimate achievement."[20]

In 1995–1996, a research group was established at the London School of Hygiene and Tropical Medicine to develop collaborations with institutions in India. As part of this process, the group conducted a review of Indian TB control activities with colleagues at the Foundation for Research in Community Health in Mumbai (FRCH). The various members of the research group came from different disciplines and perspectives. In order to address the inevitable differences and conflicts that developed, it was decided that the group would conduct its work within certain broad frameworks. These included gender, political economy and health sector reform, human rights, and public health ethics.

During the past 5 years, the group has expanded to include other members, both from within the school and from outside. Through group presentations and discussion, it has became apparent to the members that a shift in perspective was occurring or needed to occur, in order to find different approaches to the control of infectious diseases. The change was from current strategies that emphasized disease specificity

TABLE 1. The paradigm shift

From: current public health orientation	To: infectious disease policy
1. Disease specificity and verticality	Integrated/horizontal linkages
2. Standardization of interventions	Flexibility/context sensitivity
3. Short-term orientation	Longer term objectives/sustainability
4. Emphasis on product/targets	Emphasis on process
5. Limited to health sector	Linking multiple sectors
6. Focus on individual "risk"	Understanding social vulnerability: risk in the context of everyday life.
7. Operating without reference to global processes	Taking globalization as referent and context
8. Working on behalf of populations	Working in partnership with communities

and verticality, standardized interventions, and short-term orientation to an approach that looked at integration and horizontal linkages, flexibility, and context specificity with longer term objectives (TABLE 1).[21] Many of the ideas surrounding this perception arose from work on DOTS and the difficulties of implementation witnessed through work on the Revised National TB Control Programme in India, as well as work in East Africa.

CONCLUSION

The DOTS strategy is currently being revised by the World Health Organisation.[22] The draft report that is circulating demonstrates the shift in thinking about disease control that has occurred during the latter part of the 1990s. The draft document sets control activities within the field of public health and emphasizes the need for broad linkages across sectors. It constantly stresses the importance of the health care infrastructure and the importance of developing links and relationships with different groups of people, in order to support and care for the patient with TB.

An interrogation of the DOTS strategy is an opportunity to witness the creation, development, and change of a policy as it moves through time. As perspectives shift, following problems with implementation, so the policy is revised. This shift is not without its difficulties, but it is to the enormous credit of WHO that a new draft document has been created and hopefully will be soon released to assist with the implementation of TB-control activities in many countries.

ACKNOWLEDGMENTS

We would like to thank Professor Gill Walt and Dr. Louisiana Lush for their assistance with the writing of this paper and also the ESRC "Future Governance" Programme that funds the policy transfer work quoted. The Department for International Development (DFID) funded a TB Research Programme at the London

School of Hygiene and Tropical Medicine and the Nuffield Institute for Health, Leeds, between 1995 and 2001, and it was through the support of this program that many of the ideas expressed in this paper were borne.

REFERENCES

1. WORLD HEALTH ORGANISATION. 1999. What is DOTS. A guide to understanding the WHO-recommended TB control strategy known as DOTS. WHO.CDS.CPC/TB/ 99.270.
2. WALT, G. 1994. Health Policy. An introduction to process and power. Zed Books. London.
3. ANDERSON, J. 1975. Public Policy Making. Nelson. London.
4. OGDEN, J., et al. 2001. Forthcoming.
5. WORLD HEALTH ORGANISATION. 1978. Declaration of Alma-Ata. International Conference on Primary Health Care, Alma-Ata, USSR, September 6–12, 1978. World Health Organisation. Geneva.
6. MURRAY, C.J., K. STYBLO & A. ROUILLON. 1990. Tuberculosis in developing countries: burden, intervention and cost. Bull. Int. Union Tuberc. Lung Dis. **65:** 6–24.
7. CHINA TUBERCULOSIS CONTROL COLLABORATION. 1996. Results of directly observed short course chemotherapy in 112,842 Chinese patients with smear-positive tuberculosis. Lancet **347:** 358–362.
8. INTERNATIONAL UNION AGAINST TB AND LUNG DISEASE. 2000. Amsterdam Declaration to Stop TB. ISSN 1562-174X. Newsletter July 2000.
9. WALLEY, J.D., M.A. KHAN, J.N. NEWELL & M.H. KHAN. 2001. Effectiveness of the direct observation component of DOTS for tuberculosis: a randomised controlled trial in Pakistan. Lancet **357:** 664–666.
10. ZWARENSTEIN, M., J.H. SCHOEMAN, C. VUNDULE, et al. 1998. Randomised controlled trial of self-supervised and directly observed treatment of tuberculosis. Lancet **352:** 1340–1343.
11. VOLMINK, J. & P. GARNER. 1997. Directly observed therapy. Lancet **39:** 1399–400.
12. BANERJI, D. 1993. A social science approach to strengthening India's National TB Programme. Ind. J. TB **40(2):** 61–82.
13. REICHMAN, L.B. 1991. The U shaped curve of concern. Am. Rev. Res. Dis. **1444:** 741–742.
14. OGDEN, J. 2000. Improving tuberculosis control—social science inputs. Trans. R. Soc. Trop. Med. Hygiene **94:** 135–140.
15. SINGH, V., A. JAISWAL, P.P. SHARMA, et al. 1998. Patient experiences with the Revised National Tuberculosis Programme, India. (Abstract No. 367-PC) Int. J. Tuberc. Lung Dis. **2:** S354.
16. DOLOWITZ, D. & D. MARSH. 1996. Who learns what from whom: a review of the policy transfer literature. Pol. Stud. **XLIV:** 343–357.
17. SINGH, V., A. JAISWAL, P.P. SHARMA, et al. 1998. Social vulnerability and the treatment of tuberculosis in Delhi: can DOTS fill the gap? Abstract No. 368-PC. Int. J. Tuberc. Lung Dis. **2:** S364.
18. FOUCAULT, M. 1973. The Birth of the Clinic. Routledge. London.
19. TYLER, S.A. 1986. Post-modern ethnography: from document of the occult to occult document. In Writing Culture: The Poetics and Politics of Ethnography. J. Clifford & G.E. Marcus, Eds.: 122–140. University of California Press. Berkeley, CA.
20. HENDERSON, D. 1998. The siren song of eradication. J. R. Coll. Phys. **32(6):** 580–584.
21. PORTER, J.D.H., J.A. OGDEN & P. PRONYK. 1999. Infectious disease policy—towards the production of health. Health Pol. Plan. **14(4):** 322–328.
22. WHO. 2001. www.who.org

Multidrug-Resistant Tuberculosis

This Is the Cost

JOHN MOORE-GILLON

Department of Respiratory Medicine, St. Bartholomew's and Royal London Hospitals, London EC1A 7BE, United Kingdom

ABSTRACT: The costs of multidrug-resistant tuberculosis (MDR TB) reach far beyond the cost of the clinical treatment of the patient. The first impact of the discovery of MDR TB in a population is the need to recognize that all TB patients have the potential of being MDR. Public health measures to prevent the spread of MDR TB, or to control or reverse the problem where spread has already occurred, can be extremely expensive to implement. At the level of the individual patient, the second-line drugs used to treat MDR TB are more expensive, and the remaining first-line drugs will have to be used for a longer time than in drug-susceptible TB. Negative-pressure units add to the costs of treatment, as does the increased nursing intensity required. The cost to the wider economy includes lost productivity and lost tax revenue to the state as well as the cost of supporting the family if the patient is the breadwinner.

KEYWORDS: multidrug-resistant tuberculosis; economic impact of TB; clinical care costs; public health

THE FINANCIAL CHALLENGES OF MULTIDRUG-RESISTANT TUBERCULOSIS

Drug-resistant tuberculosis gives rise to challenges that go far beyond the problems associated simply with the clinical care of the patient. At the level of the individual patient with multidrug-resistant tuberculosis (MDR TB), doctors and hospital managers are having to face the fact that managing even a single case of this condition is immensely more expensive than dealing with a case of drug-sensitive disease. Just a few such additional patients may cause considerable budgetary problems, even in a well-funded institution in the developed world.

At a higher level, it has then to be recognized that, in addition to the costs associated with individual patients, the occurrence of MDR TB in *some* patients may have implications for the cost of dealing with *all* patients. Once it is acknowledged that drug resistance is a possibility, the management of all cases of TB, and in particular their initial management, must be planned with that possibility in mind. At a higher level still, spending on public health measures to prevent the spread of MDR TB, or to control and reverse the problem where spread has already occurred, can have very large financial implications, even for the wealthiest countries.

Address for correspondence: Dr. John Moore-Gillon, M.A., M.D., FRCP, Consultant Physician, Department of Respiratory Medicine, St. Bartholomew's and Royal London Hospitals, London EC1A 7BE, U.K. Voice: 0207 601 8441.

John@moore-gillon.demon.co.uk

Finally, in addition to carrying the financial burden of treating the sick and of preventing others from becoming sick, countries have to face the problem of the lost productivity of those persons. Adults who are sick for a long term are a cost to the economy in more than one way: in the cost to treat and maintain, and in the fact that they are not contributing, in taxes or productivity, to the national economy. To this must be added yet a further cost if the responsibility of supporting their dependents falls on the state rather than on the extended family—and where it does fall on the family, the impact can be devastating.[1,2]

DIFFERENT COUNTRIES, DIFFERENT PROBLEMS, DIFFERENT EXPECTATIONS

TB is a global disease and so, accordingly, is MDR TB. Self-evidently, the financial problems that MDR TB produces are different in different parts of the world: London has relatively few patients and relatively lavish resources. Sub-Saharan Africa has far more patients and far fewer resources. Facilities and finances are different, but it is often forgotten that so are expectations. Doctors in resource-rich countries can do some things beyond the dreams of their colleagues working in resource-poor countries. It must be kept in mind, though, that levels of public health protection that are—quite rightly—regarded in some countries as magnificent achievements given the resources available, could, in certain other countries, be regarded as being so far below what is expected as to amount to medical malpractice.

The expectations of doctors and other health care workers dealing with MDR TB will thus differ in different parts of the world. At least, though, health care professionals regard MDR TB as one disease, whoever it is that has the disease, and wherever they are. There may be different constraints on what we can deliver for our patients, but we all know what it is that we *ought* to deliver in an ideal world. To the policymakers and the money providers, however, MDR TB is many different diseases depending on the viewpoint.

Discussion about the cost of MDR TB in many countries is likely to be about using DOTS Plus—can it be afforded (probably yes) and can the system possibly afford drug susceptibility testing on all initial isolates of TB (almost certainly not). By contrast, in many parts of the United States and increasingly in some parts of Western Europe, the political and societal imperatives regarding the financing of MDR TB are to locate enough money to put into negative-pressure isolation every single patient coming through the door of the hospital who might possibly have pulmonary TB and keep them there until it has been proven not to be MDR.

There is, accordingly, no "one world" message: the costs of MDR TB will depend on these political and societal imperatives and the expectations that they produce.

THE INDIVIDUAL PATIENT WITH MDR TB

In managing the individual patient with MDR TB, the first and most obvious expense is the cost of drugs. Second-line drugs are more expensive, and those first-line drugs that may still be effective may need to be used for longer periods. Ethambutol,

TABLE 1. Cost of drugs used in the treatment of tuberculosis

Drug and daily dose	Annual cost £ ($)
Amikacin, 1 g	6430 (9655)
Capreomycin, 1 g	6580 (9870)
Ciprofloxacin, 1 g	980 (1470)
Clarithromycin, 1 g	1040 (1560)
Clofazamine, 300 mg	76 (114)
Cycloserine, 500 mg	1685 (2530)
Ethambutol, 1 g	356 (535)
Isoniazid, 300 mg	26 (39)
PAS, 7.4 g	5190 (7785)
Prothionamide, 750 mg	880 (1320)
Pyrazinamide, 2 g	110 (165)
Rifabutin, 900 mg	3140 (4710)
Rifampicin, 600 mg	85 (127)
Streptomycin, 1 g	2450 (3675)

for instance, is markedly more expensive than rifampicin or isoniazid. TABLE 1 shows the average U.K. costs of some of the drugs used in MDR TB.

A WHO/IUATLD survey suggests that a one-month supply of streptomycin is about $38; for amikacin, the monthly cost is $640; and for ofloxacin, the price ranges between about $88 and $200 dollars per month, with cycloserine and PAS being similarly priced. As has been pointed out, in many countries just one month's supply of just one of those drugs exceeds the entire annual per capita health expenditure.[3]

In those countries where these drugs can be (fairly) readily afforded, the expectations for levels of care are high. To the drug costs, the costs of toxicity monitoring, for example, plasma levels, audiograms, and assessments of renal impairment, must be added. But the question of drug and associated costs is only the start. The cost of managing tuberculosis really starts to escalate when in-patient care of patients is necessary.[4,5] The studies cited here reflect costs for all TB patients, not just MDR TB, but when resistant disease is being managed the costs are going to be much greater still, especially if prolonged isolation is necessary, as it often is in pulmonary disease.

Negative-pressure rooms for isolation of infectious MDR TB incur both capital building costs and annual running costs. These costs can be predicted for the anticipated useful life of the facility, and costs per room/day calculated. These calculations, however, are themselves likely to underestimate the cost of managing an individual case of MDR TB unless predictions of bed occupancy rates are robust. If a patient is placed in a negative-pressure room for two or three weeks, the institution is paying not just for the nights the patient spends there, but also is paying to be able to offer the patient that facility when it is needed: it is thus paying for those times when the room is empty and available.

Moving beyond the physical facility, there is the matter of nursing intensity. Staffing levels on the negative-pressure unit of 10 beds at Bart's Hospital in London are 50% higher than on other wards in the hospital, and this probably fairly reflects what is going on elsewhere. Quite apart from medical time and nursing staffing levels, there is the increased input of other health care professionals. Our experience is that persons experience significant psychological and indeed psychiatric morbidity with long-term isolation. Turning from the mental to the physical, cost estimates need to consider the additional medical care that may be necessary for MDR TB cases in addition to those of drug-sensitive disease: the possibility of thoracic surgical intervention is just one of these costs.

A number of figures have been produced for the total costs involved in the care of individual patients with MDR TB in resource-rich countries. Figures for individual, very expensive patients running into hundreds of thousands of pounds are well known to many of us. It has been our experience that those responsible for the allocation of resources are unimpressed by the example of single, expensive cases with many complications, so in our institution we examined a small series of patients, looking only at those with straightforward pulmonary MDR TB who were HIV-negative.[6]

In this study, we attempted to take into account all the factors mentioned above, and came up with a *minimum* mean cost of £60,000 ($90,000) per patient. We know that this underestimates the true sum, because in making the calculations reflecting facility costs we have, for instance, assumed 100% bed occupancy in our negative-pressure suite over an assumed 15-year life for the facility, and we know that full occupancy is not at 100%. These figures have been helpful in attracting the attention of our local health care planners and government and demonstrating that even though the numbers of cases are relatively small, MDR TB is a very real financial issue in our inner cities. These costs cannot be picked up easily in the standard respiratory medicine budget.

THE CONSEQUENCES FOR OTHERS

Moving beyond the individual patient, the consequences for others can be considered in at least two ways. The first of these is the relatively superficial analysis of the consequences if the patient with MDR TB passes it on to somebody else. This next person then becomes another individual with MDR TB, with all the costs that are associated with that condition. The cost of one multiinstitutional outbreak of MDR TB in New York City was estimated to be in excess of $25 million, when calculated on the basis of the number of days in the hospital alone, and the full cost is bound to be far higher than that.[7]

Further, as more than one hospital in London has discovered, the costs of transmission to others are not purely medical; hospitals have been sued when hospital inpatients have been infected by other patients with MDR TB, and the damages in some cases have been very large indeed.

But there is a second aspect to the consequences of MDR TB for others, and that is the consequences for those who do not actually have MDR TB but who *might* have it. If there is MDR TB in our community, we may have to behave differently toward all patients, at least until they have been shown to have drug-sensitive disease.

At its very simplest, this has led to subtle changes in initial drug regimens in many cases. In the United Kingdom, although superficially the national guidelines have not changed very much,[8,9] clinical practice has. Most clinicians used to use an initial three-drug regimen as a routine treatment, and four drugs were used if there was reason to suspect an increased risk of drug resistance. That has been reversed: now, use of four drugs is routine, and three are used only if the patient is regarded as being at very *low* risk for MDR TB. That increases the cost of the standard regimen by about 30%, since ethambutol—the usual fourth drug—is significantly more expensive than the others.

This has had the desirable effect of making clinicians more keen on obtaining microbiological confirmation of the disease, particularly nonpulmonary disease, because the sensitivities are so important; and data from the British Public Health Laboratory Service year on year shows an increasing proportion of microbiological confirmation.[10] Again, it must be kept in mind that this additional invasive sampling and laboratory examination represents an increased expense brought about by increased fears about drug resistance.

Additional second-line drugs may also be used initially if there is a strong clinical suspicion of resistant disease, and their use is continued until it is confirmed that the disease is, after all, fully sensitive. There is thus still more expense—for drugs, for their monitoring, and for toxicity testing—and there is increased risk to the patient. The doctor may well—in pulmonary disease—use strict isolation procedures, until it is known that the disease is drug-sensitive and the regimen is appropriate. All these consequences flow *not* from the fact that the patient has MDR TB, but purely from the fact that *others* have it and so he *might* have it.

Is there anything that can be done to reduce these costs? It is absolutely clear that if the time needed for sensitivity testing can be reduced, then there is at least the potential to save money. This should be viewed from the right direction: not much money is saved by proving somebody is drug resistant more quickly. On the other hand, because most of the patients are drug sensitive and treatment is unnecessarily expensive if patients are initially managed as possibly drug resistant, a great deal of money may be saved by proving more quickly that patients are drug sensitive. A number of publications have looked at various tests and their cost effectiveness, but one of the best analyses comes from Drobniewski and colleagues, clearly demonstrating the overall economic benefits of expenditure on molecular diagnosis of tuberculosis and drug resistance.[11]

IMPLICATIONS FOR PUBLIC HEALTH AND THE WIDER ECONOMY

The implications of the existence of MDR TB for those who may not have it relate very closely to the wider public health costs. There is a clear need to have measures in the community to control the spread of resistant disease, but even more importantly to prevent the emergence of resistant strains. Reversing the problems that developed in New York in the 1980s is estimated to have cost $1 billion.[12]

In London, a study commissioned by the Regional Public Health Office estimated that MDR TB, about 2.5% of culture-confirmed cases, accounted for 20% of spending on TB.[13] This was, as the authors acknowledged, only a fairly crude analysis, since it was not the main focus of the paper, but it does give an idea of the scale of the problem.

Beyond immediate public health issues like these is the impact of the disease in terms of the economy as a whole. Where the burden falls is dependent on national wealth and the national culture. In a country like the United Kingdom, the state's expectations of the family are essentially zero. Many families, of course, do contribute to care, but if they don't the state will more or less handle everything. The state will pay for the illness and pay for the lost work. The state will bear the burden of lost tax revenue, and the state will bear the cost of supporting the dependents if the ill person was the breadwinner. In other countries there may be no such support from the state at all.

In many places, the situation is intermediate between those two extremes. Although not specifically in the context of resistant disease, there have been numerous excellent studies from India. One such paper, by Rajeswari and colleagues, investigated a mixed population treated by government health care, nongovernmental organizations, and private practitioners and showed that the total costs, particularly indirect costs, were very high.[1] Expenditures due to TB accounted for as much as 40% of the patients' mean annual income. Strikingly, almost 20% of school-aged children of infected parents had to discontinue their school studies, either to care for their parents or to start work to contribute to the family income.

A paper from Thailand starkly demonstrates the importance of interpreting economic statistics with a full awareness of the issues that underlie them: increased expenditure on food in tuberculous households was not a reflection of an awareness of the need for good nutrition, but simply because one in six households had to sell part of their property to pay their bills and could no longer rely on home-grown produce.[2]

Turning back to industrialized nations, economic discussions about health care interventions are now commonplace. When a major pharmaceutical company puts its case to the licensing and national health care funding bodies about a new anti-influenza drug, part of the data it presents is the savings to the national economy that should result from the drug's widespread use. Similar arguments are presented for new asthma drugs and for new interventions in coronary artery disease. Are there similar arguments in developed countries for new tuberculosis interventions? There are not, but then the concept of the cost to the economy of lost productivity is harder to sell as an idea to the U.K. government, since in this and many other countries the majority of patients with TB are not employed anyway.

Can countries afford *not* to treat MDR TB? There is at present an interesting debate on this issue. It is a debate or discussion, rather than an argument, because the protagonists are all, essentially, on the same side. Greatly simplified, the arguments of Farmer and colleagues might be summed up by stating that we cannot afford not to treat MDR TB with individualized regimes however impoverished the environment in which we are trying to work.[14]

On the other hand, Espinal *et al.* argue that resources are invariably finite and often very limited and that there will be "an optimal allocation of funds that minimises current and future illness and death."[15] They will argue further that the case has not been proved that expenditure on individualized regimens rather than standardized third-line regimens will represent an optimal allocation of funds.

Iseman has addressed this debate in a short but thought-provoking editorial.[16] The utilitarian philosophers Jeremy Bentham and John Stuart Mill explored the concept of following policies that led to the greatest good or happiness to the greatest number. As Iseman puts it, "To what extent can and should we divert energies and monies to the care of the relatively small number of patients with MDR TB? Will such efforts impede the implementation of DOTS programs, the *current* utilitarian strategy favoured by the WHO?" On the other hand, would a truly utilitarian approach favor diverting the funds to MDR TB, because over the long term that will result in the greatest happiness to the greatest number, the utilitarian ideal?

IS THERE ONE WORLD MESSAGE AFTER ALL?

This paper has taken a tour around numerous and disparate aspects of tuberculosis: from costs of negative-pressure rooms in London, to the selling of the family land in Thailand, to a consideration of a school of philosophy. Earlier in the text, it was suggested there is no one world message about the cost of MDR TB: The cost of MDR TB in different countries will not just be a question of how many cases there are and how big or how small the health care budget is, it will depend on the political and societal imperatives and the expectations that they produce.

Perhaps, though, there *is* a single world message, if only it could be put across to those who need to hear it. Increased spending on TB in New York or London or Copenhagen or Paris is not motivated by concern for the poor and disadvantaged of those cities. It is driven by a combination of the fears of the middle classes and of the political unacceptability of the return of a disease that is associated with a poverty-stricken past. If policymakers could be persuaded that those fears and political threats could be reduced, not just by providing more negative-pressure rooms, but by funding TB control programs in poor countries, then some real progress might be made.

It's a tough job to persuade a government in London that putting money into Africa will eventually make voters happier about their local record on TB in the United Kingdom, not least because it will take a few years to have an effect and then the next government may get the credit. The battle against TB has to be fought in the corridors of power in Washington, London, Paris, and Berlin, as well as out in the field.

REFERENCES

1. RAJESWARI, R., R. BALASUBRAMANIAN, M. MUNIYANDI, *et al.* 1997. Socio-economic impact of tuberculosis on patients and family in India. Int. J. Tuberc. Lung Dis. **3:** 869–877.
2. KAMOLRATANAKU, P., H. SAWERT, S. KONGSIN, *et al.* 1999. Economic impact of tuberculosis at the household level. Int. J. Tuberc. Lung Dis. **3:** 596–602.
3. SCHLUGER, N.W. 2000. The impact of drug resistance on the global tuberculosis epidemic. Int. J. Tuberc. Lung Dis. **4(Suppl. 2):** S71–S75.
4. TAYLOR, Z., S.M. MARKS, N.M. RIOS BURROWS, *et al.* 2000. Causes and costs of hospitalisation of tuberculosis patients in the United States. Int. J. Tuberc. Lung Dis. **4:** 931–939.

5. MacINTYRE, C.R., A.J. PLANT & D. HENDRIE. 2001. Shifting the balance between in-patient and out-patient care for tuberculosis results in economic savings. Int. J. Tuberc. Lung Dis. **5:** 266–271.
6. WHITE, V.L.C. & J. MOORE-GILLON. 2000. Resource implications of multidrug resistant tuberculosis. Thorax **55:** 962–963.
7. FRIEDEN, T.R., L.F. SHERMAN, K. LAY MAW, *et al.* 1996. A multi-institutional outbreak of highly drug-resistant tuberculosis. JAMA **276:** 1229–1235.
8. JOINT TUBERCULOSIS COMMITTEE OF THE BRITISH THORACIC SOCIETY. 1990. Chemotherapy and management of tuberculosis in the United Kingdom: recommendations. Thorax **45:** 403–408.
9. JOINT TUBERCULOSIS COMMITTEE OF THE BRITISH THORACIC SOCIETY. 1998. Chemotherapy and management of tuberculosis in the United Kingdom: recommendations. Thorax **53:** 536–548.
10. UK MYCOBACTERIAL RESISTANCE NETWORK (MYCOBNET). 2000. Annual Report Jan–Dec 1999. Public Health Laboratory Service, London, UK.
11. DROBNIEWSKI, F.A., S.A. WATTERSON, S.M. WILSON & G.S. HARRIS. 2000. A clinical microbiological and economic analysis of a national UK service for the rapid molecular diagnosis of tuberculosis and rifampicin resistance in *Mycobacterium tuberculosis.* J. Med. Microbiol. **49:** 271–278.
12. FRIEDEN, T.R., P.I. FUJIWARA, R.M. WASHKO & M.A. HOMBURG. 1995. Tuberculosis in New York City—turning the tide. N. Engl. J. Med. **333:** 229–233.
13. NHS. 1998. Tuberculosis control in London—The need for change. NHS Executive (NT980004) December 1998.
14. FARMER, P., J. BAYONA, M. BECERRA, *et al.* 1998. The dilemma of MDR-TB in the global era. Int. J. Tuberc. Lung Dis. **2:** 869–876.
15. ESPINAL, M.A., C. DYE, M. RAVIGLIONE & A. KOCHI. 1999. Rational "DOTS plus" for the control of MDRTB. Int. J. Tuberc. Lung Dis. **3:** 561–563.
16. ISEMAN, M.D. 2000. Tuberculosis control strategies and utilitarianism. Int. J. Tuberc. Lung Dis. **4:** 95.

Drug-Resistant Tuberculosis

Concluding Remarks

PETER D.O. DAVIES

Tuberculosis Research Unit, Cardiothoracic Centre, Liverpool L14 3PE, UK

ABSTRACT: This paper summarizes the presentations of the meeting on drug-resistant tuberculosis held in London in March of 2001. Multidrug-resistant tuberculosis (MDR TB) is defined and the causes, risk factors, and recent treatment advances are briefly described. The larger social and economic environment in which MDR TB occurs is discussed.

KEYWORDS: multidrug-resistant tuberculosis; TB cure rates; prisons; TB treatment; DOTS; DOTS plus; poverty

DEFINITIONS

Multi-drug resistant tuberculosis (MDR TB) is defined as resistance to the two principal drugs used in the treatment of tuberculosis: isoniazid and rifampicin, whether there is resistance to other drugs or not. The terms "primary," and "acquired" resistance have been changed to "resistance in new patients" and "resistance in previously treated patients," respectively.

CAUSES OF MDR TB

Poor patient management, nonadherence to the prescribed regimen, a poor national TB program, or some combination of these three factors causes drug-resistant tuberculosis to emerge when patients are allowed to take a single drug. This practice results in the development of resistance to that drug.

DECREASED CURE RATES IN MDR TB

Multidrug-resistant tuberculosis is much more difficult to treat than fully susceptible disease, because treatment requires expensive second-line drugs for at least 18 months compared with a course of cheaper first-line drugs for only six months.[1] Cure rates for fully susceptible disease should exceed 90% in a well-run program. WHO provides a guideline of a minimum cure rate of 75% in order to achieve control in the community. Cure rates for drug-resistant disease vary from 60% in Hong

Address for correspondence: Dr. P.D.O. Davies, Cardiothoracic Centre, Thomas Drive, Liverpool L14 3PE, U.K. Voice: 0151293 2392; fax 01512287688.
p.d.o.davies@liv.ac.uk

Kong to as little as 5% in Russia. Variation in the incidence is widespread and ranges from 14% in new patients to 40% in previously treated patients in Estonia and Latvia to none in Northern Ireland.[2] Certain countries, such as China, Korea, and Vietnam, are seeing a decrease in MDR TB; while others, such as Russia and the Eastern European countries, are seeing an increase. In the United Kingdom, despite a 10% increase in total cases last year mainly as a result of immigration, we have had a slight fall in MDR TB cases, from about 1.5% of cases where sensitivities have been obtained to 0.8%. This compares with a steady rate of resistance to isoniazid alone of around 6%. Approximately half of these cases develop within the U.K. and half appear to be imported.[3]

RISK FACTORS FOR MDR TB

MDR TB is found much more frequently in previously treated patients. For example, a study found an incidence in Bombay of under 10% in new patients but over 50% in those who had had previous treatment.[4] MDR TB is not as common in Africa, where it remains below 5% in most countries, perhaps because most programs could not afford rifampicin until relatively recently.

HIV is the biggest risk factor for tuberculosis, increasing risk of TB infection resulting in disease by at least 100-fold. In the countries of sub-Saharan Africa, case rates have risen by up to 10-fold in a decade as HIV has spread through the community. This increase in caseload imposes a strain on the health systems and their ability to manage tuberculosis effectively, as is seen by the number of retreatment cases. This could pose a risk of an increase in drug resistance in the region.[5]

In order to prevent this, the control of tuberculosis and HIV should become a top priority. Government commitment is required to provide the necessary resources. The potential for an HIV-related increase in TB in India is even greater. Its population is at least twice that of sub-Saharan Africa. HIV levels in the community are rising rapidly; for example, the incidence in the commercial sex workers of Mumbai has risen from 5% to 50% in five years.

PRISONS

MDR in prisons poses a special problem. Too often prisoners are treated with the worst in terms of living conditions, food, and health care. Poverty and overcrowding are the rule. It is not surprising that prisons become breeding grounds for TB and MDR TB. As a rule, TB in prisons is 100 times more common than in the ouside community. But prisons are not closed systems, and whatever develops within prisons will eventually spread to the community.

Conditions are particularly bad in Russia, where 10% of her one million prisoners have active disease. In some prisons the majority of TB sufferers have MDR TB. Prisoners being treated for a susceptible strain have been known to catch a drug-resistant strain from a cellmate.

The most important long-term intervention is the move for penal reform to reduce the number of prisoners, restructure the prison buildings to ensure the passage of light and air, and create a new relationship between the Prison Medical Service and the Ministry of Health.[6]

RECENT ADVANCES IN DIAGNOSIS AND TREATMENT

Newer molecular methods of rapid diagnosis have offered some help in the management of MDR TB by providing a way to tailor drug regimens appropriately early in the treatment, particularly in response to rifampicin resistance. This has included the use of PCR-based methods, DNA sequencing, RNA-based assays, microarrays, and novel molecular phenotypic tests such as those using mycobacteriophages.[7]

The sequencing of the genome of *Mycobacterium tuberculosis* now provides us with perhaps the most important single piece of information for finding new drugs, vaccines, and diagnostic methods. The isolation of the genes providing templates for the enzymes responsible for the unique bacterial wall structure of *M. tuberculosis* should enable us to design specially targeted drugs to inhibit these enzymes and so prevent cell wall formation in the bacteria.[8] The recent discovery that the isocitrate lyase gene is necessary for the bacteria to exist in the persistent (nondividing state) may provide another way for targeted drugs to work. Synergistic mechanisms between new drugs and vaccines may provide a means of both treating disease and delivering preventive therapy to latent infection. It has been estimated that these developments will take place within five to ten years.

Discoveries within the human genome may also provide new treatments. Twin studies have shown that a genetic susceptibility to tuberculosis exists. Patients who fail to control bacterial numbers may be more likely to develop MDR TB. Certain genes such as the vitamin D receptor *tt* are associated with apparent protection from disease.[9] The HLA-D2 and the NRAMP1 gene have also shown this association. But the hunt is still on for a major gene that may provide protection or increased susceptibility. A linkage of a susceptibility gene to the X chromosome may explain why men, especially older men, have higher rates of disease. Unraveling the human genome may provide information useful in developing new vaccines or drugs that could modulate the human control mechanisms for inhibiting bacterial growth, thus reducing the likelihood of infection leading to disease.

DIRECTLY OBSERVED THERAPY (DOTS)

A more rational approach to managing the drugs we currently use until new drugs are available would be valuable. The practice of directly observed therapy (DOT), or supervised swallowing, is now insisted on by the World Health Organisation. This should not only result in the cure of the patient but in the prevention of the development of drug-resistant disease, because the patient would have no opportunity to give him- or herself monotherapy. But WHO insists that DOT be only one part of a five-part strategy, the others being a government commitment to provide resources, use of drugs with proven bioavailability, immaculate record-keeping, and fully reliable microscopy smear services. No DOTS program can be considered complete without all five components.

RESOURCE-RICH SETTINGS

Where a sophisticated laboratory service is available, culture and sensitivity testing can be done, but this will be a luxury for most services where tuberculosis is common. In the developed world drug levels may be monitored if it is thought that drug levels might be a problem, such as in renal failure. Applying a few rules here can help rational therapy: (1) Treat the whole patient, not laboratory-generated numbers. (2) Go for the highest level of drug to achieve the desired response within an acceptable level of toxicity. (3) Beware of drug–drug interactions. Studies have only been done of two-drug interactions. When a whole cocktail is being given, which is likely when HIV is being treated simultaneously with TB, the patient and health professional are sailing in uncharted waters.

TREATMENT

The treatment of MDR TB is difficult and should only be supervised by an expert TB center. Second-line drugs are less effective and more likely to cause adverse side effects. At least two, and preferably three, drugs should be given to which the bacterium is known to be susceptible upon sensitivity testing. If these are not identified at the time treatment is started, drugs should be chosen that the patient has not been treated with previously, insofar as can be determined. Risk factors for drug resistance include previous treatment, especially if prolonged; exposure to another patient with MDR TB; immigration from a country with a high incidence of MDR TB; substance abuse, including alcohol abuse; and, in the setting of an outbreak of MDR TB, the presence of HIV infection or being a child.

The older second-line drugs include cycloserine, ethionamide and prothionamide, amikacin, kanamycin and capreomycin, PAS, and thiacetazone. By serendipity, not design, a number of newer drugs have been found to be active against tuberculosis. These include the quinolones, the macrolides, clofazimine, and the combination of amoxycillin and clavulanic acid.[1]

INFECTION CONTROL

In the presence of HIV infection, MDR TB has a very high mortality. Special precautions should be taken in the hospital setting to ensure that cross infection does not occur. In the resource-rich West, MDR TB patients should be nursed in an isolation room under negative pressure, and staff should wear special sealant face masks. Patients suspected of having MDR TB should be cared for under these conditions until proven not to have MDR TB.[10]

"DOTS-PLUS"

There is much current debate as to whether the WHO DOTS strategy may lead to drug resistance. In resource-poor settings where sensitivity tests cannot be carried out, a four-drug regimen consisting of isoniazid, rifampicin, pyrazinamide, and ethambutol is given to all new patients; and the sensitivity of the bacterium to any of the drugs will remain unknown. These drugs are given under direct observation for two months, followed by administration of two drugs, usually isoniazid and rifampicin, for a further four months. Patients who relapse or fail on this regimen are given these four drugs plus streptomycin as a fifth drug. This appears to break a cardinal rule of TB treatment, which is *a single drug should never be added to a failing regimen* in case the regimen is failing because resistance to the all drugs previously used will have developed. Thus, the addition of a single drug would result in resistance arising to the newly added drug just as it does in monotherapy.

In practice, most centers have reported success with this five-drug retreatment regimen. But some areas, notably Peru, have seen an increase in drug resistance and believe the WHO treatment policy to be a possible cause. Doctors working at such centers have therefore called for a "DOTS-Plus" strategy, which includes treating patients who fail on the first-line drugs to be treated with second-line drugs such as amikacin and ciprofloxacin.

COSTS

The problem of expense arises quickly in TB treatment programs. The drug costs of first-line treatment can be as little as $10 for a six-month course. In the developed world, second-line treatment may cost $10,000. This figure is clearly beyond the scope of most countries. The proponents of DOTS-plus point out that unless we treat and cure MDR TB patients wherever they are, we may be storing up an insurmountable MDR TB mountain for the future. They also point out that the cost of second-line drugs has come down by 90% in some cases. More pressure on the pharmaceutical companies may force prices down even more. After all, they argue, these drugs have been off patent for decades. On the other hand, some say that second-line drugs will always be too expensive for the poorest countries, where TB is endemic and in any case treatment of MDR carries a low success rate even in the best hands.

ENSURING A CURE

The main problem with an extended treatment period of six months to provide a cure is that patients default. The need to ensure completion of treatment requires a team of caregivers including specially trained nurses. There is a stigma in many cultures associated with TB, which has to be overcome. Patients might be afraid that they would lose employment and income as a result of the disease. They may not appreciate the potential threat they pose in spreading disease to the rest of the community, and they might see the requirement to take their tablets as an infringement of their rights. Patients who default from treatment can usually be helped, as ways have been found to combat practical or emotional difficulties in taking medication. A skilled and motivated staff must be provided to assist such patients. Most countries have laws to enable compulsory detention in the event of a patient with potentially fatal infectious disease such as MDR TB who refuse treatment. In practice, this approach is hardly ever used, though some countries such as the United States have employed compulsory detention in as many as 1% of cases.[11]

POVERTY AND TB

Tuberculosis is a disease of poverty, and world poverty is worsening, both in terms of increasing inequality of wealth distribution and the absolute numbers of persons living in poverty. World and corporate leaders have a moral duty to reverse the continuation of world poverty. Whether by omission or commission, those of us in the developed world are benefiting materially from deprivation in the rest of the world.[12]

As Le Carre put it in his most recent novel *The Constant Gardener*, in which he gives an account of a clinical trial for a new TB drug in East Africa, "the problem with the poor is always the same. They are not rich enough to buy expensive medicines." More prophetically he adds, "[The plan] is to test the pill in Africa for two or three years, by which time KVH [the pharmaceutical company] calculates the TB will have become a *big problem* in the West."[13] For two to three years, read 20 to 30. We have been warned.

REFERENCES

1. ISEMAN, M. 1993. Treatment of multi-drug resistant tuberculosis. N. Engl. J. Med. **329:** 784–791.
2. RAVIGLIONI, M.C., C. DYE, S. SCHMIDT & A. KEESHI. 1997. The WHO Global Surveillance and Monitoring Project assessment of worldwide tuberculosis control. Lancet **350:** 624–629.
3. ROSE, A.M.C., J.M. WATSON, C. GRAHAM, *et al.* 2001. Tuberculosis at the end of the 20th century in England and Wales: results of a national survey in 1998. Thorax **56:** 173–179.
4. DAVIES, P.D.O., Z.F. UDWADIA, A. HAKIMIZON, *et al.* 1998. Drug resistant tuberculosis in Mumbai, India. Thorax **53(Suppl. 4):** A32.
5. MWINGA, A. 1998. *In* Africa in Clinical Tuberculosis. 2nd ed. P.D.O. Davies, Ed.: 619– 630. Chapman and Hall. London.
6. STERN, VIVIEN, Ed. 1999. Sentenced to Die? The Problem of TB in Prisons in Eastern Europe and Central Asia. International Centre for Prison Studies, King's College. London.
7. DROBNIEWSKI, F. 1998. Diagnosing multi-drug resistant tuberculosis in Britain. Br. Med. J. **317:** 1264–1265.
8. YOUNG, D.B. 1998. Blueprint for the white plague. Nature **393:** 537–544.
9. WILKINSON, R.J., M. LLEWLYN, Z. TOOSI, *et al.* 2000. Influence of vitamin D deficiency and vitamin D receptor polymorphism in tuberculosis among Gujarati Asians in West London: a case-control study. Lancet **355:** 618–621.
10. JOINT TUBERCULOSIS COMMITTEE OF THE BRITISH THORACIC SOCIETY. 2000. Control and prevention of tuberculosis in the United Kingdom: code of practice 2000. Thorax **55:** 887–901.
11. COKER, RICHARD J. 2000. From Chaos to Coercion: Detention and the Control of Tuberculosis. St. Martin's Press. London. pp. 304.
12. FARMER, PAUL. 1999. Infections and Inequalities. The Modern Plagues. University of California Press. Berkeley, CA. pp. 375.
13. LE CARRE, J. 2000. The Constant Gardener. Hodder and Stoughton. pp. 508.

Index of Contributors

Subject Index